T0259462

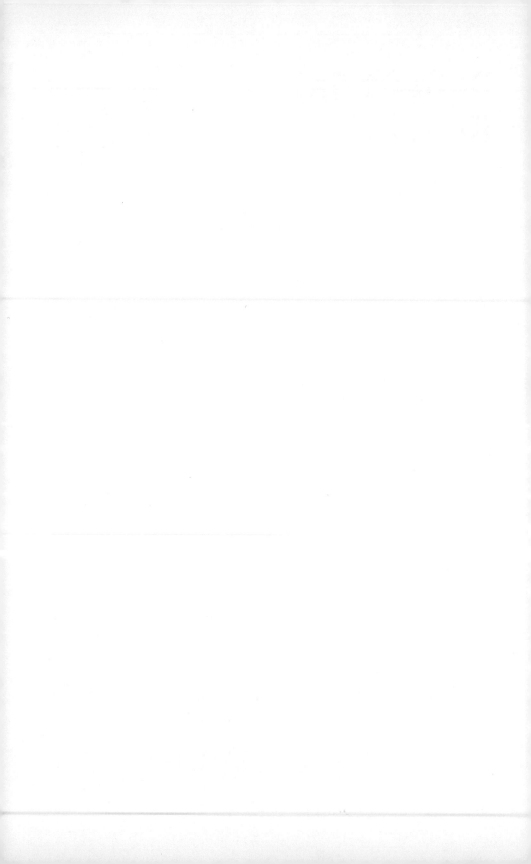

Patient Safety in Rehabilitation Medicine

Guest Editor

ADRIAN CRISTIAN, MD, MHCM

PHYSICAL MEDICINE AND REHABILITATION CLINICS OF NORTH AMERICA

www.pmr.theclinics.com

Consulting Editor
GREGORY T. CARTER, MD, MS

May 2012 • Volume 23 • Number 2

SAUNDERS an imprint of ELSEVIER, Inc.

W.B. SAUNDERS COMPANY
A Division of Elsevier Inc.

1600 John F. Kennedy Boulevard • Suite 1800 • Philadelphia, Pennsylvania 19103

http://www.theclinics.com

PHYSICAL MEDICINE AND REHABILITATION CLINICS OF NORTH AMERICA Volume 23, Number 2
May 2012 ISSN 1047-9651, ISBN-13: 978-1-4557-4210-3

Editor: David Parsons

Reprints. For copies of 100 or more of articles in this publication, please contact the Commercial Reprints Department, Elsevier Inc., 360 Park Avenue South, New York, NY 10010-1710. Tel.: 212-633-3812; Fax: 212-462-1935; E-mail: reprints@elsevier.com.

Physical Medicine and Rehabilitation Clinics of North America (ISSN 1047-9651) is published quarterly by Elsevier Inc., 360 Park Avenue South, New York, NY 10010-1710. Months of issue are February, May, August, and November. Business and Editorial Offices: 1600 John F. Kennedy Blvd., Suite 1800, Philadelphia, PA 19103-2899. Customer Service Office: 3251 Riverport Lane, Maryland Heights, MO 63043. Periodicals postage paid at New York, NY and additional mailing offices. Subscription price per year is $248.00 (US individuals), $441.00 (US institutions), $132.00 (US students), $302.00 (Canadian individuals), $575.00 (Canadian institutions), $189.00 (Canadian students), $373.00 (foreign individuals), $575.00 (foreign institutions), and $189.00 (foreign students). Foreign air speed delivery is included in all *Clinics* subscription prices. All prices are subject to change without notice. **POSTMASTER:** Send address changes to *Physical Medicine and Rehabilitation Clinics of North America*, Customer Service Office: Elsevier Health Sciences Division, Subscription Customer Service, 3251 Riverport Lane, Maryland Heights, MO 63043. **Customer Service: 1-800-654-2452 (US). From outside of the United States, call 314-447-8871. Fax: 314-447-8029. E-mail: JournalsCustomer Service-usa@elsevier.com (for print support); JournalsOnlineSupport-usa@elsevier.com (for online support).**

Physical Medicine and Rehabilitation Clinics of North America is indexed in *Excerpta Medica, MEDLINE/ PubMed (Index Medicus), Cinahl,* and *Cumulative Index to Nursing and Allied Health Literature.*

Printed and bound by CPI Group (UK) Ltd, Croydon, CR0 4YY
Transferred to Digital Print 2012

Contributors

CONSULTING EDITOR

GREGORY T. CARTER, MD, MS
Medical Director, Muscular Dystrophy Association Regional Neuromuscular Center, Providence Medical Group, Clinical Neurosciences Division, Olympia, Washington

GUEST EDITOR

ADRIAN CRISTIAN, MD, MHCM
Residency Program Director, Vice-Chairman, Department of Rehabilitation Medicine, The Kingsbrook Jewish Rehabilitation Institute, Kingsbrook Jewish Medical Center, Brooklyn, New York

AUTHORS

ELIZABETH ADAMS, MA, CCC-SLP
Department of Speech-Language Pathology and Audiology, The Kingsbrook Jewish Rehabilitation Institute, Kingsbrook Jewish Medical Center, Brooklyn, New York

LAUREL ADAMS-KOSS, OT
HSR&D RR&D Center of Excellence, James A. Haley Veterans Hospital, Tampa, Florida

BESEM AZIZ, MD
Department of Rehabilitation Medicine, Kingsbrook Rehabilitation Institute, Brooklyn, New York

FREDERICK AZIZ, MD
Department of Rehabilitation Medicine, Kingsbrook Rehabilitation Institute, Brooklyn, New York

MICHAEL BIGLOW, PharmD, BCPS, BCPP
Department of Pharmacy Services, Kingsbrook Jewish Medical Center, Brooklyn, New York

DEBORAH BRATHWAITE, MD
Department of Rehabilitation Medicine, Kingsbrook Rehabilitation Institute, Brooklyn, New York

NATASHIA T. BROWN, PhD
Neuropsychologist, Traumatic Brain Injury and Coma Recovery Unit, Department of Physical Medicine and Rehabilitation, Kingsbrook Rehabilitation Institute, Kingsbrook Jewish Medical Center, Brooklyn, New York

DAVID CANCEL, MD, JD
Resident, Department of Rehabilitation Medicine, Kingsbrook Rehabilitation Institute, Brooklyn, New York

JAISHREE CAPOOR, MD, FAAP
Children's Rehabilitation Center, White Plains, New York

ANDREA JNO CHARLES, MD
Department of Physical Medicine and Rehabilitation, Pain Therapy Group, Brooklyn, New York

HENRY COHEN, MS, PharmD, FCCM, BCPP, CGP
Department of Pharmacy Services, Kingsbrook Jewish Medical Center; Professor of Pharmacy Practice, Arnold & Marie Schwartz College of Pharmacy and Health Sciences, Long Island University, Brooklyn, New York

ADRIAN CRISTIAN, MD, MHCM
Residency Program Director, Vice-Chairman, Department of Rehabilitation Medicine, The Kingsbrook Jewish Rehabilitation Institute, Kingsbrook Jewish Medical Center, Brooklyn, New York

TAD DEWALD, BA, MPH
Department of Rehabilitation Medicine, Kingsbrook Rehabilitation Institute, Brooklyn, New York

LAURENTIU IULIUS DINESCU, MD
Department of Physical Medicine and Rehabilitation, Kingsbrook Jewish Medical Center, Brooklyn, New York

CHAUNCY EAKINS, MD
Department of Rehabilitation Medicine, Kingsbrook Rehabilitation Institute, Brooklyn, New York

ETHAN EGAN, MD
Department of Rehabilitation Medicine, Kingsbrook Rehabilitation Institute, Brooklyn, New York

CHRISTINE ELNITSKY, PhD, RN
HSR&D RR&D Center of Excellence, James A. Haley Veterans Hospital; VISN 8 Patient Safety Center of Inquiry; Colleges of Nursing and Behavioral and Community Sciences, University of South Florida, Tampa, Florida

JEFFREY S. FINE, MD
Assistant Professor, Department of Rehabilitation Medicine, Mount Sinai School of Medicine, New York, New York

CLAUDIA GIAMMARINO, MS, CCC-SLP
Department of Speech-Language Pathology and Audiology, The Kingsbrook Jewish Rehabilitation Institute, Kingsbrook Jewish Medical Center, Brooklyn, New York

JONAH GREEN, MD
Department of Rehabilitation Medicine, Woodhull Medical and Mental Health Center, Brooklyn, New York

STEPHANIE HART-HUGHES, PT, MSMS, NCS
HSR&D RR&D Center of Excellence, James A. Haley Veterans Hospital; VISN 8 Patient Safety Center of Inquiry, Tampa, Florida

ALLISON HICKMAN, DO
Resident, Department of Physical Medicine and Rehabilitation, Virginia Commonwealth University, Richmond, Virginia

M. JASON HIGHSMITH, DPT, CP, FAAOP
School of Physical Therapy & Rehabilitation Sciences, College of Medicine, University of South Florida, Tampa, Florida

ROBERT KENT, DO, MHA
Department of Neurology, College of Medicine, University of South Florida, Tampa, Florida

GAIL LATLIEF, DO, FAAPMR
Research Health Scientist, HSR&D RR&D Center of Excellence, James A. Haley Veterans Hospital; Department of Neurology, College of Medicine, University of South Florida, Tampa, Florida

EMERALD LIN, MD
Resident Physician, Department of Rehabilitation Medicine, Mount Sinai School of Medicine, New York, New York

LOU ANN LONDON, BSN, RN
Clinical Nurse Manager, SCI Unit, Mount Sinai Rehabilitation Center, The Mount Sinai Hospital, New York, New York

LISA MARTIN, PhD, RN
Senior Manager, Nursing Practice, Department of Nursing Education, The Mount Sinai Hospital, New York, New York

THOMAS R. MAYER, PsyD
Neuropsychologist, Traumatic Brain Injury and Coma Recovery Unit, Department of Physical Medicine and Rehabilitation, Kingsbrook Rehabilitation Institute, Kingsbrook Jewish Medical Center, Brooklyn, New York

SALEM MOHAMMED
Department of Rehabilitation Medicine, Kingsbrook Rehabilitation Institute, Brooklyn, New York

CHRISTINA MORIARTY, MS
Department of Speech-Language Pathology and Audiology, The Kingsbrook Jewish Rehabilitation Institute, Kingsbrook Jewish Medical Center, Brooklyn, New York

SHRUTI MURAL, BSc
Department of Rehabilitation Medicine, Kingsbrook Rehabilitation Institute, Kingsbrook Jewish Medical Center, Brooklyn, New York

VAMSI NUKULA
Medical Student, St. George's University, University Centre, Grenada, West Indies

MICHAEL OLDS, MD
Department of Rehabilitation Medicine, Kingsbrook Rehabilitation Institute, Kingsbrook Jewish Medical Center, Brooklyn, New York

BETH OLIVER, RN, MS
Associate Executive Director of Cardiac Services, Spinal Cord Injury, Lenox Hill Hospital, New York, New York

AJIT B. PAI, MD
Medical Director, Polytrauma, Hunter Holmes McGuire Veterans Affairs Medical Center; Assistant Professor, Department of Physical Medicine and Rehabilitation, Virginia Commonwealth University, Richmond, Virginia

KARISHMA PATEL, MD
Department of Pharmacy Services, Kingsbrook Jewish Medical Center, Brooklyn, New York

MARTHA T. PHAM, MS
Neuropsychology Intern, Traumatic Brain Injury and Coma Recovery Unit, Department of Physical Medicine and Rehabilitation, Kingsbrook Rehabilitation Institute, Kingsbrook Jewish Medical Center, Brooklyn, New York

SAMUEL L. PHILLIPS, PhD, CP, FAAOP
HSR&D RR&D Center of Excellence, James A. Haley Veterans Hospital; VISN 8 Patient Safety Center of Inquiry; Department of Mechanical Engineering, College of Engineering, University of South Florida, Tampa, Florida

SABINA RATNER, BS
Department of Rehabilitation Medicine, Kingsbrook Rehabilitation Institute, Kingsbrook Jewish Medical Center, Brooklyn, New York

VISHAL REKHALA, MD
Resident, Department of Physical Medicine and Rehabilitation, Kingsbrook Jewish Medical Center, Brooklyn, New York

MARC K. ROSS, MD
Department of Rehabilitation Medicine, Kingsbrook Rehabilitation Institute, Brooklyn, New York

AUDREY J. SCHMERZLER, MSN, RN
Director of Nursing, Mount Sinai Rehabilitation Center, The Mount Sinai Hospital, New York, New York

MATTHEW SHATZER, DO
Assistant Professor, Department of Physical Medicine and Rehabilitation- Hofstra- North Shore-LIJ School of Medicine, Great Neck, New York

JASON W. SIEFFERMAN, MD
Resident Physician, Department of Rehabilitation Medicine, Mount Sinai School of Medicine, New York, New York

RAJASHREE SRINIVASAN, MD
Department of Rehabilitation Medicine, Baylor University Medical Center, Dallas, Texas

ERIC C. STOBART, BS
Department of Rehabilitation Medicine, Kingsbrook Rehabilitation Institute, Kingsbrook Jewish Medical Center, Brooklyn, New York

YELENA SULER, MD
Chief, Department of Physical Medicine and Rehabilitation, Coler Goldwater Specialty Hospital and Nursing Facility, Roosevelt Island, New York, New York

SAMUEL P. THAMPI, MD
Attending Physician, Department of Physical Medicine and Rehabilitation, Kingsbrook Jewish Medical Center, Brooklyn, New York

YULIANA TODERIKA, BS, PharmD
Department of Pharmacy Services, Kingsbrook Jewish Medical Center, Brooklyn, New York

DARKO TODOROV, PharmD
Department of Pharmacy Services, Kingsbrook Jewish Medical Center, Brooklyn, New York

ANDY TRAN, MD
Department of Medical Education, Kingsbrook Jewish Medical Center, Brooklyn, New York

BRAD T. TYSON, MA
Neuropsychology Intern, Traumatic Brain Injury and Coma Recovery Unit, Department of Physical Medicine and Rehabilitation, Kingsbrook Rehabilitation Institute, Kingsbrook Jewish Medical Center, Brooklyn, New York

TRAVIS VONTOBEL, MD
Resident, Department of Physical Medicine and Rehabilitation, Kingsbrook Jewish Medical Center, Brooklyn, New York

YEVGENY ZADOV, DO
Fellow, Polytrauma, Hunter Holmes McGuire Veterans Affairs Medical Center, Richmond, Virginia

MOHAMMED ZAMAN, MD
Department of Rehabilitation Medicine, Kingsbrook Rehabilitation Institute, Brooklyn, New York

Contents

component of patient safety. The parallel concept of nurse safety cannot be ignored. Keeping nurses safe from injury helps decrease their feelings of stress and minimizes sick time. Maintaining a safe environment for patients and staff is a win–win situation for all involved.

and ethical standards. However, an emerging body of research suggests that ineffective and inappropriate care, or fatal errors, arise from the lack of productive communication between patients, families, and medical caregivers. This has prompted the evolution of a new health care discipline, patient safety, which became increasingly prominent in the 1990s. The purpose of this article is to bridge the gap between the discipline of patient safety and its relationship to the diagnosis of dysphagia.

Adrian Cristian, Claudia Giammarino, Michael Olds, Elizabeth Adams, Christina Moriarty, Sabina Ratner, Shruti Mural, and Eric C. Stobart

Communication barriers can pose a significant safety risk for patients. Individuals in a communication-vulnerable state are commonly seen in rehabilitation settings. These patients cannot adequately communicate their symptoms, wants, and needs to providers. Causes of communication barriers include neurologic impairments, such as stroke, cerebral palsy, and Parkinson disease, and language barriers. The ability of clinicians to adequately diagnose, treat, and monitor these patients is also hindered. This article identifies key communication barriers and strategies that clinicians can use to effectively communicate with these patients.

Ajit B. Pai, Yevgeny Zadov, and Allison Hickman

This article describes patient safety after traumatic brain injury (TBI). Patient safety in rehabilitation after TBI is important. Thorough assessment on initial evaluation, vigilance for medical and procedural errors, appropriate communication between medical professionals, and evaluation of systems-based practices increases patient safety. It is the responsibility of the rehabilitation treatment team to ensure that appropriate measures are taken to reduce risk of adverse events. This article is intended to promote discussion of patient safety after TBI within rehabilitation teams and to help improve outcomes throughout the spectrum of recovery.

Matthew Shatzer

There are approximately 12,000 new cases of traumatic spinal cord injury (SCI) annually. In 2010, there were approximately 265,000 individuals living with SCI. Over time, the average age of people with SCI has steadily risen, and it is now 40.7 years. There are multiple medical complications that are commonly seen in individuals with SCI. These include, but are not exclusively limited to, pneumonia, decubiti ulcers, undiagnosed fractures, urinary tract infections, autonomic dysreflexia, deep venous thrombosis, and pulmonary embolism. This article addresses the issue of patient safety in the care of adults living with an SCI.

Gail Latlief, Christine Elnitsky, Stephanie Hart-Hughes, Samuel L. Phillips, Laurel Adams-Koss, Robert Kent, and M. Jason Highsmith

This article reviews and summarizes the literature on patient safety issues in the rehabilitation of adults with an amputation. Safety issues in the following areas are discussed; the prosthesis, falls, wound care, pain, and treatment of complex patients. Specific recommendations for further research and implementation strategies to prevent injury and improve safety are also provided. Communication between interdisciplinary team members and patient and caregiver education are crucial to executing a safe treatment plan. The multidisciplinary rehabilitation team members should feel comfortable discussing safety issues with patients and be able to recommend preventive approaches to patients as appropriate.

Adrian Cristian, Andy Tran, and Karishma Patel

Cancer patients receive rehabilitation services in acute hospitalizations, rehabilitation wards, outpatient rehabilitation facilities, and home settings. Given the complexity and acuity of their medical care coupled with the long-term effects of the cancer and its treatments, patient safety is a significant concern in the delivery of rehabilitation services for this population. Cancer survivorship is growing in importance as a significant number of adults and children diagnosed with cancer are surviving beyond the 5-year mark. The goal of this article is to provide an overview to rehabilitation clinicians on the topic of patient safety in the rehabilitation of cancer patients.

PHYSICAL MEDICINE AND REHABILITATION CLINICS OF NORTH AMERICA

Preface

"First Do No Harm." These words were immortalized by Hippocrates and are part of the Hippocratic Oath taken by newly minted physicians graduating from medical school. Its profound meaning is that no harm should come to an individual receiving medical care. Regrettably, 98,000 people die each year in US hospitals due to injuries. The total cost of preventable adverse events has been estimated to range between $17 billion and $29 billion.[1]

Many explanations have been put forth as contributing factors to medical errors: (a) increasing complexity of health care delivery systems; (b) complicated medical and surgical treatments requiring specific expertise and experience; (c) advances in health care technology; (d) financial pressures placed on health care institutions; (e) shortages of key clinical staff and high patient ratios; (f) provider fatigue; (g) difficulties for physicians and other health care providers to keep up with the overwhelming amount of scientific literature; (h) cultural issues in health care institutions (culture of blame and punishment that lead to underreporting of safety risks).[2]

Adults and children living with physical disabilities have increased safety risks due to a combination of factors such as: (a) their underlying primary diagnosis and its associated impairments and disabilities; (b) existing comorbidities; and (c) social and economic challenges. In addition, they often require services across the entire continuum of health care delivery that includes both inpatient and outpatient settings. Health care facilities that provide rehabilitative services also share in the risk if medical errors occur on their premises. This is translated into increased lengths of stay, increased costs associated with the diagnosis and care for the errors, potential lost revenue if the injury occurred while the patient was on their premises, and risk for malpractice lawsuits.[2]

Medical errors are often multifactorial in origin. A culture focused on safety requires a team of dedicated health care providers whose mission is to understand the complexity of systems errors that ultimately result in an injury to an individual. This is best accomplished in a transparent, blame-free environment in which providers value learning from mistakes and seek to prevent them from happening in the first place.[2] Rehabilitation medicine clinicians are qualified to lead such teams, given that the cornerstone of rehabilitation medicine is patient-centered care.

The key element of a safety-focused culture is the close examination of failure in the rehabilitation setting. This is characterized by a dedication to the prevention, detection, and mitigation of errors.[2] Key questions to ask include (a) What is the current process?; (b) What can go wrong in this process?; (c) What is the likelihood that it will happen?; (d) What are the consequences of failure in this process? (ie, aspiration pneumonia, urinary tract infections, pressure ulcers, falls, fractures, deep vein thrombosis/pulmonary embolism, and death); and (e) What is the likelihood that significant harm will occur to the patient from them?

Phys Med Rehabil Clin N Am 23 (2012) xv–xvi
doi:10.1016/j.pmr.2012.02.016
1047-9651/12/$ – see front matter © 2012 Elsevier Inc. All rights reserved.

In the report titled, "Crossing the Quality Chasm," the Institute of Medicine outlined six dimensions of quality in health care. Care should be safe, effective, efficient, timely, patient centered, and equitable.[3] Individuals with disabilities deserve no less.

Adrian Cristian, MD, MHCM
Department of Rehabilitation Medicine
Kingsbrook Rehabilitation Institute
Kingsbrook Jewish Medical Center
585 Schenectady Avenue
Brooklyn, NY 11203, USA

E-mail address:
acristian@kingsbrook.org

REFERENCES

1. Kohn LT, Corrigan JM, Donaldson MS, editors. To err is human: Building a safer health system. Washington, DC: National Academies Press; 2000.
2. Griffin FA, Haraden C. Patient safety and medical errors. In: Ransom ER, Maulik SJ, Nash DB, et al, editors. The healthcare quality book: Vision, strategy and tools. Chicago: Health Administration Press; 2008.
3. Crossing the quality chasm: A new health system committee on quality of health care in America. Washington, DC: National Academy of Science; 2001.

Patient Safety and Quality Improvement in Rehabilitation Medicine

Adrian Cristian, MD, MHCM[a],*, Jonah Green, MD[b]

KEYWORDS

- Patient safety • Rehabilitation medicine • Quality improvement
- Cognitive biases • Systems thinking

It has been estimated that 98,000 people die each year because of medical errors.[1] Thirty-six percent of patients admitted to hospitals sustain an injury secondary to a medical error. In 9% of those admitted, the error was life threatening and in 2%, the error was thought to have contributed to the patient's death.[2] Two percent to 14% of patients admitted to hospitals have a medication-related error, and 35% to 40% of medical diagnoses are wrong according to autopsy reports, particularly in cerebrovascular disease and infections.[3–5] Approximately 1 in 10 admissions to a hospital will result in an adverse event, with about half of these being preventable.[6] It has been estimated that the average patient in an intensive care unit has 1.7 errors in his or her care per day and the average hospitalized medical patient experiences one medication error per day.[3] In addition to causing patient harm, preventable adverse events have a significant financial impact on health care. The Institute of Medicine report has estimated that the overall cost in the United States for preventable adverse events was between $17 billion and $29 billion.[1]

Medical errors occur in other health care settings besides hospitals. In 2003, a published study reported that 25% of patients in ambulatory care practices had experienced adverse drug events. Thirteen percent of these events were deemed serious. The medication classes that were most involved were the selective serotonin reuptake inhibitors (10%). Nonsteroidal antiinflammatory agents were involved in 8% of adverse drug events.[7] With the continuing trend of medicine pushing care toward outpatient settings, especially in rehabilitation medicine, the discussion and importance of patient safety must be stressed in all aspects of patient care.

Disclosures: There are no financial disclosures for the authors.

[a] Department of Rehabilitation Medicine, Kingsbrook Rehabilitation Institute, Kingsbrook Jewish Medical Center, 585 Schenectady Avenue, Brooklyn, NY 11203, USA

[b] Department of Rehabilitation Medicine, Woodhull Medical and Mental Health Center, 760 Broadway, Brooklyn, NY 11206, USA

* Corresponding author.

E-mail address: acristian@kingsbrook.org

This past year, we experienced the first member of the baby boom generation reach the age of 65 years. As more of that generation continues to age, more Americans will be undergoing rehabilitation in a variety of settings each year. These settings include (1) acute medical wards, (2) surgical wards, (3) intensive care units, (4) inpatient rehabilitation units, (5) subacute rehabilitation units in nursing homes, (6) outpatient facilities, and (7) home settings. As they are moving through this continuum of care, they are at risk of sustaining injuries that are related to their medical or rehabilitative treatments.

There are 2 goals for this article: (1) provide rehabilitation clinicians with an overview of patient safety as it applies to rehabilitation medicine and (2) provide an overview and framework for the improvement of quality in the delivery of rehabilitative care.

Patient safety has been defined as "freedom from accidental injury."[1] A distinction has to be made between patient adverse outcomes that are caused by patients' medical conditions from an adverse event, which is harm to patients as a result of medical intervention. Another distinction that needs to be made is the separation of *nonpreventable adverse events* from *preventable adverse events*. Nonpreventable adverse events are events when patients experience harm from their medical care in the absence of any errors (ie, from acceptable complications of surgery or medication side effects).[8]

The safety literature commonly defines an error as an "act of commission" (doing something wrong) or "omission" (failing to do the right thing) that leads to an undesirable outcome or significant potential for such an outcome.[9] For instance, ordering a medication for a patient with a documented allergy to that medication would be an act of commission. Failure to prescribe a proven medication with major benefits for an eligible patient (eg, low dose unfractionated heparin as venous thromboembolism prophylaxis for a patient after hip replacement surgery) would be an act of omission.[10] There are 2 types of medical errors: slips and mistakes. Slips are unconscious errors caused by an interruption in a routine while the person is not fully focused on the task. There are several reasons for the lack of focus and some examples include fatigue, lack of sleep, alcoholism, anxiety, and anger. Mistakes are errors caused by lack of knowledge; however, mistakes can be influenced by the same factors as mentioned for slips as well as unrealistic workloads and schedules and a lack of adequate training.[3] Although most preventable adverse events involve errors, not all of them do, and many safety experts prefer to highlight preventable adverse events rather than errors as their main target of the safety field.[8]

PATIENT SAFETY AND COGNITIVE BIASES IN THE PRACTICE OF REHABILITATION MEDICINE

Making good clinical decisions with patients' best interests in mind is a cornerstone of patient safety in rehabilitation medicine. Cognitive errors in decision making on the part of clinicians can lead to medical errors that can have an adverse impact on patient care. This point is especially important because there is significant variability among physicians regarding diagnosis and treatment. This next section addresses some of the cognitive biases that clinicians have in diagnosing and treating patients and general strategies to minimize them. There are several types of cognitive errors in decision making.[11,12] In the next section, some types of cognitive errors are described and some rehabilitation medicine examples are provided. They are the following:

1. Convergence: A key diagnostic dilemma that clinicians face with patient safety implications is the quick convergence on a singular diagnosis or treatment (and

excluding other possible alternatives) and then anchoring their course of action to that diagnosis or treatment, even when the outcome may not be positive. An example is assuming that the fall of an elderly patient is caused by a simple slip on a loose rug but not considering the possibility of loss of balance caused by a side effect of a medication that was recently started or orthostatic changes secondary to dehydration.

2. Over-reliance: This bias is the over-reliance and application of a limited range of diagnostic options and treatments to a broad variety of conditions when the diagnosis and treatment options are uncertain or the clinician has limited knowledge about the condition: For example, limited experience in the care of spinal cord injuries may lead a clinician to think that swelling in a paralyzed limb is a deep vein thrombosis, excluding the possibility that a recent fall may have caused a fracture in the insensate limb.

3. Pattern recognition and comparison with the current situation: In his book, *How Doctors Think*, Jerome Groopman[13] writes about how doctors are trained to think. He describes the use of prototypes in which the decision making is based on a knowledge of certain prototypes for a condition and then matching patients' symptoms and signs against that prototype. However, this way of thinking leads to the exclusion of less-common conditions (ie, zebras) when they do not fit the prototype or when patients have an atypical presentation of the condition. He describes "zebra retreat" in which doctors are not as likely to make a diagnosis of a rare condition because there is a considerable amount of effort and cost in identifying these conditions or they may not have much first-hand experience with them.[13] For example, an inexperienced physician may attribute the swelling in the arm of a patient with a history of breast cancer to lymphedema and exclude the possibility of deep vein thrombosis or metastatic disease as contributing factors. Another example is an atypical presentation of vascular claudication in a limb in a patient that also has a history of neurogenic claudication in that limb.

4. Confirmation bias: In this type of bias, data are picked that support a certain diagnosis or treatment course and data that contradict that diagnosis or treatment are discounted or excluded. Therefore, the clinician sees things that he or she wants to see. For example, a physician who commonly treats low back pain may attribute the cause of a patient's pain to a myofascial origin and not consider an alternative explanation, such as referred pain from metastatic disease to the spine.

5. Cause-and-effect bias: In this bias, a faulty assumption of cause and effect or a singular explanation (as opposed to multiple linked explanations) for a clinical condition is chosen because it supports a favored diagnosis and treatment. This bias can be linked with other types of biases, such as the confirmation bias in which more weight is assigned to data that confirm the clinician's favored diagnosis. An example is attributing a patient's inability to take pain medications as prescribed to noncompliance with the treatment plan but not taking into account the complexity of the titration schedule coupled with the patient's cognitive impairment and limited social support as contributing causes.

6. Overconfidence: This bias is the belief that a clinician's diagnosis and treatment is the right one for a patient because similar presentations in the past by other patients were also given the same diagnosis or treatment with positive outcomes. However, the fallacy here is that not all situations are exactly the same when contrasted to previous success stories. An example is a child with a history of a cancer-related lower limb amputation who presents with pain in the residual limb. The clinician thinks that the pain in the limb is caused by an ill-fitting prosthetic socket because this is what he or she typically sees in their clinic. However,

the possibility of a cancer recurrence is not entertained because that is not a common condition in the clinician's practice.

7. Recency: This bias is the tendency to emphasize the outcomes of recent diagnoses made or treatments rendered more than ones in the distant past. An example is the successful recent treatment of low back pain in several patients with acupuncture. This success would increase the likelihood that a clinician would use this type of treatment in a new patient presenting with low back pain.

8. Sunk costs: When a great deal of time, effort, and money is invested in making a diagnosis or rendering a treatment, the clinician is less likely to abandon that diagnosis or treatment if patients are not responding well clinically. An example would be a patient that has undergone joint replacement surgeries of hips and knees and extensive rehabilitative treatments and continues to complain of pain in the legs. The sunk costs are the time, surgery, and cost associated with the patient's care. Given the extent of the involvement, an alternate possible explanation, such as referred pain from lumbar spinal stenosis, is not given strong consideration.

9. Anchoring bias: In this bias, a course of action is anchored to a particular diagnosis once it has been made. This bias can be especially problematic when an expert or specialist makes the diagnosis and recommends a certain treatment that becomes a part of the patient's medical record. Any subsequent contradictory information may be ignored or minimized. Other clinicians may be less likely to challenge that diagnosis and treatment, even though it may be incorrect.[13] An example is when a pain management specialist diagnoses a patient with complex regional pain syndrome in an extremity and all subsequent treatment of the patient's arm pain is based on that diagnosis, even though there may be contradictory evidence identified by physicians who do not specialize in pain management.

10. Commission bias: This bias is based on the tendency to favor some type of action rather than inaction and monitoring a situation. This bias may be caused by pressure from patients, colleagues, or the urgency of the situation. An example is when a clinician prescribes opioid medications for chronic pain to a patient who is not an appropriate candidate for this type of medication because of pressure from the patient or his or her primary physician.

11. Context: The context of the clinical dilemma may be overlooked. An example is attributing a patient's stroke to noncompliance with antihypertensive medications. However, a closer look reveals a fragmented social support system, limited finances, and impaired decision-making capabilities secondary to prior strokes.

12. Attribution error: In this type of bias, the doctor's personal opinion of patients may influence his or her decision making. A negative impression of patients and a wish to end the patient visit quickly may lead to a narrower choice of diagnostic or treatment options and quicker convergence on a particular course of action. A positive impression of patients may lead to a bias in which positive test results are given more weight and diagnoses of serious or life-threatening conditions are minimized.[13] For example, the physician's false belief that a patient is exhibiting addictive and drug-seeking behavior in a pain clinic may have a negative effect on his or her ability to adequately treat the patient's pain.

Croskerry[12] described cognitive strategies to reduce diagnostic errors. These strategies include (1) developing an awareness of when a bias is present, (2) considering alternatives, (3) meta-cognition (reflective approach to problem solving), (4) decrease reliance on memory (use of handheld computers, algorithms), (5) develop mental simulation models of biased and nonbiased approaches, (6) provide adequate time to make good decisions, and (7) provide feedback.[12] Some strategies that can be of help in minimizing the effect of cognitive biases in rehabilitation medicine are listed in Appendix 1.

Patient Safety and Systems Thinking

Systems thinking is a framework for seeing the interrelationships and patterns that lead to events. According to Peter Senge,[14] the essence of systems thinking lies in the following: (1) seeing interrelationships rather than linear cause-and-effect chains, (2) seeing circles of causality, (3) recognizing that events are both cause and effect and nothing is ever influenced in just one direction, and (4) small actions can lead to larger consequences for better or for worse.[14]

In thinking about patient safety, it is important to understand that there can be several causes for a patient injury given the complexity of modern day health care. According to Peter Senge,[14] slow changes and a long incubation period can lead to adverse events in organizations. A problem can occur when health care providers cannot see the consequences of their individual actions in a larger system or over a long period of time. Cause and effect may not be related in time and space. Systems thinking and patient safety is about seeing the whole picture that led to the patient injury and not just the immediate cause. It is important to trace back the roots of a problem outside its immediate area and search for its presence in a larger context.[14]

Rehabilitation medicine, like any other field in medicine, needs investigation into the safety issues specific to this field and needs leaders to spearhead the changes that will improve the safety of patients receiving rehabilitative care.

Barriers, such as delays in the delivery of health care or working around obstacles in the delivery of rehabilitative care instead of addressing them, can have a significant impact on patient safety. Treating the immediate causes of a problem without addressing the fundamental flaws that led to its occurrence in the first place can lead to future patient safety events.

There are several strategies to improve patient safety through systems thinking:

1. Rehabilitation medicine leaders should create an environment in the rehabilitative setting in which clinicians are in a perpetual state of learning. This environment, which Peter Senge[14] labeled the "ideal learning organization," encourages (1) different points of view, (2) the evaluation of problems by looking at how events are interconnected, and (3) challenging the status quo.[14] In this environment, clinicians are aware of the gaps in their knowledge base and are constantly challenging themselves to improve the ways in which they deliver rehabilitative care. Rehabilitation managers and supervisors see errors in rehabilitative care as opportunities to learn and improve rather than opportunities to punish. Clinicians are encouraged to seek a deeper understanding of the fundamental causes of events that led to the patient injury in the provision of rehabilitative care. They develop and use a skill set in which they see their actions in a broader context of interrelationships of events.
2. Constantly evaluate current systems of delivery of rehabilitative care. There are constant changes in the way that rehabilitation is provided in a health care system. These changes could be caused by internal or external influences or both. They may be related to staffing models, level of expertise of rehabilitation clinicians in caring for people with disabilities, financial constraints, and types of disabilities, to name just a few examples. These changes can gradually affect the quality of care being provided and, therefore, systems that may have worked in the past may not be as effective in the present or the future. A constant vigilance for the

complexity of the rehabilitative care and a proactive approach to changes that emphasize patient safety and quality is important. Reflection on what works and what does not work and then comparing it with how it should work in an ideal system is an important tool for rehabilitation clinicians. Some common strategies to prevent errors in rehabilitation settings are outlined in Appendix 2.

3. Develop a unified belief, culture, and practice among all rehabilitation clinicians that patient safety is a fundamental cornerstone in the provision of rehabilitative services. This development is evidenced in all aspects of rehabilitative practice, such as (1) orientation and mentoring of new staff, (2) diagnosis and patient-specific safety practices in the provision of rehabilitative services in a variety of settings (inpatient, outpatient, and home settings), (3) selection of equipment used in patient care, and (4) continuous attention to quality and patient safety through multidisciplinary reflection, analysis of current practices, and quality improvement.

4. Plan for failure. Rehabilitation providers should anticipate patient safety failures through constant vigilance and assessment of patient care practices and the environment in which rehabilitative services are provided. They should see what failure looks like and work backward from that potential negative outcome to minimize its risk of occurring in the first place. For example, the admission of a high-fall-risk patient to an inpatient rehabilitation unit should trigger a process in which several team members involved in the patient's care work in unison to prevent it from happening: The physiatrist would review the medications and eliminate medications that can increase the risk of disorientation and sedation; Rehabilitative nurses can offer the patient prompted toileting before bedtime to reduce the need for the patient to get up in the middle of the night to attempt to go to the bathroom; Physical therapists and occupational therapists can evaluate for environmental risk factors in the patient's room and in his or her home and provide appropriate training and assistive devices at the patient's bedside.

In addition to falls, other examples of potential adverse outcomes seen in a rehabilitative setting include (1) contractures, (2) pressure ulcers, and (3) urinary tract infections and aspiration pneumonias. The rehabilitation team should implement strategies that minimize the risk of these adverse events from occurring in the first place but, once they have occurred, should identify strategies that minimize their risk of progression.

5. A simulated scenario of a potential patient safety event and rehearsal among team members is an effective tool used to foster effective communication in the likelihood that a true event should occur. For example, life-threatening emergencies on inpatient rehabilitation units may not occur frequently; however, when they do occur, it is important that team members communicate and act in a coordinated manner. Team members can rehearse a simulated life-threatening emergency scenario with discussion following the event on areas that went well and areas in need of further improvement.

6. Conduct constant surveillance of the delivery of rehabilitation services for systems barriers and constraints that can have an adverse effect on patients undergoing rehabilitation and removal of barriers as they arise. For example, changes in staffing levels or expertise coupled with an increase in the number of daily admissions and discharges and a higher diagnostic complexity of patients can all potentially increase the risk of errors in the provision of care to patients admitted to an inpatient rehabilitation unit. One strategy to make managers aware of this trend is to establish internal scorecards that collect this information for review by rehabilitation managers on a regular basis.

7. Focus on long-term, multidisciplinary solutions for fundamental causes of systems-based problems rather than only on temporary symptomatic solutions and evaluate the potential intended and unintended consequences of the solutions.
8. Design safe processes. Griffin and Haraden[6] described the development of a "safety conscious culture" in health care organizations. Key elements of this culture include (1) safeguards that take into account the variability in the provision of care by different providers, (2) decreasing the complexity of a process by reducing the number of steps in that process, (3) constantly reviewing a process and eliminating steps that are no longer needed, (4) standardizing processes and minimizing variability because variability can increase the risk for error, (5) equipment should be used that minimizes the reliance on human memory, and (6) safety programs should simultaneously address the prevention, detection, and lessening the risks of injuries.

ROOT-CAUSE ANALYSIS

Unfortunately, errors will occur. Once an error has occurred, several questions arise: (1) How did the error occur? (2) What factors contributed to the error? (3) How can a similar error be prevented in the future? The root-cause analysis (RCA) is a process whereby these questions are addressed in a systematic manner to identify the root causes of the error so that corrective actions can be put into place.

To ensure that RCAs are maximally productive, certain elements are important according to Wachter.[8]

1. Strong leadership and facilitation: Leadership needs to make sure that discussion is based on fixing systems as opposed to assigning blame.
2. An interdisciplinary approach: When forming a committee for the RCA, there should be representatives from all relevant disciplines focusing on identifying system factors that led to the error and what can be done to prevent recurrence in the future.
3. Individuals who participated in the case should be invited to tell their stories in an open, blame-free environment.

QUALITY-IMPROVEMENT METHODOLOGY

The process of quality improvement can be divided into 7 basic components: (1) definition of the problem, (2) identification of appropriate data to be collected, (3) mapping out the current process and identifying the barriers to the process, (4) selection of interventions, (5) implementation of interventions, (6) studying the effect of the interventions, and (7) reflecting on lessons learned. This section briefly describes these steps. A detailed description of each of the tools commonly used in this process is beyond the scope of this article; however, the reader is referred elsewhere for this information.[15]

Team Members

One of the most important aspects of the quality-improvement process is the selection of the right members for the quality-improvement team. Team members should evaluate the process and interventions from different perspectives and be able to work well as a group. Team members may include physiatrists, physical therapists, occupational therapists, rehabilitation nurses, psychologists, social workers, administrators, and patients.

Definition of the problem
In this step, the problem is identified and placed in the context of the organization and its challenges and goals. Once the problem has been clearly defined, the goals for the successful resolution of the problem also need to be clarified.

Data
To fully understand the problem, it is important that appropriate and relevant data are identified, collected, and analyzed. Team members should also identify objective benchmarks against which the effectiveness of the interventions can be measured.

Process and barriers
It is important to obtain a good understanding of the process contributing to the problem from a multidisciplinary perspective. First and foremost, what should the process be under ideal circumstances? Secondly, what is the process in its current state (as is)? A mapping of the steps in the process can be helpful to visualize the process. Third, what are the barriers to the process? There are several different types of barriers to a process. Some broad categories include people, plant/equipment, and policies/procedures. A fishbone cause-and-effect diagram can be useful in grouping barriers into one or more of these categories and identifying core causes for a problem.

Interventions
Once the barriers have been identified, it is important for the team members to brainstorm for all possible interventions and then to rank them with respect to a variety of factors, such as the importance of the intervention to solving the problem and the ease of implementation.

Implementation
Interventions that are ranked the highest are implemented.

Data collection and analysis
Data that were identified in step 2 as being important to evaluating the effectiveness of the interventions are collected and analyzed.

Lessons learned
In this final phase, team members reflect on the process, effectiveness of the interventions, and identification of future areas in need of improvement.

Institute for Healthcare Improvement

Because of the rising number of medical errors in the health care setting, in a time of growing technology and innovations, an organization known as the Institute for Healthcare Improvement (IHI) was formed. It is an independent not-for-profit organization based in Cambridge, Massachusetts that thinks everyone deserves safe and effective health care. The IHI originally developed the 100,000 Lives Campaign, which has now expanded to the 5 Million Lives Campaign. The goal of the campaign is to prevent 5 million incidents of medical harm over a period of 2 years (from December 12, 2006 to December 9, 2008). At the end of 2008, the IHI had signed up 4050 hospitals and more than 2000 facilities as participating members to their campaign.

The IHI encouraged hospitals and other health care providers to implement a series of interventions to reduce infections (methicillin-resistant *Staphylococcal aureus*, ventilator-associated pneumonia, central-line infections), pressure ulcers, medication-related errors, surgical complications, and use evidence-based care in the management of patients (ie, congestive heart failure, myocardial infarctions) in their facilities.[16]

Donald Berwick explained the aim of the 5 Million Lives Campaign and what can also be used to describe the ideology of patient safety with the following statement:

"The names of the patients whose lives we save can never be known. Our contribution will be what did not happen to them. And, though they are unknown, we will know that mothers and fathers are at graduations and weddings they would have missed, and that grandchildren will know grandparents they might never have known, and holidays will be taken, and work completed, and books read, and symphonies heard, and gardens tended that without our work would never have been."[16]

SUMMARY

Patient safety is a cornerstone of high-quality rehabilitative care. Rehabilitation clinicians should be aware of cognitive biases that can influence decisions in making a diagnosis or implementing a treatment plan and implement strategies to minimize their influence. Rehabilitation clinicians should also recognize the importance of systems thinking about errors and have a good working knowledge about quality-improvement methodology.

REFERENCES

1. Kohn LT, Corrigan JM, Donaldson MS, editors. To err is human: building a safer health system. Washington, DC: National Academies Press; 2000.
2. Steel K, Gertman PM, Crescenzi C, et al. Iatrogenic illness on a general medical service at a university hospital. N Engl J Med 1981;304:638–42.
3. Leape L. Error in medicine. JAMA 1994;272(23):1851–7.
4. Lesar TS, Briceland LL, Delcoure K, et al. Medication prescribing errors in a teaching hospital. JAMA 1990;263:2329–34.
5. Cameron HM, McGoogan E. A prospective study of 1152 hospital autopsies: inaccuracies in death certification. J Pathol 1981;133:273–83.
6. Griffin FA, Haraden C. Patient safety and medical errors. In: Ransom ER, Maulik SJ, Nash DB, et al, editors. The healthcare quality book: vision, strategy and tools. Chicago: Health Administration Press; 2008.
7. Gandhi TK, Weingart SN, Borus J, et al. Adverse drug events in ambulatory care. N Engl J Med 2003;348(16):1556–64.
8. Wachter RM, Foster NE, Dudley RA. Medicare's decision to withhold payment for hospital errors: the devil in the details. JT Comm J Qual Patient Saf 2008;34(2): 116–23.
9. White F, Nanan D. Clinical decision making part 1: errors of commission and omission. J Pak Med Assoc 2003;53(4):157–9.
10. Available at: http://www.ahrq.gov. Accessed February 15, 2012.
11. Roberto M. "Lessons from Everest: the interaction of cognitive bias, psychological safety and systems complexity" Harvard Business School California management [review]. Fall 2002;45(1).
12. Croskerry P. The importance of cognitive errors in diagnosis and strategies to minimize them. Acad Med 2003;78:775–80.
13. Groopman J. How doctors think. New York: Houghton Mifflin Company; 2007.
14. Senge P. The fifth discipline: the art and practice of the learning organization. New York: Currency Doubleday; 1990.
15. The memory jogger-healthcare edition: a pocket guide of continuous improvement and effective planning-first edition. Salem (NH): GOAL/QPC; 2008.
16. Available at: http://www.ihi.org. Accessed March 11, 2012.

APPENDIX 1: STRATEGIES TO MINIMIZE COGNITIVE BIASES IN THE PRACTICE OF REHABILITATION MEDICINE

1. Clinicians should be aware of the different types of cognitive biases and be able to recognize their presence in patient care.
2. Clinicians should also be aware of their own vulnerabilities to certain types of biases.
3. Clinicians should ask patients, and other clinicians involved in the patients' care, open-ended questions that can be used to generate a broad list of possible diagnoses. Patients should also be encouraged to ask questions because this can help prompt the consideration of other diagnostic and treatment options.
4. Clinicians should evaluate the clinical presentation from multiple perspectives and understand them in a broader context.
5. Clinicians should consider multiple possible explanations for the clinical presentation.
6. Clinicians should resist the temptation of quickly converging on one diagnosis.
7. Clinicians should identify the worst possible diagnosis and its outcome, the likelihood of its occurrence, and strategies that can be used to minimize that risk.
8. Clinicians should evaluate the primary data set and draw their own conclusions to avoid the biases and preconceptions of other clinicians involved in the care of patients.
9. Clinicians should give equal consideration to data that both support and negate a diagnosis.
10. In matching signs and symptoms against a prototype of prior similar diagnoses treated, it is helpful to consider how this clinical situation is both similar and different from the prototypes.
11. Clinicians should consider how their own personal opinion of the patient may be a cause of bias in diagnosis and treatment.
12. Clinicians should be aware of the pitfalls of over-reliance on matching against a prototype in establishing a diagnosis. They should consider atypical presentation of common conditions and unusual conditions (ie, zebras) in their differential diagnosis.

APPENDIX 2: PREVENTION OF MEDICAL ERRORS IN THE REHABILITATION SETTING

1. Standardize treatment protocols to minimize variability in care wherever possible and rehearse these protocols on a regular basis.
2. Use checklists whenever possible.
3. Orient and mentor new staff in the treatment protocols.
4. Have a built-in redundancy and duplication of protocols and processes.
5. Have appropriate, safe environments for staff and patients undergoing rehabilitation.
6. Have appropriate work schedules and clear descriptions of work to be performed by rehabilitation staff.
7. Have adequate staffing for the number of patients requiring treatment, taking into account the complexity of their care.
8. Use electronic medical records whenever possible.

Safety Precautions in the Rehabilitation Medicine Prescription

Deborah Brathwaite, MD[a],*, Frederick Aziz, MD[a],
Chauncy Eakins, MD[a], Andrea Jno Charles, MD[b],
Adrian Cristian, MD, MHCM[a]

KEYWORDS

• Rehabilitation precautions • Heat therapy • Cold therapy

The rehabilitation medicine prescription is a communication tool between the referring physician and the rehabilitation team in both the inpatient and outpatient settings. This instrument is critical in both directing a course of treatment as well as minimizing risk to the patient during the treatment sessions. The goal of this article is to provide an overview of the rehabilitation prescription with an emphasis on safety.

MEDICAL HISTORY

A thorough review of the patient's medical history is the foundation for the rehabilitation medicine prescription. Information is typically obtained from the patient, family members, clinicians with knowledge about the patient's medical condition, and the patient's medical record.

In the body of the history of present illness, the details of the chief complaint for which the patient is seeking medical attention should be emphasized. Here the physiatrist should allow the patient or if possible a family member to express the history and symptoms in his or her own words. A review of the chart should also be done to summarize all of the important medical or surgical information needed for treatment. It should be organized in a chronologic narrative manner, including onset, location, duration, severity, modifying factors, associating symptoms, treatment, and functional status.

PRECAUTIONS—GENERAL CONSIDERATIONS

Patients referred for rehabilitation often have several comorbid medical conditions. It is important to think systematically about these conditions and their potential impact

Disclosures: None.
[a] Department of Rehabilitation Medicine, Kingsbrook Rehabilitation Institute, 585 Schenectady Avenue, Brooklyn, NY 11203, USA
[b] Department of Physical Medicine and Rehabilitation, Pain Therapy Group, 856 Dekalb Avenue, NY 11221, USA
* Corresponding author.
E-mail address: dbrathwaite@kingsbrook.org

Phys Med Rehabil Clin N Am 23 (2012) 231–239
doi:10.1016/j.pmr.2012.02.002
1047-9651/12/$ – see front matter © 2012 Published by Elsevier Inc.

pmr.theclinics.com

on the patient during his or her rehabilitation treatments. For example, if a lower extremity amputee with diabetes, coronary artery disease, peripheral vascular disease, and neuropathy is referred for rehabilitation, what are the specific risks posed to the patient while undergoing rehabilitation, and how can they be minimized? The rehabilitation medicine prescription should address the risks associated with each of these medical conditions in the context of rehabilitation. In addition, one should also take into consideration the main condition for which the patient is being referred and its own risks to the patient's safety.

Precautions in the general prescription should take into consideration the various interventions that are commonly used by members of the rehabilitation team such as modalities and exercise.

Modalities are of added benefit to many therapy programs. In prescribing modalities, it is important to take into consideration various patient specific factors such as:

Sensory deficits
Decreased vascular supply
Underlying scars
Underlying malignancy
The patient's ability to communicate
Cognitive impairments
Presence of metal objects in the body (eg, joint replacements, bullets, shrapnel)
Presence of implanted electronic devices (ie, pacemakers, baclofen pumps, spinal cord stimulators
Pregnant uterus
Presence of superficial infections
Active joint diseases (ie, rheumatoid arthritis).

The choice of modality should also be carefully considered (ie, heat, cold, electrical stimulation), as well as the frequency, intensity, duration, and type of modalities.

Cold Therapy

General precautions to the use of cold modalities include history of cold intolerance, arterial insufficiency, impaired sensation, Raynaud disease, cryoglobulinemia, and cognitive and communication deficits.[1]

Heat Therapy

When applying a heat modality, care must be taken not to apply it over: areas of acute trauma or sites of active inflammation, areas with impaired sensation, edema, scars, areas that are poorly vascularized, or areas that are malignant. Additionally, it should not be used in people with impaired communication or cognition.[1] Similar general heat precautions apply to use of ultrasound as well with additional precautions.Ultrasound should not be applied over the brain, eyes, reproductive organs, the pregnant uterus, the spine or laminectomy sites, and areas with skeletal immaturity.[1] Shortwave diathermy should not be used in patients with metallic devices such as pacemakers, intrauterine devices, deep brain stimulators, or surgical implants, near contact lenses, or with skeletal immaturity.[1] Patients using hot packs should never lie on the pack. Since transcutaneous electrical nerve stimulation can cause skin irritation, stimulus areas should be rotated. The duration for most modalities is 20 the 30 minutes except for ultrasound, which is 5 to 10 minutes per site.

Exercise

The choice of exercises should also be carefully considered in the rehabilitation medicine prescription, since different types of exercises carry their own specific risks. Commonly prescribed exercises include resistive, endurance, and balance training exercises. Strengthening exercises including isometric, isotonic, and isokinetic exercises should be rhythmic, performed at low-to-moderate speed, and done through a full range of motion. The patient should maintain full breathing, since heavy resistance training associated with a patient holding his or her breath can result in dramatic rises in systolic and diastolic blood pressure.[2] Recommended guidelines for strength training include; performing a minimum of 8 to 10 exercises that train the major muscle groups, 1 set of 8 to 12 repetitions resulting in volitional fatigue for each exercise, and exercise for no more than 1 hour. Exercises should be performed at least 2 days per week.[2] Isometric exercises should be used with caution in individuals with hypertensive and cardiac disease. Isotonic exercises can be performed with free weights or an exercise machine. Proper lifting techniques should be used to avoid injury. The equipment used should be maintained in good condition to prevent injury. Exercise machines are safer to use when compared with free weights. They require less training and stabilize the body. Additionally, it is easier to control the exercise throughout the range of motion. Patients should also be instructed to perform the exercise in a pain-free range.[2]

EXERCISE IN SPECIAL POPULATIONS
Pregnancy

Exercise in pregnancy is contraindicated if the patient has significant heart or lung disease or incompetent cervix; is at risk for preterm labor; or has persistent second or third trimester bleeding, ruptured membranes, preeclampsia, vaginal bleeding, or decreased movements of the fetus. Relative contraindications include severe anemia, poorly controlled diabetes, morbid obesity or extremely underweight, or poorly controlled hypertension.[2]

In the following sections an overview of some specific precautions will be provided.

Cardiac precautions

Cardiac precautions are parameters provided to the therapist to safely administer therapeutic exercise to patients with various cardiac conditions. Depending on the cardiac condition, precautions may require modification. Patients with uncontrolled arrhythmias, unstable angina, resting stays depression greater than 2 mm, critical aortic stenosis, resting systolic blood pressure (SBP) greater than 200 mm Hg or diastolic blood pressure greater than 110 mm Hg, orthostatic SBP drop 10 to 20 mm Hg, or fall in SBP greater than 10 mm Hg with exercise, must not be allowed to exercise until these conditions are properly treated. The patient with a resting heart rate greater than 120 beats per minute (BPM) at rest or greater than 140 BPM with light activity should not exercise until the heart rate is adequately controlled.

During the acute phase of cardiac rehabilitation, the intensity of exercise must be monitored and the intensity gauged by the patient's heart rate. There are 2 methods of determining the target heart rate. One method is 220 minus the age of the patient or Karvonen method. The Karvonen method calculates the training heart rate (THR) by taking into account the resting heart rate (RHR) and the maximal heart rate (MHR). The MHR can be based on stress test results. The formula is: (THR = RHR + (MHR - RHR) × I).[3]

The Borg scale is often used to gauge the effort that a patient is exerting during aerobic exercise sessions. It has 2 key elements: a numerical scale that ranges from 0 to 20 and descriptors of perceived exertion by the patient during the exercise session. The American College of Sports Medicine (ACSM) recommends exercise intensity within a range of 12 to 16 on the Borg Scale.[4] The ACSM recommends that people who are less conditioned exercise at a lower intensity, for shorter durations of time and at at higher frequencies per day or per week.[4] For progression of exercise duration, the ACSM recommends a 5- to 10-minute increase every week to 2 weeks over the first 4 to 6 weeks of an exercise program for healthy adults.[4]

Patients who have undergone coronary artery bypass or heart transplant surgery often require additional precautions related to the type of surgery performed. One example is sternal precautions. Sternal precautions are meant to reduce exertion across the sternum. They include: lifting less than 10 lbs of weight bilaterally, active bilateral shoulder flexion less than 90°, active bilateral shoulder adduction less than 90°, and no hand-over-head activities.[5]

Additionally, for patients receiving beta blockers, the THR should be set at 10 to 20 beats above RHR. Patients also should be instructed to avoid valsalva maneuvers while performing resistive exercises.

Pulmonary precautions

Oxyhemoglobin saturation should be maintained at a level greater than 88% during exercise. Resting oxyhemoglobin saturation less than 88% on room air or while breathing the prescribed level of supplemental oxygen is an absolute precaution in which the referring physician should be notified, and exercise testing or therapeutic exercise should be terminated. Caution should be taken with resting heart rates greater than 125 BPM 10 minutes following exercise. The referring physician should be notified with systolic blood pressure greater than 200 mm Hg plus or minus diastolic blood pressure greater than 100 mm Hg.[6,7]

Precautions for patients with pulmonary hypertension include low resistance exercise (such as dumbells, cuff weights, or elastic band); higher intensity resistance training is not recommended. Forward bending from the waist, with the head in a lowered position, is not recommended, as this may exacerbate symptoms of lightheadedness and produce a valsalva effect. Performing positional changes such as lying to sitting position is acceptable after instructing to patient in pace breathing.[6]

Hypoglycemia and hyperglycemia Patients with a history of diabetes are at risk for hypoglycemia during exercise. Specific precautions in this population include: adjusting the insulin dose or carbohydrate intake before exercise, refraining from exercising during the peak hours of insulin hypoglycemic effect, eating snacks during exercise, refraining from exercises that raise blood pressure if the patient has retinopathy, and wearing appropriate shoes if the patient has peripheral neuropathy.[2]

Blood sugar levels must be tested before and after exercising to check for hypoglycemia. If the sugar level is less than 100 mg/dL before exercise, a carbohydrate snack should be given and the glucose level should be monitored during exercise. The patient should not exercise if the glucose level is greater than 350 mg/dL to 400 mg%.[2] Patients should also be monitored when exercising later in the day to watch for the somoygi effect while exercising.

Rehabilitation medicine staff should be knowledgeable for the signs and symptoms of hypoglycemia. It is also important to note that the use of heart rate to establish exercise intensity may be inappropriate in those diabetics with autonomic neuropathy. Rate of perceived exertion should be used to establish intensity of training.[2]

Orthopedic precautions

It is very important when treating patients after any orthopedic procedure to have good communication with the orthopedic surgeon involved in the patient's care to determine appropriate orthopedic precautions. These can include range of motion restrictions, weight bearing precautions, exercise precautions, and modality-specific precautions. The treating staff must be aware of the following weight bearing precautions:

Nonweight bearing (NWB)—0% of the body weight
Toe-touch weight bearing (TTWB)—up to 20% of the body weight
Partial weight bearing (PWB)—20% to 50% of the body weight
Weight bearing as tolerated (WBAT)—50% to 100% of the body weight
Full weight bearing (FWB)—100% of the body weight.[8]

Range of motion restrictions, resistive exercise, and modality precautions are often specific to the patient's underlying orthopedic condition and surgical treatment rendered, and a detailed description is beyond the scope of this article. Rehabilitation medicine clinicians are advised to clarify these precautions with the orthopedic surgeon. Concerning lower limb joint replacement, it is important to check with orthopedist on patient-specific precautions following joint replacement surgery.

The patient with a cemented hip, can be WBAT by day 2 with an assistive device. Several positions should be avoided after total hip arthroplasty. These include: no hip flexion past 90°, no adduction of the leg past midline (do not cross leg), and no internal rotation of hip. It is recommended that an abduction pillow be used while patient is in bed or wheelchair and that the patient uses a bedside commode. These hip precautions should be observed for at least 12 weeks.[8]

NEUROLOGIC DISEASES

Patients with neurologic diseases pose unique safety challenges to the rehabilitation team due to the complexity and variety of their impairments. In this section, a brief overview is provided with respect to 3 commonly encountered conditions in the rehabilitation setting. They include: brain injury, multiple sclerosis, and stroke.

Brain Injury Precautions

Given the extent of injuries that can occur in a traumatic brain injured patient, it is important that all rehabilitation team members are aware of the specific impairments affecting these patients. These can include

Communication and swallowing deficits
Cognitive impairments—decreased level of alertness, decreased memory, attention, and executive function
Seizures
Behavior-related (ie, agitated)
Impaired Vision And Hearing
Visual–spatial impairments
Cardiac and pulmonary disease related to trauma
Fractures
Spinal cord injury
Burns
Pressure ulcers
Incontinence of bowel and bladder
Contractures
Amputations.

The rehabilitation team should be aware of the extent of these deficits and medical/surgical treatments to date.

The precautions should be specific and include

Vital sign parameters (ie, blood pressure, heart rate, respiratory rate, and pulse oximetry ranges)
Weight-bearing restrictions
Seizure risk
Recommendations on management of behavior issues
Visual–spatial deficits
Positioning concerns (ie, risk for aspiration pneumonia—head of bed kept elevated)
Pressure ulcer-related recommendations (ie, number of minutes that patient can sit in a wheelchair)
Prosthetic- or orthotic-specific recommendations (number of minutes that the patient should wear an orthotic device)
Restrictions to range of motion, types of exercise and modalities
Risk for falling.

Treating therapists should check vital signs, monitor the patient, and communicate with the referring physician changes in the patient's status while undergoing therapy sessions so that he or she can be promptly evaluated and treated. These changes can include a change in mental status, seizures, difficulty breathing, pain, shortness of breath, change in vocal quality, and difficulties managing secretions.

Multiple Sclerosis

Important safety considerations in patients with multiple sclerosis include: falls, exacerbations secondary to heat or exercise, progression of disease, or diverse impairments (ie, visual impairments, unilateral weakness, generalized weakness, and cognitive impairment).

Falls are an important sequela of gait and balance disturbances in multiple sclerosis patients. The use of assistive device has also been implicated as another fall risk.

Fatigue is the most common symptom impairing activities of daily living and the most common complaint by multiple sclerosis patients. Caution must be taken when prescribing exercise and modalities in this population, as symptoms can temporarily worsen on exposure to heat or exercise.[7,8]

Progression of disease in multiple sclerosis can lead to new impairments or worsening of previous impairments, thereby changing the patient's safety risk level. For example, new-onset visual and cognitive symptoms in a patient with existing unilateral lower extremity weakness can increase his or her risk for falling. It is recommended that rehabilitation clinicians caring for patients with multiple sclerosis monitor them closely for change in their condition.

The diverse presentation of impairments described previously can pose additional safety risks in which the combination of impairments poses a greater safety risk than each one of them would have posed on its own.

Stroke

Impairments commonly seen after stroke include: communication deficits, cognitive deficits, swallowing deficits, hemi-paresis, incontinence, visual–spatial deficits, impaired balance, seizures, and sensory loss. Patients commonly referred for stroke rehabilitation often also have comorbidities that may have contributed to the stroke such as diabetes, hypertension, and heart disease. In addition, patients may have had prior strokes that left them with residual deficits before the most recent stroke.

Therefore, safety precautions should address the stroke-specific impairments as well as those of the associated conditions.

The combination of impairments described previously increase the risk for falls, aspiration pneumonia, deep vein thrombosis, pressure ulcers, seizures, and contractures to name a few.

The rehabilitation prescription should include any or all of the following precautions as they apply to the patient:

Fall risk
Seizure risk
Aspiration risk
Visual–spatial deficits
Cardiac and hypertensive precautions
Exercise and modality restrictions secondary to sensory-, balance-, and weakness-related impairments
Hypoglycemic risk if the patient is diabetic
Orthopedic precautions (ie, weight bearing status, range of motion restrictions).

It is important that all rehabilitation staff abides by the rehabilitation precautions. For example, if a physical therapist identifies a fall risk factor in a stroke patient during transfers, he or she should share that information with other disciplines such as occupational therapy, speech pathology, and rehabilitation nursing, since the risk for falling is also present when the patient is seen by the other disciplines.

SPECIAL CONSIDERATIONS

Spasticity, a motor disorder resulting from hyperexcitability of the stretch reflex is seen in many areas of rehabilitation (eg, traumatic brain injury, spinal cord injury, multiple sclerosis, strokes), and it can be very disabling, resulting in weakness, pain, decreased dexterity, slowing of cognition, and fatigue. The decision to treat must consider the pros and cons of treatment, and the causes for an increase in tone must be determined before initiating treatment. Patients should be treated when the spasticity interferes with function. Potential benefits of treatment should outweigh the possibilities of adverse effects or toxicity due to the drugs used. Noxious stimuli such as pressure ulcers, distended bladders, fecal impaction, ingrown toe nails, or tight clothing should all be avoided. Patients with intrathecal pumps must be monitored, as there are concerns for catheter dislodgment, cerebral fluid leak, or the development of seroma.[9] There are health risks with the abrupt withdrawal of such medication like baclofen. Patients receiving medications such as baclofen, tizanidine, and dantrolene should be monitored, since too little medication will inadequately suppress spasticity, and too much may cause reduced limb tone that is less than adequate for optimal function.

The rehabilitation medicine prescription should include a section on spasticity related safety concerns. These should include: medications being used to treat the spasticity and most recent dosage, presence of an intrathecal baclofen pump, and surgeries performed for the treatment of spasticity.

Venous Thromboembolic Disease

Prevention of a deep vein thrombosis (DVT) is very important in rehabilitation medicine, since many rehabilitation patients are at high risk for developing DVT due to their underlying diagnoses (ie, stroke, brain injury, joint replacement, cancer, medical deconditioned state). The rehabilitation prescription should include information about the presence of a DVT, its location, date that it was diagnosed, and the treatment rendered. In addition, specific information should be provided with respect to restrictions to exercise, range of motion, and weight bearing status. Rehabilitation medicine staff should also have working knowledge of this condition, including risk factors, prophylactic regimens, clinical presentation, and treatment. Prophylactic medications commonly used include subcutaneous heparin, warfarin, and aspirin, and these should be instituted if not contraindicated.[1] In patients with hemorrhagic bleeds, the placement of sequential compressive devices on extremities (without contraindications such as recent surgery or ulcers on extremities) is an alternative for pharmacologic DVT prophylaxis.[2]

Heterotopic Ossification

This condition is commonly seen following a variety of conditions such as traumatic brain injury, spinal cord injury, stroke, total hip arthroplasty, and burns. Common locations include hips, knees, shoulders, and elbows. The presence of heterotopic ossification can significantly limit the range of motion in the affected joint, thereby impacting on mobility and activities of daily living. Diagnostic radiographs can aid in the confirmation of heterotopic ossification. Since heterotopic ossification can mimic DVT, it is very important to carefully examin the patient and perform the appropriate work up so as not to miss a diagnosis, which can be more detrimental to the patient.

The rehabilitation prescription should include the following information with respect to heterotopic ossification: location, medical treatments being rendered, and range of motion restrictions.

Pressure Ulcers

Patients with neurologic diagnoses such as stroke, spinal cord injury, brain injury, and medical debility who are referred for inpatient rehabilitation are at risk for developing pressure ulcers. Specific risk factors include: immobility, shearing forces, prolonged pressure over a bony prominence, incontinence, and malnutrition.[8] Prevention is the cornerstone of good medical, nursing, and rehabilitative care in high-risk populations. Nutritional support should always be implemented for stage 3 or 4 nutrition—30 to 35 kcal/kg/d, 1.2 to 1.5 g/kg/d protein, fluids 1 mL/kcal.[2] The patient should be turned every 2 hours, and the lateral decubitus (90°) position should be avoided. The patient should be assessed weekly. Heel protectors, appropriate mattress, and frequent debridement for necrotic areas can all be of help. The rehabilitation prescription should include the following information with respect to pressure ulcer \specific precautions: risk level for pressure ulcers, location of existing pressure ulcer, stage of pressure ulcer, treatments being rendered for the pressure ulcer, pressure relief strategies that need to be followed.

CANCER PRECAUTIONS

In cancer patients, hematological complications can adversely affect a patient's morbidity and mortality. In rehabilitation, programs should be individualized to accommodate the hematological limitations. The treating therapist should be instructed to withhold any therapy sessions if the hemoglobin is less than 8 g/dL. Aerobic or progressive resistance programs should be avoided. For patients with thrombocytopenia, the platelet count should be monitored regularly. Since a platelet count of 20,000/µL is a critical value, therapy should be withheld for values below this level. General guidelines for physical activity are as follows: less than 20,000/µL, functional mobility/activities of daily living; 20,000 to 30,000/µL, light exercise, active range of motion and functional mobility: 30,000 to 50,000/μL, moderate exercise, stationary bike; 50,000 to 150,000/μL, progressive resistive exercise, bicycling; greater than 150,000/μL, unrestricted normal activity.[10]

REFERENCES

1. Weber DC, Hoppe KM. Physical agent modalities. In: Braddom RL, editor. Physical medicine and rehabilitation. 4th edition. Philadelphia: Elsevier-Saunders; 2011. p. 449–63.
2. Wilder RP, Jenkins JG, Seto CK, et al. Therapeutic exercise. In: Braddom RL, editor. Physical medicine and rehabilitation. 4th edition. Philadelphia: Elsevier-Saunders; 2011. p. 403–24, 706, 1205.
3. David SP. Exercise presciption: a case study approach to the ACSM guidelines. 2nd edition. Champaign (IL): Human Kinetics; 2007.
4. American College of Sports Medicine. Guideline for exercise testing and prescription. 4th edition. Philadelphia: Lea & Febiger; 1991.
5. Chahalin LP, Lapier TK, Shaw DK. Sternal precautions: is it time for change? Precautions versus restrictions—a review of literature and recommendations for revision. Cardiopulm Phys Ther J 2011;22(1):5–15.
6. AACVPR. Pulmonary rehabilitation programs. 4th edition. Champaign (IL): Human Kinetics; 2011.
7. Cuccurullo SJ. Physical medicine and rehabilitation board review. 2nd edition. New York: Demos Medical Publishing; 2010.
8. O'Young B, Young M, Steins S. Physical medicine and rehabilitation secrets. 2nd edition. Philadelphia: Hanley & Belfus; 2002.
9. Stetkarova I, Yablon SA, Kofler M, et al. Procedure and device-related complications of intrathecal baclofen administration for management of adult muscle hypertonia: a review. Neurorehabil Neural Repair 2010;24(7):609–19.
10. Stampas A, Smith RG, Savodnik A, et al. Hematologic complications of cancer. In: Stubblefield MD, O'Dell MW, editors. Cancer rehabilitation, principles and practice. New York: Demos Medical; 2009. p. 401–2.

Patient Safety at Handoff in Rehabilitation Medicine

Jason W. Siefferman, MD*, Emerald Lin, MD, Jeffrey S. Fine, MD

KEYWORDS

- Handoff • Handover • Communication • Transfer • Discharge
- Admission • Rehabilitation

Improve the effectiveness of communication among caregivers.[1]
—National Patient Safety Goal 2, The Joint Commission

The Joint Commission (TJC) Center for Transforming Healthcare has cited communication as the most frequent root cause in sentinel events, with failed patient handoffs playing a "role in an estimated 80% of serious preventable adverse events."[2] Beyond the identification of this prominent culprit, there is limited consensus about what leads to communication failures or how to prevent them.[3,4] Handoff, or transfer of patient care information, occurs formally and informally many times each day. Handoff takes place within and between care teams, across all levels of care providers, and between institutions. Handoff at rehabilitation admission is at a particularly high risk for communication failure, and this review of the patient handoff literature discusses handoff safety, barriers, specific requirements and recommendations, and improvement methodologies.

As part of the postacute care (PAC) continuum, patients admitted to rehabilitation medicine settings, including acute rehabilitation (AR) and subacute rehabilitation (SAR) facilities, are often transferred with insufficient or inaccurate information from the referring hospital.[5–7] This presents a significant safety issue, especially as rehabilitation units accept many multimorbid and acutely postoperative patients who frequently require ongoing acute-level care.[5] These patients have a potentially higher risk of complications than patients discharged home,[6,8] and certain information is essential for providing safe and effective care.[9–11]

Handoff has been defined as, "The transfer of responsibility and accountability for some or all aspects of care for a patient, or group of patients, to another person or

Department of Rehabilitation Medicine, Mount Sinai School of Medicine, New York, NY, USA
* Corresponding author. One Gustave L. Levy Place, Box 1240, New York, NY 10029.
E-mail address: jsiefferman@gmail.com

Phys Med Rehabil Clin N Am 23 (2012) 241–257
doi:10.1016/j.pmr.2012.02.003
1047-9651/12/$ – see front matter © 2012 Elsevier Inc. All rights reserved.

professional group on a temporary or permanent basis."[12] Admission to a rehabilitation unit may represent the most dramatic transfer of care in our health care system, as full responsibility and accountability for possibly all aspects of care change. Other types of transfers, such as from one hospital intensive care unit (ICU) to another, might involve more critical patient scenarios, but there is often more commonality between those units than exists between any medical or surgical ward and a rehabilitation facility.

With a rehabilitation admission, changes often include the level of care (ICU vs step-down vs ward), individual members of the primary team, specialty of the primary team (physicians and nurses), the addition of other team players (therapists), and even a change of the hospital center itself. Less obvious are changes in pharmacy formulary, team structure and hierarchy (including presence or absence of residents or physician extenders), reimbursement algorithms, and the availability of subspecialty consultants familiar with the patient. The rehabilitation admission handoff, therefore, presents a tremendous opportunity for miscommunication, communication deficits, and inaccuracies.

Despite the potential patient safety risks of inadequate patient handoff, published research is limited and best practices have yet to be universally established.[3,13-15] Most studies have focused on inpatient intershift handoffs (ie, nursing shift change), intrafacility handoffs (ie, emergency room [ER] to ward) and discharge to home.[3] To our knowledge, there are no peer-reviewed articles reporting the state of handoff practices to the acute rehabilitation setting, although studies have been presented at national meetings.[5,16] Unfortunately, many quality improvement projects and studies are performed for institutional advancement rather than academic enterprise, and are not submitted for publication.[17]

As the science of handoff remains in its formative stages, no universal standardized handoff protocol for admission to AR or SAR hospitals has been established. TJC and the World Health Organization (WHO) have identified handoff standardization as a key element in improving patient safety[18,19]; however, specific handoff elements and methods of standardization have not yet been firmly established in daily clinical practice.

To determine the most appropriate content for handoff, the purpose and importance of handoff must first be reviewed. The definition cited previously is broad, and specific clinical scenarios require tailored handoffs.[3,13,20] For example, an orthopedic patient may have specific weight-bearing restrictions or deep vein thrombosis (DVT) prophylaxis instructions that have direct implications for therapy and medical management. Even if the patient does not have any restrictions, simply because the patient is on a service with such a high prevalence of such restrictions, this becomes a very relevant pertinent negative for handoff. Case-specific criteria, such as these, both reinforce the need for standardization and render it a challenging process.

IMPORTANCE OF HANDOFF

Each patient handoff poses a potential safety risk,[4] and a TJC study found that handoffs were defective 37% of the time.[2] Defective handoffs may lead to treatment delays, inappropriate treatment, increased length of stay, and even serious adverse events.[2,4] An Australian study found that 11% of 30,000 preventable adverse events resulting in disability were a result of poor communication, compared with only 6% that were a result of practitioner oversight.[21] In the United States, one malpractice insurance company reported that the leading cause of claims resulting from patient transfer was communication breakdown.[22]

Among all points of transfer, communication breakdown at discharge has been found to be a leading cause of adverse events.[9-11] Discharge summaries are often not available at the time of the first outpatient follow-up (<34%), and those completed by the time of follow-up often lacked important content, such as discharge medications, test results, and tests pending at discharge.[9,23,24] The latter has been directly associated with adverse events.[24–26] In addition, an absent discharge summary at outpatient follow-up has been found to increase the risk of hospital readmission.[11] A medical reconciliation that lacks explanations for any changes in home medications may also result in adverse events.[27]

As discharge information from the acute hospital often forms the basis for admission orders in a rehabilitation facility, this becomes a focus of concern for patient safety.[6] Any deficits or inaccuracies in discharge paperwork present a significant safety issue, especially considering that patients on admission to AR facilities are generally less medically stable than those discharged home.[6,8] Disturbingly, our study of information received at the time of admission to AR found that the more medically complex patients (greater number of medical comorbidities) arrived with significantly less complete information.[5] Similarly, an evaluation of discharge paperwork received by SAR facilities found that only 33.5% of packets contained all applicable measures, with a defect rate ranging from 24.0% to 39.0% across 5 hospitals.[6]

HANDOFF ELEMENTS

Although poor communication is prevalent and associated with negative outcomes, the delineation of handoff elements and types of handoff information that are most important remains unresolved. Other than the association between omitted pending test results and adverse events,[24–26] we found no other study that linked the absence of a particular element to an adverse event. Our previously mentioned AR study failed to correlate the absence of any one piece of relevant information with adverse events, although there were very few adverse events overall.[5]

The criteria for evaluating handoffs or discharge packets vary among studies. The core elements include TJC requirements with additional elements determined by the study authors. TJC requires a medical reconciliation and 6 discharge summary elements.[1] Additional elements apply if the hospital uses an electronic medical records (EMR) system and wishes to qualify for federal benefits.[28]

The discharge summary, according to TJC Standard RC.02.04.01,[1] should state:

- Reason for hospitalization
- Procedures performed
- Care, treatment, and services provided
- Condition at discharge
- Information provided to patient and family
- Follow-up care.

Although not explicitly required, others have thought it reasonable to expect activity restrictions, weight-bearing status, and diet instructions to be included also.[29]

Instructions reviewing all medications are also among the information required to be provided to the patient.[1] The medication reconciliation is meant to clarify discrepancies between discharge medications and medications taken before admission. TJC National Patient Safety Goal (NPSG 03.06.01) states that the process should include medication name, dose, frequency, route of administration, and reason for starting or changing doses.[1] Beyond these defined elements, this NPSG also provides for the inclusion of other information that may be required to safely administer medications in the future: "Organizations should identify the information that needs to be collected to reconcile current and newly ordered medications and to safely prescribe medications in the future."[1] This infers the inclusion of recent international normalized ratio (INR) values for patients on warfarin, or serum drug levels for patients on antiepileptics.

Although anticoagulation information is not explicitly required, NPSG 03.05.01 is to "reduce the likelihood of patient harm associated with the use of anticoagulant therapy."[1] Routine short-term prophylactic anticoagulation is excluded, but only when "the patient's laboratory values for coagulation will remain within, or close to, normal values." Although heparin 5000 units subcutaneously every 12 hours would be excluded, warfarin with a goal INR of 1.8 to 2.2 would not. There is, therefore, some embedded responsibility placed on the discharging service to ensure that the admitting service receives all the information necessary to safely continue anticoagulation.

The federal certification criteria for "meaningful use" of an EMR require that other relevant clinical data elements be documented and shared. To qualify for financial incentives, the hospital, via its EMR, must "provide patients with an electronic copy of their health information (including diagnostic test results, problem list, medication lists, medication allergies, discharge summary, procedures) on request."[28] An additional criterion states that when a facility "transitions their patient to another setting of care...[it] should provide summary of care record."[28]

Despite these requirements, discharge summaries were absent or incomplete in 42.0% of admissions to AR[5] and 21.0% to 29.7% of admissions to SAR.[6,29] Medication reconciliation was absent or incomplete in 39% of admissions to AR,[5] and information was missing in up to 35% on admission to SAR.[6] Follow-up instructions, which were absent in 2.0% to 43.0% of a larger review of discharge summaries,[9] were missing in 60.0% of AR admissions,[5] and 11.1% of SAR admissions.[6]

Additional nonrequired data elements that have been screened for on admission to AR and SAR facilities include:

- Laboratory results[5,6]
- Radiology results[5,6]
- Test results pending at transfer[6]
- Anticoagulation instructions/relevant data[5,7]
- Weight-bearing status/therapy precautions[5,16]
- Steroid instructions[5,16]
- Seizure treatment/prophylaxis instructions[5]
- Antibiotic instructions/duration[5,16]
- Wound care instructions[16]
- Dietary restrictions.[16]

A review of discharge-to-home paperwork by Kriplani and colleagues[9] found diagnostic test results, including laboratory and radiology results, absent in 33% to 65% of discharge summaries. Laboratory results were missing from only 12.0% of AR[5] and 17.9% of SAR[6] admissions. Similarly, radiology results were missing from 20.0% of AR[5] and 10.7% of SAR[6] admissions. Our AR study found that radiology results were most likely to be omitted for trauma cases, and were included less frequently for patients who later suffered adverse events (60% vs 81%, nonsignificant).[5] Information about test results pending at transfer was absent in 65.0% of general discharges[9] and 47.2% of SAR admissions.[6]

Anticoagulation instructions and pertinent information was specifically studied on admission to SAR by Gandara and colleagues.[7] For their study, the Anticoagulation

Task Force at Massachusetts General Hospital determined that the following elements are essential for safely prescribing warfarin:

- Indication
- Target INR range
- Treatment duration
- Last 3 INR values with dates
- Last 3 warfarin doses
- Recommended dose until next INR
- Responsible follow-up provider.

The same panel determined that to safely prescribe unfractionated heparin (UH) or low-molecular-weight heparin (LMWH), the following elements are essential:

- Indication
- Agent
- Dose
- Treatment duration
- Required monitoring (if indicated).

They found that discharge summaries contained all of the required information for only 16.4% of patients on warfarin and 45.4% of patients on UH or LMWH.[7] The most common missing elements for UH of LMWH were duration of therapy (50.6%) and monitoring parameters (90.3%). For warfarin, recent INR (59.9%) and prior warfarin doses (55.0%) were most often absent, followed by identification of the follow-up provider.[7] Interestingly, community hospitals and surgical services were more likely to provide this required information. Our AR study found that DVT treatment/prophylaxis instructions were missing in 40% of admissions, most frequently among those with a brain or spine diagnosis.[5]

Weight-bearing status and therapy precautions, including brace and immobilization instructions, were missing in 52% of AR admissions.[5] Similarly, steroid, antiepileptic, and antibiotic recommendations were missing in 56% to 62% of AR admissions.[5] Of patients admitted with a brain diagnosis, steroid instructions (when indicated) were provided for only 11%, and antiepileptic instructions for 42%.[5]

Although this information is absolutely necessary to continue the patient's care, empiric evidence that the inclusion of these data in admission handoff improves patient safety has yet to be produced (with the exception of test results pending at transfer).[24–26] Our study found that medical reconciliation, therapy precautions, and imaging results were missing among patients with adverse events more often than among those without adverse events, but these results were not statistically significant.[5] Evidence supporting the inclusion of additional rehabilitation-specific handoff elements, which presumably improve patient safety, will endorse the need for and better clarify the standardization of rehabilitation admission handoffs. Please see Appendix 1 for a list of rehabilitation-specific handoff elements.

BARRIERS TO HANDOFF

For patient handoff to be effective, "both the sender and the receiver achieve a shared understanding and perceive the content in the same way."[30] This includes the concrete data elements (ie, vitals, laboratory tests), as well as the emphasis placed on them and their role in the decision making process. Although communication tools and frameworks have been recently introduced, no standardized formula has been developed that consistently results in such a shared mental model. Many of the obstacles that prevent effective handoff have been identified, though, and these may be minimized or avoided.

Some of the more insidious barriers to effective communication arise from individual means of filtering and processing information.[30] As autonomy and individual performance are rewarded by the health care system,[4] these factors may play a larger role. Our individuality arises from the sum of our personal experiences, which is influenced by the following[4]:

- Identity (race, ethnicity, gender, age, and so forth)
- Culture
- Personality
- Language
  - Regional vernacular
  - Health literacy
  - Verbal expression and comprehension education
- Fears/Insecurities.

Considering the potential disparity between caregiver demographics and the community they serve,[31] these variables require particular attention when providing education and handoff to patients and their families.

Previous health care experiences also affect our delivery and interpretation of handoff, and may be shaped by the following[4]:

- Institutional protocols
- Prior cases (similar patients)
- Specialty or subspecialty focus
- Goals of care
- Hierarchy within the care team.

Perhaps easier to address, though, are some of the systematic barriers to handoff. These include workflow, institutional, and educational barriers. Workflow barriers refer to the challenges of finding appropriate time and space for handoff. For example, nurses have ongoing patient care requirements, unpredictable staffing shortages, time constraints, and possibly even simultaneous administrative responsibilities that form unique daily barriers to handoff.

Anesthesiologists reported handoff occurring in the midst of other attention-demanding activities.[32] Furthermore, they may have been only transiently involved in the patient's care and are therefore unable to provide a comprehensive handoff.[32] A study of ER physicians reported that high workloads prevented them from reassessing a patient between handoff and transfer, and so the admitting service was rarely notified of any interim changes.[33] This potential for communication failure may be amplified if there are long boarding times combined with provider shift changes.

Workflow barriers to handoff on admission to AR or SAR might often include a combination of the barriers mentioned previously. Physician-to-physician handoff is uncommon, and handoff more likely follows a path of discharging provider to social worker to admissions coordinator to physician. This complexity presents many opportunities for communication breakdown:

- The discharging provider may not be the primary provider and may not know the pertinent elements for that patient's handoff (ie, mobility restrictions or anticoagulation instructions).[5]
- Discharge paperwork is often completed in advance, and updates are not made while the patient is awaiting a vacant rehabilitation bed.[5]

- The discharging social worker and provider may be overworked, making coordination for discharge planning difficult.[5]
- The discharging provider may not be aware of the handoff elements that are most important for a rehabilitation provider to know on admission.
- When the patient arrives, which may be later in the evening, the discharging service may be unavailable to answer questions.

Institutional support and intervention with the goal of improving handoff could potentially address many of the workflow barriers. Historically, there has been limited oversight, standardization, and training of staff regarding proper handoff.[4] This is likely related to a combination of caregiver resistance to practice change, the cost of implementing new handoff procedures, and the lack of research demonstrating the economic benefit of improved handoff.[4] Although TJC Leadership Standards require that leaders "provide for an infrastructure that enables effective communication,"[34] they do not specify the methodology or means by which this should be accomplished. Similarly, discrete outcome measures and goals are not set.

METHODS OF IMPROVING HANDOFF

Handoff should ideally occur in a setting with minimal distractions, at a time dedicated to the transfer of care. In one study, precise, unambiguous, face-to-face communication produced the best handoff results.[35] Handoff is most effective as a dialogue, where both parties establish common ground for understanding the information conveyed and interpreting its significance.[13] In addition, according to TJC, any type of handoff communication should include "an opportunity to clarify any ambiguous information," as this improves the effectiveness of handoff.[18]

In August 2009, The Joint Commission Center for Transforming Care initiated the Handoff Communication Project to develop a model to assist health care organizations overcome barriers to effective handoff. The resulting handoff solution helps to reduce process variation and is summarized by the acronym SHARE[36]:

- Standardize critical content: includes details of patient history; emphasis on key information; synthesizing patient information from separate sources
- Hardwire within your system: includes standardizing forms, tools methods, checklists; quiet workspace that is conductive to sharing information; stating expectations about how to conduct a successful handoff; use new and existing handoff technologies
- Allow opportunities to ask questions: includes critical thinking skills when discussing patient care; expecting to receive all key information; scrutinizing and questioning the data; sharing information as an interdisciplinary team; exchanging contact information in the event there any additional questions
- Reinforce quality and measurement: includes demonstrating leadership commitment to successful handoffs; holding staff accountable for managing patient's care; monitoring compliance using standardized forms and methods; using data to determine a systematic approach for improvement
- Educate and coach: includes teaching staff what constitutes successful handoff; standardizing training on how to conduct a handoff; providing real-time performance feedback to staff; making successful handoffs an organizational priority.

Standardization of handoffs reduces variation in the amount of information and style of presentation, and has been shown to improve handoff safety.[18] An NPSG is to "implement a standardized approach to handoff communications, including an opportunity to ask and respond to questions."[18] It ensures that essential information is included and potentially distracting extraneous information is excluded. It also establishes a predictable flow of the information from the presenter, providing structure and consistency.[3] A standardized handoff, although structured, cannot be rigid. It must be flexible enough to apply to diverse patient scenarios.[13]

In 2009, the American College of Physicians, Society of Hospital Medicine and American Geriatrics Society among others, developed consensus standards to improve the quality of transitions between inpatient and outpatient settings. These guidelines, the Transitions of Care Consensus Conference (TOCCC) Policy Statement, include recommendations for effective care plan transition records including a minimum set of data elements that are irreducible, and an additional set of elements that should be included in an "ideal transition record."[37] Kripalani and colleagues[9] investigated deficits in communication and information transfer between hospital-based discharging physicians and community-based primary care physicians. Their recommendations included structured discharge summaries with subheadings to organize the information most relevant to follow-up care in the outpatient setting. Please see Appendix 2 for the compiled recommendations.

Another standardized tool that may aid in communication at transitions of care is the Continuity Assessment Record and Evaluation (CARE) tool. It was designed partly to unify admission and discharge assessment tools currently used in AR and SAR settings, namely the Inpatient Rehabilitation Facility Patient Assessment Instrument and the Minimum Data Set, respectively. The CARE tool incorporates many of the transition elements previously outlined and includes many pertinent rehabilitation items, measured in the following 4 domains:

- Medical, including changes in disease severity, current health status
- Functional, including performance of activities of daily living
- Cognitive
- Social/Environmental factors.

It is designed to be administered on admission and discharge from all ACH and PAC settings.

Several verbal communication tools have been developed to "standardize and hardwire" content, including the sequence and reporting of information elements at handoff in a variety of settings. The SBAR handoff was developed at Kaiser Permanente of Colorado and initially developed as a tool to be used in urgent care settings where promptness and accuracy are critical to immediate patient care decisions.[38] SBAR has also been successfully applied in other care settings including AR.

- Situation: "What is going on with the patient?" Identify self, location, patient, and reason for concern; briefly identify the problem with onset and severity.
- Background: "What is the clinical background or context?" Pertinent medical history, including admitting diagnosis and admission date, current medications, allergies, intravenous fluids, vital signs, laboratory results (date and time test was done and results of previous tests for comparison), and code status.
- Assessment: "What do I think the problem is?" Provide your assessment of the current clinical situation.
- Recommendation and Request: "What should we do to correct it?" Provide your recommendation, including a management plan that will immediately follow, such as laboratory tests, imaging, medications, specialist consultation, or transfer to a different level of care.

The Department of Health and Human Services, Department of Defense, and Agency for Healthcare Research and Quality (AHRQ) developed an "evidence-based framework to optimize team performance across the health care delivery system": Strategies & Tools to Enhance Performance and Patient Safety (TeamSTEPPS).[39] This program is based on 4 core teachable-learnable skill modules: leadership, situation monitoring, mutual support, and communication. A recommended TeamSTEPPS communication strategy designed to enhance information exchange during transitions in care, is IPASStheBATON.[39] It is designed to be used for more comprehensive handoffs as an alternative to SBAR.

(I) Introduction: Identify yourself and your role
(P) Patient: Name, identifiers, age, sex, and location
(A) Assessment: Chief complaint, vital signs, symptoms, diagnosis
(S) Situation: Current condition/situation, level of diagnostic certainty, recent changes, response to treatments and code status
(S) Safety concerns: Pertinent laboratory/imaging results, allergies, precautions (falls, isolation, and so forth), and socioeconomic factors
the
(B) Background: Pertinent medical history, including prior episodes, current medications, family history
(A) Actions: Care currently provided or newly required, with concise rationale
(T) Timing: Convey level of urgency, including explicit timing and prioritization of next actions to be taken
(O) Ownership: Identify person(s) responsible for the actions in the next interval of care; may be patient or family/caregivers
(N) Next: Next steps to be taken, anticipated changes, primary plan and backup plans

Despite the amount of ongoing research and tools under development, there remains a lack of consensus and robust evidence on best handoff practices.[3,13–15] Furthermore, valid standardized tools for evaluating handoff quality are lacking.[3] Based on the available evidence, WHO has made the following handoff recommendations[4]:

1. Use a standardized approach
   a. Use SBAR (or similar tool)
   b. Allow enough uninterrupted time for questions
   c. Include patient status, medications, treatment plans, advance directives, and significant status changes
   d. Limit information exchange to what is necessary for safe patient care
2. Implement systems that ensure the patient and next health care provider receive information at discharge, including discharge diagnoses, treatment plans, medications, and test results
3. Educate caregivers on effective handoff communication
4. Encourage interorganizational communication.

Standardization has been shown to improve critical thinking while minimizing time spent away from direct patient care.[40] Discharge summaries have been improved by implementing standardized content.[11] One study showed that a standardized operating room to ICU handoff protocol significantly decreased technical errors and information omissions, along with improving teamwork.[41] In another study, pharmacists combined a standardized form with verbal handoff, reducing errors and omissions at transfer ($P<.0001$) and interventions required because of errors or omissions ($P = .001$).[42] Success has also been demonstrated with a standardized intershift ER physician protocol.[14] Standardization of rehabilitation admission forms, including many of the previously mentioned handoff elements, have been proposed and implemented (see Appendix 1), but no data on effectiveness are currently available.[5–7]

Patient safety experts advocate for design improvements in care delivery systems, which would facilitate handoff standardization.[19] Technology can improve accuracy by[4]

- Accounting for human factors (error prediction)
- Incorporating appropriate redundancies
- Forced functions/elements
- Simplifying the process (reducing opportunity for error).

Among infrastructural supports for handoff, electronic sign-outs have been shown to reduce rates of preventable adverse events.[43] In one study, the use of an electronic discharge summary resulted in improved quality and timeliness over dictation, with more frequent documentation of follow-up issues, pending test results, and patient-family handoff.[23] For physician-physician handoff, a Veterans Affairs hospital designed software that provided readable and complete handoffs.[44] One caution, though, is that design for such systems should be driven by the intended users. "Top-down deployment of informatics systems that doesn't consider real-time work flow results in work-arounds, frustration, and failure."[45]

An often overlooked resource for safety and quality improvement is the actual patient and his or her family. Patient and family involvement in handoff at discharge has been shown to reduce rates of rehospitalization, as well as the overall cost of hospitalization.[46,47] Caregivers may include patients and their families in the handoff process in the following ways[4,47]:

- Educate patients about their conditions, using teach-back techniques
- Provide information about medical conditions and surgical procedures
- Discuss the current plan of care, including formal family meetings
- Review current medications and instructions
- Allow patients to review their medical record
- Create opportunities for questions and answers.

Please see Appendix 3 for a comprehensive patient handoff model.

Incorporating new handoff methodologies is undoubtedly challenging. Kind and Smith[29] suggested that "Modification of the Joint Commission discharge summary component standards might be instrumental in changing U.S. discharge summary documentation practices." Position statements by professional organizations stating key handoff elements for their specialty may also be helpful. Others promote the involvement of institutional administration in the implementation of handoff protocol improvements.[48,49] Improvements beyond policy changes, however, such as infrastructure upgrades with associated costs, require articulate qualitative and quantitative (ie, financial) analysis to garner institutional support.[50] Further research in this area will be necessary for effective change to occur.

SUMMARY AND FUTURE TRENDS

Standardization of handoff communication has improved operational safety in commercial industries and similarly yielded patient safety improvements in many medical settings. Cited studies demonstrate that improvements are necessary in rehabilitation medicine, particularly on admission to AR and SAR.

Comprehensive Acute Care Hospital (ACH) discharge summary information, such as content outlined by TOCCC, translates across all settings and forms a foundation for best practices. Providers receiving patients in rehabilitation settings require inclusion of additional key elements to accomplish the ideal handoff, as demonstrated in part by the CARE tool. Effective handoffs enable rehabilitation clinicians to develop safe interdisciplinary treatment plans with a medically stable foundation to achieve expected functional goals. Successful rehabilitation preadmission and admission handoffs ensure continuity of all care plans and treatment timelines, including on specialist follow-up and eventual discharge to subsequent community providers.

Institutional support is essential for workflow adjustments, infrastructure, training, oversight, and feedback for ongoing and dynamic handoff performance improvement. Providing a structured environment and an institutional culture that expects complete and accountable handoffs are part of the recommended standardization and hardwiring of the transition process. Communication tools, such as SBAR and IPASStheBATON, provide a checklist framework to preserve content completeness despite workflow distractions or changes in setting. These tools can be further customized and appended to meet rehabilitation specialty or discipline-specific needs.

Ongoing research evaluating clinical, financial, and patient satisfaction outcomes will provide future direction for effective handoffs. Eventual universal EMR, maturation of medical home models, and transition to the tenth revision of the International Classification of Diseases (with complementary reference to the International Classification of Functioning, Disability and Health [ICF] framework) all provide rich opportunities for communication and patient safety improvements. Thorough and effective discharge communications avoid fragmentation of information and care. Standardization of handoff content and process will create a virtual discharge planner for all care transitions.

Arising technologies, such as cloud-based personal medical records and patient-specific education materials and discharge instructions, will allow patients to access their own health care information anywhere. Combined with integrated home-based medical monitoring equipment, patients and their families will be able to participate in their care more actively than ever. Although these tools could not replace direct provider-provider handoffs, patient involvement in the process is empowering, and will allow them to assume some interim responsibilities between provider encounters. Patient involvement will likely also help prevent information loss or inaccuracies during transitions of care.

Rehabilitation settings are traditionally recognized as models of effective interdisciplinary team communication. Rehabilitation providers are creative, adaptable and optimistic clinicians and empathetic communicators who are well accustomed to coordinating care for their patients. These patient-centered skill sets and accommodating philosophy will certainly be practical in navigating the patient safety and communication horizon, perhaps generating leaders in this growing and important field.

REFERENCES

1. Joint Commission on Accreditation of Healthcare Organizations. Comprehensive accreditation manual for hospitals. Oakbrook Terrace (IL): The Joint Commission; 2012.
2. Joint Commission Center for Transforming Healthcare announces hand-off communications solutions. Joint Commission Online. 2010. Available at: http://www.jointcommission.org/assets/1/18/jconline_Oct_21_10_update.pdf. Accessed December 5, 2011.
3. Ong MS, Coiera E. A systematic review of failures in handoff communication during intrahospital transfers. Jt Comm J Qual Patient Saf 2011;37(6):274–84.

4. Communication during patient handovers. Patient safety solutions. World Health Organization; 2007. Available at: http://www.ccforpatientsafety.org/common/pdfs/fpdf/presskit/PS-Solution3.pdf. Accessed December 5, 2011.

5. Siefferman J, Lin E, Ambrose FA. Improving patient handoff for acute rehabilitation admission. Orlando (FL): American Academy of Physical Medicine and Rehabilitation; 2011.

6. Gandara E, Moniz T, Ungar J, et al. Communication and information deficits in patients discharged to rehabilitation facilities: an evaluation of five acute care hospitals. J Hosp Med 2009;4(8):E28–33.

7. Gandara E, Moniz TT, Ungar J, et al. Deficits in discharge documentation in patients transferred to rehabilitation facilities on anticoagulation: results of a systemwide evaluation. Jt Comm J Qual Patient Saf 2008;34(8):460–3.

8. Prvu Bettger JA, Stineman MG. Effectiveness of multidisciplinary rehabilitation services in postacute care: state-of-the-science. A review. Arch Phys Med Rehabil 2007;88(11):1526–34.

9. Kripalani S, LeFevre F, Phillips CO, et al. Deficits in communication and information transfer between hospital-based and primary care physicians: implications for patient safety and continuity of care. JAMA 2007;297(8):831–41.

10. Moore C, Wisnivesky J, Williams S, et al. Medical errors related to discontinuity of care from an inpatient to an outpatient setting. J Gen Intern Med 2003;18(8): 646–51.

11. van Walraven C, Seth R, Austin PC, et al. Effect of discharge summary availability during post-discharge visits on hospital readmission. J Gen Intern Med 2002; 17(3):186–92.

12. Bywaters E, Calvert S, Eccles S, et al. Safe handover: safe patients. Guidance on clinical handover for clinicians and managers. British Medical Association; 2011. Available at: http://www.bma.org.uk/images/safehandover_tcm41-20983.pdf. Accessed December 5, 2011.

13. Gibson SC, Ham JJ, Apker J, et al. Communication, communication, communication: the art of the handoff. Ann Emerg Med 2010;55(2):181–3.

14. Cheung DS, Kelly JJ, Beach C, et al. Improving handoffs in the emergency department. Ann Emerg Med 2010;55(2):171–80.

15. Cohen MD, Hilligoss PB. The published literature on handoffs in hospitals: deficiencies identified in an extensive review. Qual Saf Health Care 2010;19(6):493–7.

16. Neufeld NJ, González Fernández M, Cabahug P, et al. Pre and post analysis of a lean six sigma quality improvement project to increase discharge paperwork completeness to a comprehensive integrated inpatient rehabilitation program. Orlando (FL): American Academy of Physical Medicine and Rehabilitation; 2011.

17. Davidoff F, Batalden P. Toward stronger evidence on quality improvement. Draft publication guidelines: the beginning of a consensus project. Qual Saf Health Care 2005;14(5):319–25.

18. Croteau R. JCAHO comments on handoff requirement. OR Manager 2005;21(8):8.

19. WHO. Communication During Patient Handovers. Patient Safety Solutions 2007. Available at: http://www.ccforpatientsafety.org/common/pdfs/fpdf/presskit/PS-Solution3.pdf. Accessed December 5, 2011.

20. Van Eaton E. Handoff improvement: we need to understand what we are trying to fix. Jt Comm J Qual Patient Saf 2010;36(2):51.

21. Zinn C. 14,000 preventable deaths in Australian hospitals. BMJ 1995;310(6993):1487.

22. Andrews C, Millar S. Don't fumble the handoff. Inpatient providers, specialists, and the primary care physician: a medical care delivery system with benefits and complex risks. J Med Assoc Ga 2007;96(3):23–4.

23. O'Leary KJ, Liebovitz DM, Feinglass J, et al. Creating a better discharge summary: improvement in quality and timeliness using an electronic discharge summary. J Hosp Med 2009;4(4):219–25.

24. Apker J, Mallak LA, Gibson SC. Communicating in the "gray zone": perceptions about emergency physician hospitalist handoffs and patient safety. Acad Emerg Med 2007;14(10):884–94.

25. Roy CL, Poon EG, Karson AS, et al. Patient safety concerns arising from test results that return after hospital discharge. Ann Intern Med 2005;143(2):121–8.

26. Moore C, McGinn T, Halm E. Tying up loose ends: discharging patients with unresolved medical issues. Arch Intern Med 2007;167(12):1305–11.

27. Schnipper JL, Kirwin JL, Cotugno MC, et al. Role of pharmacist counseling in preventing adverse drug events after hospitalization. Arch Intern Med 2006;166(5):565–71.

28. Department of Health and Human Services. Health information technology: initial set of standards, implementation specifications, and certification criteria for electronic health record technology. Fed Regist 2010;75(144):44589–654.

29. Kind AJ, Smith MA. Documentation of Mandated Discharge Summary Components in Transitions from Acute to Subacute Care (vol. 2: Culture and Redesign). 2008.

30. Chatman IJ, editor. Joint commission guide to improving staff communication. Oakbrook Terrace (IL): Joint Commission Resources; 2009.

31. Office of Minority Health. National Standards on Culturally and Linguistically Appropriate Services in Health Care. 2001. Available at: http://minorityhealth.hhs.gov/assets/pdf/checked/finalreport.pdf. Accessed December 27, 2011.

32. Smith AF, Pope C, Goodwin D, et al. Interprofessional handover and patient safety in anaesthesia: observational study of handovers in the recovery room. Br J Anaesth 2008;101(3):332–7.

33. Horwitz LI, Meredith T, Schuur JD, et al. Dropping the baton: a qualitative analysis of failures during the transition from emergency department to inpatient care. Ann Emerg Med 2009;53(6):701–10, e704.

34. Schyve PM. Communication: the bond to patient safety. Joint Commission guide to improving staff communication. Oakbrook Terrace (IL): Joint Commission Resources; 2009.

35. Solet DJ, Norvell JM, Rutan GH, et al. Lost in translation: challenges and opportunities in physician-to-physician communication during patient handoffs. Acad Med 2005;80(12):1094–9.

36. Facts about the Hand-off Communications Project. Joint Commission Center for Transforming Healthcare; 2011. Available at: http://www.centerfortransforminghealthcare.org/assets/4/6/CTH_HOC_Fact_Sheet_9_29_11.pdf. Accessed February 6, 2012.

37. Snow V, Beck D, Budnitz T, et al. Transitions of Care Consensus Policy Statement American College of Physicians-Society of General Internal Medicine-Society of Hospital Medicine-American Geriatrics Society-American College of Emergency Physicians-Society of Academic Emergency Medicine. J Gen Intern Med 2009;24(8):971–6.

38. Institute for Healthcare Improvement. SBAR technique for communication: a situational briefing model. 2011. Available at: http://www.ihi.org/knowledge/Pages/Tools/SBARTechniqueforCommunicationASituationalBriefingModel.aspx. Accessed January 10, 2012.

39. TeamSTEPPS (R) strategies & tools to enhance performance and patient safety. Agency for Healthcare Research and Quality; 2011. Available at: http://teamstepps.ahrq.gov. Accessed February 6, 2012.

40. Hansten R. Streamline change-of-shift report. Nurs Manag 2003;34(8):58–9.

41. Catchpole KR, de Leval MR, McEwan A, et al. Patient handover from surgery to intensive care: using Formula 1 pit-stop and aviation models to improve safety and quality. Paediatr Anaesth 2007;17(5):470–8.
42. Coutsouvelis J, Corallo CE, Dooley MJ, et al. Implementation of a pharmacist-initiated pharmaceutical handover for oncology and haematology patients being transferred to critical care units. Support Care Cancer 2010;18(7):811–6.
43. Petersen LA, Orav EJ, Teich JM, et al. Using a computerized sign-out program to improve continuity of inpatient care and prevent adverse events. Jt Comm J Qual Improv 1998;24(2):77–87.
44. Anderson J, Shroff D, Curtis A, et al. The Veterans Affairs shift change physician-to-physician handoff project. Jt Comm J Qual Patient Saf 2010;36(2):62–71.
45. Nikula RE. Why implementing EPR's does not bring about organizational changes—a qualitative approach. Stud Health Technol Inform 2001;84(Pt 1):666–9.
46. Forster AJ, Clark HD, Menard A, et al. Adverse events among medical patients after discharge from hospital. CMAJ 2004;170(3):345–9.
47. Coleman EA, Parry C, Chalmers S, et al. The care transitions intervention: results of a randomized controlled trial. Arch Intern Med 2006;166(17):1822–8.
48. Reason J. Understanding adverse events: human factors. Qual Health Care 1995;4(2):80–9.
49. Sutcliffe KM, Lewton E, Rosenthal MM. Communication failures: an insidious contributor to medical mishaps. Acad Med 2004;79(2):186–94.
50. Mourad M, Cucina R, Ramanathan R, et al. Addressing the business of discharge: building a case for an electronic discharge summary. J Hosp Med 2011;6(1):37–42.

APPENDIX 1: REHABILITATION-SPECIFIC HANDOFF ELEMENTS

- Laboratory results with dates
- Radiology results with dates
- Test results pending at transfer with contact number at discharging institution
- Anticoagulation instructions
  - Prophylaxis versus treatment
  - Duration of prophylaxis or treatment
  - Goal (ie, partial thromboplastin time [PTT], INR)
  - Last 3 INR or PTT values with dates/times
  - Last 3 doses with dates/times
  - Recommended dose until next INR
  - Responsible follow-up provider
- Steroid instructions
  - Indication
  - Dose/Taper instructions
  - Duration
  - Glucose monitoring
- Seizure instructions
  - Prophylaxis versus treatment
  - Antiepileptic dose
  - Recent and target serum levels
  - Duration of prophylaxis or treatment
- Antibiotic instructions/duration
  - Indication: source and culture results
  - Duration of treatment

- Therapy precautions, as indicated
  - Cardiac limitations
  - Weight-bearing status of each limb
  - Mobility with/without brace
    - Brace at all times versus out of bed
    - Duration of brace use
    - Contact information for brace supplier
- Ventilator instructions
  - Settings/Schedule
  - Recent blood gas results
- Wound care instructions
  - Dressing
  - Suture removal
- Diet instructions
  - Swallowing status
  - Diet order.

APPENDIX 2: DISCHARGE SUMMARY RECOMMENDATIONS

Transitions of Care Consensus Conference (TOCCC) Transition Record Data Elements[37]
- Minimum transition data set that should always be part of any transition record
  - Principal diagnosis and problem list
  - Medication list with reconciliation including over-the-counter, herbals
  - Allergies and drug interactions
  - Clear identification of medical home/coordinating physician/institution with contact information
  - Patient cognitive status
  - Test results/pending results.
- Ideal transition record includes the following in addition to those listed above
  - Emergency plan, contact person, and phone number
  - Treatment and diagnostic plan
  - Prognosis and goal of care
  - Advanced directives, power of attorney, consents
  - Planned interventions
  - Durable medical equipment
  - Wound care
  - Assessment of caregiver status
  - Patients and/or caregivers must receive, understand, and be encouraged to participate in the development of their transition record, which should take into consideration the patient's health literacy and insurance status, and be culturally sensitive.

Information Transfer at Hospital Discharge[9]
- Discharge summaries should be structured with subheadings to organize and highlight the information most pertinent to follow-up care, including
  - Primary and secondary diagnoses
  - Pertinent medical history and physical findings
  - Dates of hospitalization, treatment provided, brief hospital course
  - Results of procedures and abnormal laboratory test results

o Recommendations of subspecialty consultants
o Information given to patient and family
o The patient's condition or functional status at discharge
o Reconciled discharge medication regimen, with reasons for any changes and indications for any newly prescribed medications
o Details of specific follow-up arrangements made
o Specific follow-up needs, including appointments or procedures to be scheduled, and tests pending at discharge
o Name and contact information of the responsible hospital physician.

APPENDIX 3: PATIENT EDUCATION ABOUT INFORMATION THAT PATIENTS SHOULD HAVE WITH THEM BETWEEN TRANSITION POINTS

Acute Care to Rehab, Subacute, Home	Patient/Family Should Understand:
Brief hospital course List of medical problems with brief explanations Surgical procedure(s) with date(s) and surgeon(s) Patient should leave with copy of discharge summary	What happened to them in the hospital, including surgical dates, complications, and their current medical problems
Activity restrictions Weight-bearing status Brace/immobilization requirements and duration Review equipment patient is to receive	What precautions they have to take because of their condition/surgery, ie, restricted use of a limb, instructions for using a brace
Medication reconciliation List of medications linked to medical problems Instructions on how to take medications Reasons for new medications or changes in home medications Include instructions for anticoagulation, seizure, corticosteroid, or antibiotics if applicable Wound care instructions Bowel routine/urethral catheterization instructions Glucose monitoring and treatment instructions Diet instructions, including feeding tube care	What medications are they on now and instructions for taking, ie, corticosteroid taper instructions, antibiotic duration Are there any changes from the home medications and if so, why was the change made? Who will provide assistance when it is needed for each self-care task?
Key imaging and laboratory findings	Important laboratory tests and imaging, ie, INR levels if patient is on warfarin. Provide electronic copies of imaging if available
Follow-up instructions linked to medical problems Prognosis	Who are they following up with for each problem: specialists and primary care? Side effects or adverse events to

Adverse events to watch out for and action to take	watch out for and what to do: ie, fever, seizure, headache, blurry vision
Contact information: Provider, HHA, visiting nurse service, equipment supplier	Attending physician at discharge, medical records office, specialists and primary care follow-up, vendors expected to deliver equipment

Safety in the Rehabilitation Setting: A Nursing Perspective

Audrey J. Schmerzler, MSN, RN[a],*, Lisa Martin, PhD, RN[b], Beth Oliver, RN, MS[c], Lou Ann London, BSN, RN[d]

KEYWORDS

- Patient safety • Patient outcomes • Rehabilitation
- Rehabilitation nursing

OVERVIEW OF PATIENT SAFETY

It is a new era for rehabilitation centers. Patients admitted have significant comorbidities. Insurance companies are denying appropriate patients admission to the rehabilitation center. It is becoming increasingly difficult to maintain occupancy. Administration is watching their bottom line and the contribution of rehabilitation to margin. Governmental regulations threaten the survival of rehabilitation centers. These factors together result in fiercer competition for patients among rehabilitation centers.

Patients and families, as consumers, have many tools at their disposal to help them choose a rehabilitation center. The public can access www.hospitalcompare.hhs.gov to see how well an institution is doing in terms of patient satisfaction scores and safety. They want facilities that have physiatrists with great reputations, appropriate nurse/patient ratios, and a place that has excellent patient outcomes in function and safety. As a consequence, there is now increased attention and emphasis on patient safety.

Safe patient care is also vital to an institution's financial well-being. A decreased incidence of patient falls, pressure ulcers, medication errors, and wrong-site surgery means a shorter patient length of stay. This translates into increased revenue for the institution (hospitals receive monies per patient discharge).

[a] Mount Sinai Rehabilitation Center, The Mount Sinai Hospital, One Gustave Levy Place, Box 1169, New York, NY 10029, USA
[b] Nursing Practice, Department of Nursing Education, The Mount Sinai Hospital, One Gustave Levy Place, Box 1144, New York, NY, USA
[c] Spinal Cord Injury, Lenox Hill Hospital, New York, NY 10075, USA
[d] SCI Unit, Mount Sinai Rehabilitation Center, The Mount Sinai Hospital, One Gustave Levy Place, Box 1169, New York, NY 10029, USA
* Corresponding author.
E-mail address: audrey.schmerzler@mountsinai.org

Phys Med Rehabil Clin N Am 23 (2012) 259–270
doi:10.1016/j.pmr.2012.02.004
1047-9651/12/$ – see front matter © 2012 Elsevier Inc. All rights reserved.
pmr.theclinics.com

Definitions of Safety

According to the Oxford Dictionary safety is defined as "the condition of being protected from or unlikely to cause danger, risk, or injury."[1] "The prevention of harm to patients" is how the Institute of Medicine defines patient safety.[2]

The Joint Commission standards outline general guidelines for safety in describing the appropriate environment of care. Elements include the actual building or space for patients, visitors, and staff; the equipment used to support patients and maintain the building or space; and all people who enter the environment. **Table 1** outlines the general categories related to patient safety and some examples of risk prevention.[3]

Other Joint Commission safety topics include a detailed description of life safety standards as described in the National Fire Protection Association Life Safety Code. The life safety chapter lists specific criteria for the physical environment, protection during construction or when the Life Safety Code is not met, building and fire protection features integrity of means of egress, the maintenance of fire alarm systems, systems for extinguishing fires, and other very specific requirements.

The Joint Commission introduced the National Patient Safety Goals program in 2002 with the goal of assisting organizations to focus on important areas of patient safety. The goals are continuously evaluated so that they may represent current best practices. For example, elements for attainment of the goals are reexamined and may be revised to pinpoint specific risk areas. Goals may also be dropped from the safety goal list and added to elements of overall standards. A goal for implementation in 2012 addresses catheter-associated urinary tract infection (CAUTI).[4] This

Table 1
Joint Commission general categories related to patient safety

Aspects of the Environment	Description	Examples of Risk Prevention
Safety and security	Physical environment, access to security-sensitive areas, smoking, product recalls	Appropriate security measures, prohibition of smoking with policy
Hazardous materials and waste	Chemicals, radioactive materials, hazardous energy sources, hazardous medications, hazardous gases, hazardous vapors	Inventory of hazardous items, proper labeling of hazardous materials, choice of safe equipment
Fire safety	Fire, smoke, other products of combustion, fire response plans, fire drills, management of fire detection, alarms and suppression equipment and systems, measures to implement during construction or when life safety code cannot be met	Free and unobstructed exits, fire response plan, fire drills at least once per shift per quarter in each building with documentation, monthly inspection of fire extinguishers with documentation
Medical equipment	Selection, testing, maintenance of medical equipment and contingencies when failure occurs	End user participation in choice of equipment, plan for inspecting, testing, and maintaining equipment, reporting and analysis of failures
Utilities	Inspection and testing of operating components, control of airborne contaminants, management of disruptions	Availability of emergency power, testing and management of medical gas systems

particular goal is extremely relevant to rehabilitation nursing as a nurse-sensitive indicator. In one staff nurse–initiated study on rehabilitation units,[5] ownership of the process of prevention by nurses was described as the major factor in decreasing CAUTI.

The other National Patient Safety Goals are also closely related to the work of rehabilitation nurses, including patient identification, effective communication, safety in medication administration, reducing the risk of health care–associated infections, medication reconciliation, and the universal protocol.[3]

Suicide prevention has been recognized as another goal for healthcare settings, including the rehabilitation patient population. In a recent retrospective cohort study,[6] the authors evaluated the mortality, life expectancy, risk factors for death, and causes of death after traumatic brain surgery rehabilitation. They identified that persons experiencing traumatic brain surgery are three times more likely to commit suicide than persons in the general population.

In 2010, the Joint Commission issued a sentinel event alert related to the prevention of suicide in nonpsychiatric settings. The focus of the alert was to urge staff in nonpsychiatric settings to screen for suicidal risk. The Joint Commission alert highlighted the fact that suicide ranks in the top five events reported to the Joint Commission and that 2.45% occurred in nonpsychiatric settings, such as "home care, critical access hospitals, long term care hospitals and physical rehabilitation hospitals."[7] Among the risk factors described in the alert were "physical health problems, including central nervous system disorders such as traumatic brain injury, chronic pain or intense acute pain; poor prognosis...disability."[7] The Joint Commission alert urged all facilities to consider what additional risk reduction strategies are appropriate for their particular setting.

The National Quality Forum Update[8] identified 34 safety practices for healthcare organizations to adopt to improve patient safety. The categories of practices include a culture of safety, communication, medication management, prevention of infections, and others. These standard safety practices can be used to guide rehabilitation settings in goals for safety improvement.

Rehabilitation nurses are primary stakeholders in the application of these Joint Commission and other quality standards for the rehabilitation setting. One commonly mentioned idea for the identification of safety issues is clinical safety rounds. In a randomized study of clinical safety rounds,[9] a rounding intervention by hospital executives and others demonstrated improvement in the nurses' perception of safety culture. Executive Walk Rounds was conducted by leadership staff trained in the method; staff reported safety concerns for follow-up. Campbell and Thompson[10] described an application of clinical safety rounds in an academic medical center. Rounds centered on small groups of staff on individual hospital units. A standard approach was created and used by the rounding team. For example, specific questions were asked on rounds to stimulate discussion about safety and the identification of salient concerns and worries about patient safety. The data resulting from the rounds were analyzed and led to changes in general processes of care and the resolution of specific local problems.

Although nurses were involved in these two rounding initiatives, nurses were not identified as the primary leaders. It is possible that nurses conducting their own local safety rounds could provide additional information regarding their organization's safety vulnerabilities. Nurse rounding on patients has been advocated as a patient satisfaction strategy with a safety component. The results of a quasiexperimental study[11] suggested that hourly rounding on patients decreased falls and led to greater patient satisfaction. Rehabilitation nurses may be able to further elaborate processes and strategies for the identification of safety issues and interventions in the rehabilitation population.

Patient Safety Education and Competencies

The current emphasis on patient safety has stimulated an examination of nurse competencies related to patient safety. A national initiative called the Quality and Safety Education for Nurses adapted the competencies identified by the Institute of Medicine and formulated key nurse competencies, all of which relate to safety for the patient.[12] For example, patient-centered involves developing an active partnership with patients and families. Teamwork and collaboration target the ability to effectively communicate with team members. Evidence-based practice focuses on need to use high-quality evidence for information. The safety competency emphasizes standardized practice, communication of hazards and errors, and reporting of near misses and risk events. Finally, the informatics competency values technology to effectively prevent errors and coordinate care.[13] Although this initiative began as an academic endeavor and has also included clinical partnerships as described by Fater and Ready,[14] these key competencies should be threaded through nurse orientation and clinical continuing education for rehabilitation nurses.

A review article[15] evaluated patient safety assessment tools, including nine tools for nursing professionals. The nursing tools included the following: quality improvement knowledge, skills, and attitudes; patient safety attitudes, skills, and knowledge scale; essay; situation awareness checklist; clinical simulation evaluation tool; knowledge, skills attitudes criterion, clinical performance evaluation tool; and two unnamed checklists. Of these tools, only the quality improvement knowledge, skills, and attitudes and the patient safety attitudes, skills, and knowledge scale were reported to have content validity. Although it may not yet be practical to use these evaluation tools, other outcome measures already part of rehabilitation nursing can be the focus at this time, such as decreased falls, decreased pressure ulcers, and decreased infection, all of critical and practical importance to rehabilitation patients.

Patient Populations in Rehabilitation Centers

The patient population in rehabilitation units and centers are individuals who not only have a disability but who still require medical attention and 24-hour nursing monitoring and care. Consequently, discharge from the acute setting to home or a subacute facility is not a viable option. Common disabilities seen in the rehabilitation setting include brain injury (traumatic and nontraumatic); spinal cord injury (traumatic and nontraumatic); stroke; amputation; debility; and persons having undergone hip or knee replacement. By nature of these disabilities many patients have cognitive or memory deficits, problems with perception, gait disorders, swallowing difficulties, or other significant functional deficiencies. In addition, because of the push to shorten length of stays in acute hospitals, patients are entering rehabilitation centers with an increased number of comorbidities and are sicker than in previous years.

The goal of rehabilitation is for the person with a disability to increase their functional or cognitive level of independence and, when appropriate, how to direct their care. The patients attend therapy and are taught strategies to overcome physical, psychological, or cognitive deficits. In this nursing plays a large part. Nurses not only direct and advocate for the patient to practice what they have learned in therapy but are also instrumental in education of the patient and their family. Areas of educational focus include bowel and bladder management, skin care, respiratory function, and health promotion and wellness.

The combination of high acuity, physical and cognitive impairments, and emphasis on increasing independence mandates an increased awareness of safety issues by the rehabilitation nurse. The rehabilitation patient is at risk for falls, pressure ulcers, and aspiration pneumonia.

Elements of creating and maintaining a safe patient environment include effective communication; a sound education program (for patients and staff); and adequate staffing. Communicating at change of shift reports or at hand off before breaks informs one's colleagues about patient status and potential problems. Being up to date on the latest technology or new medications not only helps improve the patient's medical and functional status, but alerts the nurse to any potential errors in medication orders or inappropriate use of a product. Adequate staffing prevents staff fatigue, which can lead to poor judgment and decision making and ensure timely answering of the call bell. This prevents patients from putting themselves in harm's way because they become impatient waiting for help and try to do for themselves.

The focus on patient safety is not a new issue or concern in health care. Keeping patients safe while in the hospital has always been the priority for nursing. This dates back to Florence Nightingale, who wrote "It may seem a strange principle to enunciate as the very first requirement in a hospital that it should do the sick no harm."[16]

Over the years, landmark studies by the Institute of Medicine, Agency for Healthcare Research and Quality, National Quality Form, Institute for Healthcare Improvement, and regulatory agencies, such as The Joint Commission and Centers for Medicaid and Medicare (CMS), have identified strategies to improve health care and keep patients safe.

IDENTIFICATION OF TOP SAFETY ISSUES: PROBLEM AND PREVENTION STRATEGIES
Medication Safety

According to the Institute of Medicine, medication errors are among the most common medical errors. It is estimated that at least 1.5 million people are harmed every year as a result of a medication error. These medication errors result in extra medical costs of $3.5 billion a year to treat drug-related injuries.[17] Efforts to decrease the number of medication errors consist of increased communication and education. Consumer-friendly pamphlets highlighting and outlining medication routes, purpose, and side effects should be made and given to patients. These pamphlets should be written in a way that patients understand what is being communicated. The standard is for the information to be written at the fourth grade level. In addition, pamphlets in other languages, those that are prevalent in one's area, should be readily available.

All nurses know about the five rights of medication administration. However, most do not know that some experts advocate eight rights of medication (**Table 2**).

Pressure Ulcers

There have been many estimates made of pressure ulcer–related costs. A CMS estimate in 2007 placed the average cost of preventable pressure ulcers at $43,180 per hospital stay.[18] Another estimate placed pressure ulcer–related costs between $5 and $8.5 billion annually, with per patient costs estimated at more than $10,500 per patient.[19] Length of stay is increased for patients with pressure ulcers (30.4 vs 12.8 days), with subsequent increases in cost.[19]

The incidence of pressure ulcers in hospitalized patients in the United States is reported to range from 1.5% to 10.3%.[19] A consensus paper from the International Expert Wound Care advisory panel also reported pressure ulcer incidence in this range, with incidence of new pressure ulcers in acute-care patients approximately

Table 2
The five rights of medication administration

	Number	Right	Components
Known five rights	1	Right patient	Use two identifiers
	2	Right medication	Check medication label
	3	Right dose	Check order
	4	Right route	Check order and appropriateness of route
	5	Right time	Check frequency of ordered medication and time of last dose
Lesser known rights	6	Right documentation	Document after medication is given
			Chart all pertinent information including time, dose, route, response
	7	Right reason	Confirm rationale for medication
	8	Right response	Was desired response achieved? Document response

7%, with wide variation among institutions.[18] CMS reported 257,412 cases of preventable pressure ulcers as secondary diagnoses in 2007.[18]

The National Pressure Ulcer Advisory Panel defines a pressure ulcer as "localized injury to the skin and/or underlying tissue usually over a bony prominence, as a result of pressure, or pressure in combination with shear and/or friction" (http://npuap.org/pr2.htm). This panel defines six classifications of pressure ulcer, stages I-V, suspected deep tissue injury, and unstageable ulcers.

A number of conditions place individuals at risk for the development of pressure ulcers. These risk factors include prolonged immobility; friction (rubbing); shearing; decreased sensation to the area or decreased cognition; excessive moisture or dryness; inadequate nutrition; and reduced tissue elasticity.

Immobility creates pressure buildup at bony areas because patients are unable to redistribute pressure. Shearing occurs when layers of the skin slide over one another and the underlying tissues. It is mostly caused by pulling linen from beneath patients while the patients are still lying on it or when patients slide down in bed or chair (http://www.molnlycke.com/patient/en/Wound/wounds/Pressure-ulcer/r). Friction occurs when the skin is dragged across a surface because it causes damage to skin cells and minute blood vessels. Use of a draw sheet (during turning) helps to prevent friction. Decreased sensation to the area under pressure causes a pressure ulcer to develop; decreased cognition is also a factor because in both instances the patient is unaware of what is happening. Excessive moisture or dryness makes the skin highly susceptible to damage, because in both cases the skin becomes more fragile and breaks easily. Poor nutrition intake, especially vitamin C, protein, and zinc, can contribute to the possibility of skin breakdown. Reduced tissue elasticity, usually seen in the geriatric population, causes the skin to be thinner, making it much easier for tissue and blood vessel damage (http://www.mayoclinic.com/health/bedsores/DS00570/DSECTION=risk-factors).

Many patients in rehabilitation are at risk of skin breakdown because of immobility, insensate skin, impaired circulation, impaired cognition, and altered nutrition. Preventing pressure ulcers and preventing existing pressure ulcers from worsening is a hallmark of rehabilitation nursing (**Table 3**). Rehabilitation nurses know the importance of positioning and turning patients, weight shifts when in the wheelchair, the use of specialized cushions and mattresses, the importance of good nutrition, and the importance of education.

Table 3 Measures to prevent pressure ulcers	
Measure	**Explanation**
Turning and positioning	When in bed, the patient should be repositioned every 2 hours and not left to lie in one position. When seated in a chair pressure relief should be given every 20 minutes for 2 minutes.
	The use of specialized mattresses, specialized cushions, and specialized wheelchairs is very instrumental in preventing pressure ulcers. Patients must first be assessed for the most appropriate surface to prevent skin breakdown because there are many varieties to choose from, such as foam, air, and gel. Pressure mapping done in bed or while seated determines the areas of skin most susceptible for pressure ulcer development and is a good indicator as to the type of surface to choose.
Keep skin dry	Lotions and powder should be used sparingly so as to allow the skin to be cool and dry. Too much lotion causes the skin to remain moist and in turn causes the skin to break easily. Incontinent patients should be cleaned as soon as they have an accident and not left lying in the urine or stool because bacteria predisposes the skin to infection and breakdown.
Minimize friction and shear	When moving the patient in bed or in a chair, lift the patient and do not drag them. The patient should be moved as a unit and pillows or padding should be used to prevent skin surfaces from rubbing against each other. Avoid massaging over bony prominences because this may cause damage to underlying blood vessels.
Watch out for pressure-inducing objects	Catheter tubes, tight articles of clothing, tight shoes, bunching of bed linen or diapers.

This area has taken on added importance because the CMS has determined that beginning October 1, 2012, all inpatient rehabilitation facilities (IRFs) must submit a measure for new or worsening pressure ulcers. Any IRF that does not comply with this mandate will see their payments reduced by 2% in fiscal year 2014. Data for the pressure ulcer measure will be collected by the IRF-Patient Assessment Instrument.

Falls Prevention

Rehabilitation centers are populated with patients with a variety of disabilities, including brain injury, spinal cord injury, debility, amputations, and hip or knee replacements. Not only do many of these patients have cognitive deficits that may manifest as poor insight into their own impairments, but they also have deficits in judgment and memory and limitations in physical functioning. These limitations coupled with the goal of rehabilitation, for patients to increase their functional independence, results in a population extremely vulnerable to falls and injury from falls.

Historically, it is not unusual for the falls rate on a rehabilitation unit to be higher than that of an acute care unit. Approximately 3% to 20% of inpatients fall at least once during their hospital stay; these falls result in injuries, increased lengths of stay, malpractice lawsuits, and more than $4000 in excess charges per hospitalization.[20] Fall rates in general rehabilitation settings range from 12.5% to 39% depending on the setting compared with 1.4% in a general hospital.[21]

In 2009 the CMS adopted the practice of not paying for hospital-acquired conditions, which includes injuries from falls. In addition, the Joint Commission has a patient safety goal devoted to reducing harm from falls and a standard that discourages the use of restraints because of the incidence of deaths related to restraint use.

The combination of a vulnerable population with the recent CMS and Joint Commission initiatives has placed an increased emphasis on rehabilitation centers to find innovative ways to increase patient safety, decrease the incidence of falls, and decrease the number and severity of injuries that result from falls. The added challenge is to remain fiscally prudent while implementing these programs.

To provide a safe environment for this patient population, rehabilitation centers institute various falls-prevention programs. These programs comprise a number of methods to decrease the incidence of falls, including the use of constant observation (CO) and high–low beds. CO is the use of a staff member to provide CO of a patient. Types of CO include one-to-one or two-to-one. One-to-one CO is when one staff member observes one patient and two-to-one is one staff member is assigned to observe two patients at the same time. There are hospital-specific policies and procedures that guide the practice of CO and the use of high–low beds and clearly define what it entails for that center.

Safety huddles and communication are also important components of fall prevention. During change of shift reports staff members (RN to RN, ancillary to ancillary, RN to ancillary) should discuss any patients who are a fall risk. The discussions should entail measures taken to prevent a fall for the patient at risk. If a patient has fallen, this should be discussed during the change of shift report. In addition, after a patient fall a huddle should also occur. At this huddle, the staff discusses what factors led to the fall, what the patient stated was the reason for the fall, and if the fall could have been prevented. Interventions should then be implemented to prevent further falls.

Additional interventions to prevent falls include placing at-risk patients closer to the nursing station, using amber lighting in the room, additional grab bars in the room to allow for support when ambulating, low-gloss floors to increase depth perception, appropriate footwear, and constant patient and staff education about fall risks.

CAUTI

Urinary tract infections, the most common acquired hospital infection, account for 40% of all hospital-acquired infections; 80% of those infections are associated with indwelling urethral catheters.[5] Healthcare-associated infections are the eleventh-leading cause of death in the United States and cost more than $4.5 billion per year.[22]

CMS has determined that beginning October 1, 2012, all IRFs must submit data for a urinary CAUTI measure. Any IRF that does not comply with this mandate will see their payments reduced by 2% in fiscal year 2014.

The Guideline for the Prevention of Catheter Associated Urinary Tract Infections 2009 (**Table 4**) states that inappropriate catheter use occurs when the catheter is in place to maintain continence or because of inadequate staffing. An indwelling catheter is appropriate in those patients with healing sacral or perineal wounds or for those patients immobilized for long periods because of immobile thoracic or lumbar spine.

This is an area where rehabilitation nurses will have a huge impact. Bladder programs, whether intermittent catheterization schedules or trial voiding, are a practice well known to rehabilitation practitioners. Nurses should advocate for early catheter removal and then implement the appropriate bladder program. In addition, use of bladder ultrasound is recommended to measure postvoid residuals in place of catheterizing for residual urine. An effective bladder management program helps preserve

Table 4		
Examples of appropriateness versus inappropriateness of indwelling catheter use		
Situation	Appropriate Use of Indwelling Catheter	Inappropriate Use of Indwelling Catheter
Need for accurate measurements in acutely ill patients	√	
To improve comfort at end of life	√	
To assist in healing of sacral or perineal wound	√	
Acute urinary retention or bladder outlet obstruction	√	
Substitute for nursing care for the patient with incontinence		√
Obtaining urine samples of patient who can void voluntarily		√
Prolonged postoperatively without appropriate indicators and documentation (eg, received large volumes of diuretics during surgery or urologic surgery)		√

the upper tracts of the bladder, prevents further complications, and establishes effective and complete emptying of the bladder at regular intervals. This in turn helps decrease the likelihood of urinary tract infections.

Dysphagia and Aspiration Pneumonia

Because of poor head, lip, and tongue function, neuroinsult to the central nervous system, and altered levels of consciousness dysphagia is often seen in individuals after brain injury (stroke and traumatic brain injury) and in several neurologic conditions (eg, amyotrophic lateral sclerosis and spinal cord injury). As a result of dysphagia the risk for aspiration pneumonia and nutritional compromise is increased.

Safety interventions to prevent aspiration pneumonia and poor nutritional intake in the patient with dysphagia include assessing swallowing and nutritional status; implementation of alternate means of feeding and nutrition (feeding tubes or parenteral nutrition); supervision of meals; providing a quiet distraction-free environment during meal time; ensuring that the patient eats small quantities of food at a time in an upright position and that the patient does not pocket their food; and instituting a dysphagia diet (**Table 5**). Liquids are divided into thin (water, apple juice, Italian ices, and broths) and thickened liquids (pear nectar or tomato juice). There are many versions of a dysphagia diet. Check with the dietary department or hospital policies and procedure manual for the type of dysphagia diet practiced in one's place of work.

OVERVIEW OF NURSE SAFETY

No discussion on safety is complete without addressing the issues of nurse safety. In 2011, the American Nurses Association surveyed 4614 nurses and asked about their health and safety concerns in relation to their work environments and exposure to hazards.[23] The respondents overall stated that conditions have improved but still expressed concern about musculoskeletal injuries, stress, overwork, and on-the-job assaults.

Table 5
Elements of a generic dysphagia diet

Level/Stage	Examples of Food
Level/Stage I Dysphagia diet or aspiration precautions diet Food that is homogenous, very cohesive, pudding-like, requiring very little chewing ability	Pureed foods, pudding, mashed potatoes, thinned cooked cereals, pureed noodle recipes, mousse, plain yogurt, sauces and gravies
Level/Stage II or mechanical soft Cohesive, moist, semisolid foods, requiring some chewing	Minced poultry and meat, cooked cereals, flaked fish, vegetable soup, minced cakes and minced potatoes, minced ripened bananas
Level/Stage III or soft (advanced) Soft foods that require more chewing ability	Ground fish and meat, scrambled eggs, custard, ice cream, ground potatoes and noodles, cottage cheese, creamed soups and ripe bananas
Regular	Finely chopped foods, some of which are chopped poultry and meat, chopped potatoes, cream cheese, vegetable soup, flaked fish and omelets; no restrictions

Rehabilitation nurses are especially vulnerable in these areas. Messages on rehabilitation Listserves highlight that although patients admitted to rehabilitation centers have a much higher acuity than in the past, staffing levels have not changed. Nurses are now dealing with patients with significant medical issues in addition to their rehabilitation disability and needs. Other nursing responsibilities include increased paperwork, working with distraught family members, and interacting with consultants. The result is stress and overwork.

Many rehabilitation patients are physically dependent requiring increased hands-on care. Although rehabilitation nurses are experts in proper transfer techniques and proper body mechanics staff injuries can and do occur. In recent years, many facilities have implemented no-lift policies or minimal-lift policies to reduce the risk of injury to patients and nurses associated with manual lifting, transferring, repositioning, or movement of patients. Several states have passed legislation requiring hospitals to establish and implement programs on safe patient handling. However, because of the cost not all rehabilitation facilities have overhead lifts and other safe patient handling equipment. The rehabilitation nurse must advocate for these items. In lieu of the more expensive overhead lifts, alternate equipment, such as mobile transfer lifts, could be purchased to maintain and safeguard staff safety.

Patients and families faced with devastating and life-changing disabilities often have a difficult time dealing with the reality of their situation. Consequently, the nurse is often the recipient of their anger and frustration. This may be exhibited by verbal and physical abuse. The rehabilitation facility must have policies and programs in place to address issues of staff abuse. Educational sessions must be regularly scheduled that teach staff how to de-escalate volatile situations and defend themselves. In addition, counseling sessions must be available to allow the staff to express their feelings and concerns.

Unfortunately, in the nursing literature there are a limited number of articles that address safety from a nursing perspective. The lack of effective communication is essential and has been cited as the root cause in almost every sentinel event reported by the Joint Commission.[24] Teams that focus on collaboration, communication, and goal achievement must be formed. It is time for nursing as a group to invite other disciplines to participate in safety discussions to cultivate a common ground of patient safety.

SUMMARY

Maintaining a safe environment for patients and staff is a win–win situation for all involved. Patients feel secure and can rehabilitate without fear of falls, pressure ulcers, aspiration pneumonia, or medication errors. Nurses work in a center that is highly regarded for its promotion of staff safety and overall quality care. The institution is not penalized financially for poor quality and poor patient outcomes and reaps fiscal benefits and an enhanced reputation.

REFERENCES

1. Available at: http://oxforddictionaries.com/definition/safety?region=us. Accessed February 22, 2012.
2. Institute of Medicine. To err is human: building a safer health system. Washington, DC: National Academy Press; 1999.
3. Joint Commission. 2012. Hospital accreditation standards. Oakbrook Terrace (IL): Joint Commission Resources; 2012.
4. Joint Commission. 2011. Facts about national patient safety goals. Available at: http://www.jointcommission.org. Accessed January 6, 2012.
5. Salamon L. Catheter-associated urinary tract infections: a nurse-sensitive indicator in an inpatient rehabilitation program. Rehabil Nurs 2009;4(6):237–42.
6. Harrison-Felix CL, Whiteneck GG, Jha A, et al. Mortality over four decades after traumatic brain injury rehabilitation: a retrospective cohort study. Arch Phys Med Rehabil 2009;90:1506–13.
7. Joint Commission. 2010. The joint commission sentinel event alert, Issue 46. 2010. Available at: http://www.jointcommission.org. Accessed January 6, 2012.
8. National Quality Forum. 2009. Safe practices for better healthcare—2009 update: a consensus report. Available at: http://www.qualityforum.org. Accessed January 6, 2012.
9. Thomas EJ, Sexton JB, Neilands TB, et al. The effect of executive walk rounds on nurse safety climate attitudes: a randomized trial of clinical units. BMC Health Serv Res 2005;5(1):28.
10. Campbell D, Thompson M. Patient safety rounds: description of an inexpensive but important strategy to improve safety culture. Am J Med Qual 2007;22:22–6.
11. Meade C, Bursell A, Ketelsen L. Effects of nursing rounds on patients' call light use, satisfaction, and safety. Am J Nurs 2006;107(9):58–70.
12. Cronenwett L, Sherwood G, Barnsteiner J, et al. Quality and safety education for nurses. Nurs Outlook 2007;55(3):122–31.
13. Jarzemsky P, McCarthy J, Ellis N. Incorporating quality and safety education for nurses competencies in scenario design. Nurse Educ 2010;25(2):90–2.
14. Fater K, Ready R. An education partnership to achieve safety and quality improvement competencies in nursing. J Nurs Educ 2011;50(12):693–6.
15. Okuyama A, Martowirono K, Bignen B. Assessing the patient safety competencies of healthcare professionals: a systematic review. BMJ Qual Saf 2011; 20(11):991–1000.
16. Nightingale F. Notes on nursing: what it is, and what it is not. Available at: http://digital.library.upenn.edu/women/nightingale/nursing/nursing.html. Accessed February 22, 2012.

17. Institute of Medicine. Preventing medication errors. Washington, DC: National Academy Press; 2007.
18. Infection Control Today. Available at: http://www.infectioncontroltoday.com/articles/2008/08/cms-to-put-pressure-on-providers-for-decubitus-ul.aspx. Accessed January 6, 2012.
19. Allman RM, Goode PS, Burst N, et al. Pressure ulcers, hospital complications, and disease severity: impact on hospital costs and length of stay. Adv Wound Care 1999;1(12):22–30.
20. Inouye SK, Brown CJ, Tinetti ME. Medicare nonpayment, hospital falls, and unintended consequences. N Engl J Med 2009;360(23):2390–3.
21. Lee JE, Stokic DS. Risk factors for falls during inpatient rehabilitation. Am J Phys Med Rehabil 2008;87:341–53.
22. Newman DK. The indwelling urinary catheter principles of best practice. J Wound Ostomy Continence Nurs 2007;34(6):655–61.
23. 2011 Health and Safety Survey. Available at: http://www.nursingworld.org/MainMenuCategories/WorkplaceSafety/workplaceviolence. Accessed January 6, 2012.
24. Nadzam DM. Nurses' role in communication and patient safety. J Nurs Care Qual 2009;24(3):184–8.

Medication Safety in Rehabilitation Medicine

Laurentiu Iulius Dinescu, MD[a], Darko Todorov, PharmD[a],
Michael Biglow, PharmD, BCPS, BCPP[a], Yuliana Toderika, BS, PharmD[a],
Henry Cohen, MS, PharmD, FCCM, BCPP, CGP[a,b,*], Karishma Patel, MD[a]

KEYWORDS

- Medication errors • Medication reconciliation
- Venous thromboembolism prophylaxis
- Medication-related falls • Pain management
- NSAID-induced gastropathy

CHARACTERISTICS OF THE REHABILITATION MEDICINE POPULATION

Rehabilitation medicine is practiced in a variety of settings such as acute medical and surgical wards, inpatient rehabilitation facilities, nursing homes, outpatient clinics, and even the patient's home. Physiatrists are an integral part of the care provided in many of these settings and are often consulted to provide diagnostic and therapeutic services and expertise to individuals with a variety of diagnoses such as spinal cord injury (SCI), traumatic brain injury, stroke, and musculoskeletal pain syndromes. In this role, it is imperative that physiatrists have a working knowledge of various medications as well as the principles of medication safety. This article provides the reader with a foundation in the general and specific aspects of medication safety as they apply to the practice of rehabilitation medicine.

ADVERSE DRUG EVENTS

Adverse drug events (ADEs) are a consequence of pharmacotherapy in patient care. The average rate of ADEs in a hospital setting range from 2 to 7 events per 100 admissions, giving an annual occurrence of 770,000.[1] The estimated average direct cost to a hospital is $5.6 million dollars per year.[1] The true cost, which includes hospital

[a] Department of Pharmacy Services, Kingsbrook Jewish Medical Center, 585 Schenectady Avenue, Brooklyn, NY 11203, USA
[b] Arnold & Marie Schwartz College of Pharmacy and Health Sciences, Long Island University, Brooklyn, NY, USA
* Corresponding author. Department of Pharmacy Services, Kingsbrook Jewish Medical Center, 585 Schenectady Avenue, Brooklyn, NY 11203.
E-mail address: hcohen@kingsbrook.org

Phys Med Rehabil Clin N Am 23 (2012) 271–303
doi:10.1016/j.pmr.2012.02.005
1047-9651/12/$ – see front matter © 2012 Published by Elsevier Inc.
pmr.theclinics.com

readmission, lost productivity, and legal proceedings and settlements, is much greater and difficult to assess.

The definition of an ADE is any injury from the use of a drug.[2] This avoids the labeling of a reaction as an ADE. A distinction should be made between ADEs and adverse drug reactions (ADR), which are events or injuries occurring in normal prescribing practices (ie, normal doses and frequencies). ADR include side effects that are known reactions to medication and are listed in the detailed prescribing information as well as allergic reactions, which are unexpected and unpredictable immune responses. Other than ADRs, ADEs are also secondary to medication errors, as discussed later. ADEs secondary to medication errors are more common but may or may not result in patient harm. These types of ADEs should be listed as preventable ADEs.[3]

Reporting ADEs is the single most important aspect to identifying and assessing process failures within a health care system. When reporting an ADE, it is important to supply as much information regarding the patient and situation as is needed to allow an understanding of not only what happened but why the event occurred. An ADE should also be listed in the patients' medical record and appropriate updates to allergy and medication intolerance profiles should be made to prevent the same reaction from recurring, if applicable. Reporters should understand that the process is nonpunitive and is meant to identify process failures. ADEs can be classified by severity: mild, moderate, and severe, with descriptions noted in **Table 1**.[2]

Administrative bodies such as a medication safety committee or a pharmacy and therapeutics committee are hospital-specific organizations that evaluate ADEs on a regular basis. The multidisciplinary committees meet either monthly or quarterly and, based on observed trends, can initiate further inquiries into medication use at the facility. Actions taken by these committees can include initiation of a medication-specific protocol, drug restriction, and/or removal from the institution's formulary. On a wider level, MedWatch is a reporting system set up by the US Food and Drug Administration (FDA) to track approved medications. Voluntary submissions are assessed to determine whether regulatory actions are required, which can include mandatory warnings, labeling changes, requests for postmarketing studies, or withdrawal of a medication from the market.

MEDICATION ERRORS

As mentioned earlier, medical errors, and in particular medication errors, are rigorously scrutinized, reported, and investigated in the health care industry, and by state and

Table 1 Definition of ADE severity levels	
ADE Severity Level	**Description**
Mild	A transient reaction that may or may not require an intervention (ie, drug discontinuation)
Moderate	Requiring active treatment of the event as well as further laboratory and diagnostic assessment to determine the extent of the nonserious reaction
Severe	Life-threatening or organ-threatening events that result in prolonged hospitalization, transfer to a higher level of care, significant or permanent disability, and/or death

Data from Nebeker JR, Barach P, Samore MH. Clarifying adverse drug events: a clinician's guide to terminology, documentation, and reporting. Ann Intern Med 2004;140:795–801.

federal governments. The FDA (www.fda.gov/medwatch.htm), Institute for Safe Medi-cation Practices (www.ismp.org), US Pharmacopeia (www.usp.org), and MedMARX (www.medmarx.com) are some of the bodies that track medication errors in the United States. Medication errors represent the largest single cause of errors in the hospital setting, accounting for more than 7000 deaths annually.[4]

Common types of errors are caused by (1) inadequate knowledge about the drug, (2) insufficient knowledge about the patient, (3) rules violations, (4) slips and memory lapses, (5) transcription errors, (6) faulty drug identity checking, (7) faulty com-munication with other services, (8) inadequate monitoring, and (9) drug stocking and delivery.

Leape and colleagues[5] reported more than 15 types of medication errors: wrong dose, wrong choice, wrong drug, known allergy, missed dose, wrong time, wrong frequency, wrong technique, drug-drug interaction, wrong route, extra dose, failure to act on test, equipment failure, inadequate monitoring, preparation error, and others. Of the 130 errors for physicians, most involved the wrong dose, wrong choice of drug, and known allergy. Among the 126 nursing administration errors, most were associ-ated with wrong dose, wrong technique, and wrong drug. Each type of error occurred at various stages, although some occurred more often during the ordering and admin-istration stages.

High-risk Medications[6]

Although every medication poses risks, the following list identifies some common classes of high-risk medications associated with errors:

- Medications with a low therapeutic index: a low ratio between the toxic dose and the therapeutic dose (eg, digoxin)
- Concentrated electrolyte solutions: solutions such as potassium chloride and sodium chloride solutions can be inadvertently administered in their undiluted strengths (concentrated solutions of electrolytes should not be kept on the floor where they can be administered without dilution)
- Anticoagulants: coumarin anticoagulants, like Coumadin, are metabolized differ-ently by patients and subject patients to drug interactions that may increase or decrease the therapeutic effect
- Narcotics/patient-controlled analgesia: combined with sedatives/hypnotics (anti-histamines Phenergan, Benadryl, hydroxyzine) can augment the risk for falls and the respiratory-depressant and depressant properties of these drugs, increasing the risk of respiratory depression or arrest
- Insulin: there are several types of insulin with a variety of rates of onset and dura-tion, as well as different concentrations that may create confusion
- Chemotherapeutic agents: these are highly toxic and can cause morbidity and death when administered incorrectly.

Strategies that can be used to Minimize the Patient Safety Risk:

1. Use tracking and trending to identify problems.
2. Reinforce policies and procedures to ensure that staff understand and follow appropriate protocols for dispensing medications (correct drug, dose, route, patient, time). Schedule periodic policy reviews to ensure staff/physician compli-ance with those policies.
3. Make medication information easily available to physicians and staff (using the help of a pharmacist, software, or Internet access to drug information).

4. Identify high-risk medications used in the facility.
5. Implement medication reconciliation at critical changes in patients' conditions and settings.
6. Educate patients about their medications and their intended effect, and encourage them to ask questions that could help prevent medication errors.

MEDICATION RECONCILIATION

Medication reconciliation is an important practice at all points along the health care continuum of care. Given that more than half of all hospital admissions have at least 1 medication discrepancy, with 33% having mild to moderate harm potential, and 6% severe harm potential, there is significant room for improvement.[7] Common errors include incorrect doses/frequencies, missing medications, and inappropriate durations of use.

Medication reconciliation is described as the process of avoiding inadvertent inconsistencies across transitions in care by reviewing the patient's complete medication regimen at the time of admission, transfer, and discharge, and comparing it with the regimen being considered for the new setting of care.[8] How that process is determined is up to the specific institutions and vary in several features but there are some basic recommendations for what the process should entail. The Institute for Healthcare Improvement (IHI) suggests at least 3 steps to the process: verify by collecting the list of medications, vitamins, nutritional supplements, over-the-counter drugs, and vaccines; verify that the medications and dosages are appropriate; reconcile and document any changes.

Other aspects to this process include (1) specifying responsibilities for each health care discipline; (2) using a standardized form for regimen evaluation; (3) determining an explicit time frame for completion that is relevant to the setting (eg, ambulatory vs acute care); (4) implementation of educational programs for health care professionals as well as patients and caregivers, and designing a monitoring process to ensure compliance and evaluate for improvement.[8,9]

Strategies for improving medication reconciliation compliance vary from basic health care provider education to implementation of advanced information technology. However, it is not yet agreed as to what is an effective implementation. Studies investigating the impact of a pharmacist-led intervention or the implementation of electronic medical records show improvement in the reduction of preventable ADEs but the results are mixed and inconsistent.[10,11]

Currently, The Joint Commission (TJC) has suspended the enforcement of the National Patient Safety Goal (NPSG) #8, which requires health care systems to accurately and completely reconcile patients' medications across the continuum of care. As medication reconciliation becomes more standardized and monitoring processes are better refined, this aspect of patient care will be enforced with as much emphasis as the other NPSGs.

PATIENT AND FAMILY EDUCATION

Poor compliance with a medication regimen is a long-standing problem, leading to unnecessary disease progression or complications, decline in the functional abilities, increased numbers of visits to the emergency room, increased hospital readmission rates, reduced quality of life, and even death.

According to the World Health Organization (WHO), only about 50% of patients who suffer from chronic diseases take their medicines as prescribed.[12] In the United States, nonadherence affects Americans of all ages, both genders, and involves higher-income, well-educated people just as much as those at lower socioeconomic levels.[13] Between 12% and 20% of patients take other people's medicines[14]; following a heart attack, only 45% of patients regularly take β-blocker (BB) medications during the first year after leaving the hospital[15]; less than 2% of adults with diabetes follow the American Diabetes Association recommendations.[16]

In its report "To Err is Human; Building a Safer Health System," the Institute of Medicine (IOM) encouraged clinicians to educate their patients about (1) the medications they are taking, (2) reasons why they are taking them, (3) what the medications look like, (4) time of day that the medications should be taken, (5) potential side effects, (6) what to do if they experience side effects, and (7) need for regular testing.[17]

Strategies for improving patient adherence include increasing patient and family awareness about medications through discussions at the time that the health professional (1) writes the prescription and (2) at the time that the patient fills the prescription at the pharmacy. These discussions are best accomplished by relaying the most important information first, repeating key points, having the patient restate key instructions,[18] and encouraging the patient to ask questions and share information.[19] Most individuals want from their physicians all information concerning possible adverse effects of the prescribed medication and do not favor physician discretion in these decisions.[20]

Patients forget more than half of the information obtained from a verbal explanation immediately after hearing it.[21] Because many patients commonly seen by physiatrists suffer from diseases manifested by cognitive impairment, such as stroke or brain injury, a partner or caregiver who accompanies the patient to doctor visits should be welcomed and encouraged to take notes during the discussion, and written information about the treatment should be provided to them.

Other ways to improve adherence include (1) tailoring the medication regimen to the patient's daily schedule, (2) decreasing the number of doses to once or twice daily,[21,22] (3) eliminating unnecessary medications or using combination products, (4) changing the route of administration, and (5) decreasing the overall cost of the medication regimen if necessary. In a study published in *JAMA* comparing compliance rates for daily dosing versus twice a day, 3 times a day, and 4 times a day, compliance rates averaged 76% during 3428 days observed; 87% of the once daily, 81% of the twice daily, 77% of the 3 times a day, and 39% of the 4 times a day dosages were taken as prescribed.[23]

MEDICATION SAFETY IN PATIENTS WITH DYSPHAGIA

Dysphagia is a clinical syndrome defined as an inability to swallow, or a sensation that solids or liquids do not pass easily from the mouth to the stomach.[24] This condition can occur in patients with structural deficits or dysfunction of the oral cavity and/or pharynx secondary to neurologic or muscular disorders. Some common and potentially life-threatening consequences of dysphagia include choking, aspiration, pneumonia, malnutrition, and dehydration. These consequences are of increased importance in the rehabilitation unit, where the patients commonly present with impaired mobility and tend to remain in a supine position for prolonged periods of time.

Certain medications can cause or even exacerbate an existing dysphagia. Sedatives may affect swallowing by acting on the central nervous system. Anticholinergics or diuretics can make chewing and swallowing difficult because of decreased saliva production. Other medications, such as nonsteroidal antiinflammatory drugs (NSAIDs), bisphosphonates, potassium chloride, quinidine, tetracyclines, clindamycin, and iron products, can result in esophageal injury when not taken properly or when esophageal motility is impaired.[24]

Patients after endotracheal intubation or tracheostomy may have different degrees of dysphagia caused by soft tissue injuries at the oropharyngeal level. Older patients are also at higher risk for dysphagia caused by decreased oropharyngeal motility and reduced saliva production. The type of diet (eg, pureed, chopped, regular), fluid thickness, and other techniques to improve the patient's dysphagia need to be implemented on an individual basis. Changes may be necessary in the medication regimen or in the way medications are administered because some may be difficult to swallow or are potentially dangerous if crushed or chewed, whereas others should not be crushed (enteric coated, extended release, long acting, controlled release, and sustained release). Liquid and capsules are the preferred form of medication for patients with dysphagia.

THE ROLE OF THE CLINICAL PHARMACISTS IN MEDICATION MANAGEMENT

Clinical pharmacists are experts in the therapeutic use of medications and have the ability to provide recommendations on the safe, appropriate, and cost-effective use of medications. They are involved in direct care patient rounds, medication order review, patient counseling, medication therapy management, participation in procedures that use high-risk medications, medication procurement, providing drug information services, and documentation of interventions. Clinical pharmacists play an integral role in preventing medication errors as part of the health care multidisciplinary team.

MEDICATION-INDUCED FALLS

Medication-induced falls in the geriatric or rehabilitation population are a significant concern. The most recent American Geriatrics Society (AGS) and British Geriatrics Society (BGS) clinical practice guidelines on the prevention of falls in older persons note 3 specific medication-based recommendations[25]:

- Minimization or withdrawal of psychoactive medications when possible
- Reduction in total number of medications or dose in individual medications
- Review all medications for possible minimization or withdrawal.

The main focus of these recommendations is on the unnecessary use of medication or overprescribing practices that can be noted as polypharmacy. Studies have shown that the number of drugs a patient is on is a significant predictor of falls, with the greatest risk occurring in patients with regimens of 4 or more medications.[26–28]

Medications that have been identified that increase risk for falls are listed in **Table 2**. Multiple meta-analyses have been published evaluating the specifics of drug classes and their fall-risk potential.[29–31] These analyses identified neuroleptics/antipsychotics, antidepressants, benzodiazepines, and sedatives/hypnotics as high risk for falls. Narcotic agents were not associated with an increased risk of falls

Table 2		
High-risk falls medication		
Psychotropics	**Cardiac Medications**	**Antihypertensives**
Sedative hypnotics	Class IA antiarrhythmics	Antihistamines
Benzodiazepines	Diuretics	Anticonvulsants
Antidepressants		NSAIDs
Antipsychotics		Corticosteroids
		Muscle relaxants
		Digoxin
		Nitrates
		Hypoglycemics
		Anti-Parkinson drugs

and antihypertensives, with the exception of diuretics, were not consistently associated with an increased risk.[29–31]

The mechanisms behind drug-induced falls are multifactorial and range from alterations in hemodynamics (specifically orthostatic hypotension) to sedation via multiple mechanisms and receptor activities. Antihypertensives work in multiple fashions but all medications of this class can cause falls via syncope secondary to orthostatic hypotension. Orthostatic hypotension, or postural hypotension, is defined as a reduction in the following within 3 minutes of changing position from sitting to standing or laying down to sitting[32]:

- Systolic blood pressure of at least 20 mm Hg; or
- Diastolic blood pressure of at least 10 mm Hg.

Chronic antihypertensive therapy has not been associated with an increased risk for fall but rapid titration of drugs in this class can predispose a patient to falls. A recommendation for preventing this occurrence is to allow an adequate time between dose increases to allow the medication to reach its maximal effect.

Sedation by centrally acting medications is the major concern for the higher-risk medications, particularly the antipsychotics that act on multiple receptors. This reduction in wakefulness increases the risk for fall by impairing balance and reducing response time. It can occur via multiple mechanisms via receptor activity, predominantly antagonism of histamine, α-1, and muscarinic receptors or agonism of γ-aminobutyric acid (GABA) and opioid receptors.

Interventions to reduce medication-induced falls continue to be difficult to apply to clinical practice because of a lack of details of the medications taken in the study population as well as variability of practice settings.[33] One clinical trial by Campbell and colleagues[27] noted a 66% reduction in the risk of falling (hazard ratio 0.34, 95% confidence interval 0.16–0.74) after a gradual withdrawal of psychotropic medications. However, 47% of these patients required restarting the medication after only 1 month.[27] Pharmacist-led medication review as an intervention was studied as a fall-preventative measure and showed a significant improvement compared with the control group in the number of falls per patient (0.8 vs 1.3 falls per patient, $P<.0001$).[34] Another retrospective study evaluating the collaboration of a consultant pharmacist, research nurse, and a physician in a rehabilitation unit showed reductions in cardiovascular (CV) drugs, analgesics, psychotropics, and sedatives that correlated with a 47% reduction in falls in the intervention group.[35]

These studies emphasize the need for regular medication profile monitoring performed by a pharmacist or any other health care practitioner. Other general prescribing practices that may aid in reducing or limiting the potential for falls is to use the lowest effective dose, avoid unneeded polypharmacy, evenly divide fall-risk medications that require multiple doses per day (ie, use dosing every 12 hours instead of twice a day), avoid the use of multiple sedating medications on an as-needed basis, and shift to bedtime dosing of sedating medication if possible.

Clinical pearls

- Avoid the use of high-risk fall medications if possible. (eg, sedatives, neuroleptics, benzodiazepines)
- Fall risk is increased in patients on 4 or more medications
- Interventions to reduce fall risk include using the lowest effective dose, avoiding unnecessary polypharmacy, adjusting dosing times to avoid overlap and/or daytime sedation

GERIATRIC PHARMACOKINETICS AND PHARMACODYNAMICS

Pharmacokinetics and pharmacodynamics are more unpredictable in the elderly than in the younger population because of natural body changes that are caused by aging. In addition, there are limited data regarding the use of medications in the elderly because of extensive exclusion criteria in research studies.

Pharmacokinetics refers to the processes of absorption, distribution, metabolism, and excretion. As people age, certain physiologic changes occur: decrease in total body water and muscle mass, but an increase in body fat. Organ function starts to decrease by the third decade, and by the sixth decade the reduction reaches 25%.[36] Medication regimens need to be tailored accordingly.

Absorption

With increase in age, the elderly experience a decrease in gastric acid secretion, delayed gastric emptying, reduced intestinal transit time, and reduced gastrointestinal (GI) blood flow. These changes delay the onset of the first dose of the medication (ie, pain medication), but are less visible with chronically taken medications.[37] Achlorhydria or hypochlorhydria can also be caused or exacerbated by long-term use of proton pump inhibitors (PPIs) or histamine-2 blockers. It leads to decreased absorption of certain medications such as itraconazole, ketoconazole, iron, calcium carbonate. A way to improve medication absorption is to take azoles with an acidic beverage (eg, cola), iron with vitamin C on empty stomach, and calcium carbonate with meals.[38]

Delayed gastric emptying may contribute to furosemide resistance in worsening heart failure. Elderly dry skin with decreased lipid content and reduced blood flow may lead to decreased absorption of topical agents, especially lipophilic medications (ie, fentanyl, testosterone, and estradiol). Intramuscular and subcutaneous routes of administration are less preferred compared with the oral route in frail elderly because of decreased muscle mass and resultant decreased absorption. Transbuccal absorption of fentanyl was found to be unchanged with older age.[36–38]

Distribution

Because of the increase in body fat and decrease in muscle mass and total body water in the elderly, lipophilic medications like diazepam and chlordiazepoxide have prolonged duration of action. Lower doses of lipophilic medications with longer intervals in between are preferred.[36,37] Hydrophilic medications like aminoglycoside, digoxin, and lithium have decreased volume of distribution, which may increase serum concentration; therefore, reduction in dose is advisable.[37]

Protein Binding

In malnourished and frail elderly, albumin levels are decreased. This decrease leads to an increased free fraction of highly albumin-bound medications and, in turn, to an exaggerated transient (except phenytoin) pharmacologic effect (ie, diazepam [98%], ibuprofen [90%–99%], furosemide [90%], phenytoin [0%–95%], warfarin [99%], valproic acid [80%–90%]). Doses of these medications should be titrated carefully.[36,37]

Metabolism

Liver blood flow as well as its mass decreases with age by 20% to 40%.[36] Because of decreased blood flow, medications with high first-pass extraction rate have higher bioavailability (ie, metoprolol, propranolol, verapamil, morphine), therefore reduction in dose is advisable. Phase I metabolism (oxidation, reduction, and hydrolysis) that involves the CYP 450 enzyme system varies among elderly; for safety, decreased phase I metabolism should be expected. Some example of phase I metabolized medications include diazepam, quinidine, and theophylline. Phase II metabolism (glucuronidation, acetylation, sulfation) stays unchanged with age in most cases. Examples of phase II metabolized medications include lorazepam and oxazepam.[36,37,39]

Excretion

As with liver, the elderly have a decreased renal mass, renal blood flow, glomerular filtration rate (GFR), filtration fraction, and tubular secretion. GFR declines by 25%–50% by 90 years of age.[38] Most medications need to be renally adjusted (ie, carbapenems, fluconazole, vancomycin, aminoglycosides, acyclovir, most angiotensin-converting enzyme inhibitors [ACEIs], atenolol, digoxin, gabapentin, pregabalin, allopurinol).[36,37]

Pharmacodynamics

Physiologic changes in the elderly lead to an increased or decreased response to certain medications. Orthostatic hypotension is common in the elderly because of decreased capacity of baroreceptors to react to a decrease in blood pressure on rising. Some of the medications that could contribute to this process are α-blockers, diuretics, opioids, direct vasodilators, tricyclic antidepressants (TCAs), antipsychotics, and ACEIs. Possible solutions are to administer the offending medication at night, if appropriate, and to educate the patient about slow rising and staying hydrated.

As catecholamine levels increases, downregulation of β1 receptors occurs: expect decreased response to β1 agonists and increased response to BB and calcium channel blockers (CCB). Consider starting at the lowest dose of BB or CCB and titrate carefully based on patient's response. **Box 1** describes other major pharmacodynamic changes that are expected in the elderly.[36–38] **Table 3** is useful for rehabilitation clinicians because it lists commonly used drugs that predispose the patient to cardiac arrhythmias like torsades de points[40] or seizure activities.[41]

DRUG INTERACTIONS

Clinicians should be aware of potential drug interactions because they are common (about 7%–25%), underreported, result in dissatisfaction with care, and frequent emergency department visits. Predisposing risk factors include polypharmacy, multiple comorbidities, use of drugs with narrow therapeutic ranges, and increased age.[42] The goal of medication metabolism is to make the drug more polar and readily

---

Box 1
Pharmacodynamic changes in elderly and recommendations

1. Increased risk of developing corrected QT interval (QTc) prolongation and torsades de pointes (avoid combination of medications that prolong QTc, a list of which is given later)

2. Increased risk of electrolyte abnormalities (caution with selective serotonin reuptake inhibitors [SSRIs], sulfamethoxazole and trimethoprim, diuretics, ACEI)

3. Increased susceptibility to anticholinergic side effects, increased sensitivity to benzodiazepines, and increased chance of extrapyramidal side effects with dopamine-blocking agents (starting with lower doses and monitoring for side effects is advisable)

4. Increased response to warfarin (starting with lower dose and slower titration is advisable)

5. Increased chance of GI bleeding with NSAIDs or aspirin

6. Increased response to lower serum levels of antiseizure drugs and immunosuppressants but increased chance of side effects

Table 3
Medications associated with corrected QT interval (QTc) prolongation, lowering seizure threshold, and warfarin interactions

QTc Prolongation	Lowering Seizure Threshold	Warfarin Interactions
Amiodarone	Tramadol	Metronidazole (↑INR)
Quinidine	Carbapenems	Trimethoprim-sulfamethiazole (↑INR)
Haloperidol	Meperidine	Amiodarone (↑INR)
Methadone	Bupropion	Carbamazepine (↓INR)
Erythromycin	Amphetamines	Barbiturates (↓INR)

Abbreviation: INR, international normalized ratio.

available for excretion. Most of the drugs are metabolized through the liver. Phase I metabolism (oxidation, reduction, and hydrolysis) is predominantly catalyzed by the cytochrome P450 superfamily of mixed oxidases (CYP), which is organized into 18 families (ie, CYP3) and 43 subfamilies (ie, CYP3A4). Primary CYP 450 enzymes include 3A4, 2D6, 2C9, 2C19, 1A2, and 2E1. More than 50% of all hepatic reactions occur through CYP3A4. Drug interactions occur through various mechanisms such as induction/inhibition of metabolism of the medications, reduced absorption, altered gastric pH, and inhibition of renal tubular transport. Dose adjustments are advisable to avoid subtherapeutic or supratherapeutic effects of interacting medications.[43,44]

Warfarin is one of the most common medications seen in rehabilitation practice because of its wide indications. It is metabolized to S and R enantiomers. S enantiomer is 3 to 5 times more potent than R enantiomer, thus drug interactions with S enantiomer are more significant. S enantiomer is metabolized through CYP 2C9, whereas R enantiomer is primarily metabolized by CYP 1A2 and CYP 3A4. Significant drug interactions of warfarin are shown in **Table 3**. Bleeding risks increase with addition of aspirin at more than 1.5 g/d, NSAIDs, penicillins at high doses, tamoxifen, rivaroxaban, and natural supplements (Ginkgo biloba or St. John's wort). The combinations mentioned earlier should be avoided.[45,46]

ANTICOAGULANT PHARMACOLOGY
Venous Thromboembolism

Venous thromboembolism (VTE) is a serious but preventable cause of morbidity and mortality in hospitalized patients in rehabilitation that can be reduced by means of mechanical or pharmacologic thromboprophylaxis. Treatment options include early ambulation, use of stockings and alternating pressure devices, and antithrombotic agents (**Tables 4–6**). Although early mobilization is recommended for mildly affected patients, seriously ill patients or those with severe motor impairments often cannot return to walking. For patients who are at high risk of bleeding and patients with intracranial or active GI bleeding, compression stockings and intermittent compression devices are reasonably effective options. Pharmacologic agents should be initiated as soon as it is medically safe. The anticoagulation type, intensity, and duration should be adjusted on an individual basis depending on bleeding risk.

Recent literature has shown that, even after developing VTE, early, and even immediate, ambulation after initiation of appropriate anticoagulation therapy in conjunction with compression therapy does not increase development of pulmonary embolism (PE), contrary to the old belief that bed rest for several days is safest for preventing PE in patients with proximal deep vein thrombosis (DVT).[53,54] Initiation of early ambulation results in faster decrease of swelling and pain. Below-knee stockings with 30 to

40 mm Hg pressure at the ankle are indicated after proximal DVT and have been shown to reduce the development of postthrombotic sequelae by approximately 50% when worn for at least the first 2 years.[55]

The risk of thromboembolism should be assessed and classified into low, moderate, or high risk, and the prophylactic or therapeutic treatment should be started accordingly. Anticoagulant therapy is initiated with either unfractionated heparin (UFH) or subcutaneous low-molecular-weight heparin (LMWH) followed by oral anticoagulation.

DVT treatment with LMWH is preferred because it does not require laboratory monitoring. If UFH is used, it is initiated with an intravenous bolus dose followed by continuous infusion. Patients require regular monitoring of activated partial thromboplastin time (aPTT), with heparin dose adjusted to achieve an aPTT target range of 1.5 to 2.5 times the normal for 2 consecutive measurements. LMWH or UFH should be continued for at least 5 days to minimize risk of extension of thrombosis or recurrence of PE. Warfarin therapy is started within 24 hours of heparin treatment. The initial starting dose is 5 to 7.5 mg/d. The dosage is subsequently adjusted according to the patient's International Normalized Ratio to a therapeutic range of 2.0 to 3.0. Warfarin therapy should overlap heparin therapy for at least 3 to 5 days, bridging to long-term therapy for at least 3 months with oral anticoagulant. Bleeding is the main complication of anticoagulation and requires careful monitoring depending on the clinical condition of the patient and the drug used.

- For patients after total hip or knee replacements, at least 10 days and up to 35 days of LMWH or fondaparinux or warfarin and intermittent pneumatic compression devices are recommended by the American College of Chest Physicians for VTE prophylaxis in patients in rehabilitation.[47] Routine screening for DVT or PE in asymptomatic postoperative orthopedic patients is not recommended.
- Patients with SCIs are prone to stasis of the venous circulation, hypercoagulability of the blood, and intimal vascular injuries (known as the Virchow triad). DVT develops in approximately one-half to three-quarters of those with SCI who do not receive DVT prophylaxis, with the highest risk 7 to 10 days after injury,[56–59] especially in patients with motor complete injuries and injuries at or below the thoracic level. Although it is not considered standard of care, screening with a duplex ultrasound is a common practice by some physicians because most persons with SCI who develop DVT do not have clinical signs or symptoms such as swelling, warmth, or pain.[58–60]

DVT prophylaxis is the standard of care because of the high incidence of DVT and the potential fatal outcome of a PE. Studies have shown subcutaneously administered LMWH to be more effective in preventing both DVT and PE after SCI, compared with fixed-dose UFH.[61–63] No difference has been found between once-daily and twice-daily LMWH administration regimens.[64] Prophylaxis should continue until the time of discharge for those with motor incomplete SCI, for 2 months for those with uncomplicated complete injuries, and for 3 months for those with complete motor injuries with additional risk factors (previous thrombosis, cancer, heart failure, lower limb fracture, obesity, or age greater than 70 years). During the first 2 weeks after injury, pneumatic compression devices are also recommended.[65]

The treatment regimen for DVT or PE typically involves treatment doses of LMWH, UFH, or fondaparinux, followed by the oral anticoagulant warfarin, unless anticoagulation is contraindicated, for 6 months after the first DVT is diagnosed.[66,67] If there is DVT recurrence or progression, then indefinite anticoagulation is recommended.

Removable inferior vena cava (IVC) filters are indicated for persons who have failed anticoagulant prophylaxis with the development of DVT or PE despite adequate

Table 4
Anticoagulants for deep vein thrombosis (DVT) prophylaxis and their properties

	Mechanism of Action	Route	Pharmacokinetics	Common Adverse Events	Common Drug Interactions	Monitoring	Reversal
Dabigatran[a]	Direct thrombin inhibitor (factor IIa)	By mouth	Elimination: renal (80%) Half-life (normal renal function): 12–17 h	Hemorrhage, dyspepsia (abdominal/epigastric discomfort/pain), nausea, vomiting, constipation, abnormal liver enzymes	Substrate of P-glycoprotein: ketoconazole, verapamil, amiodarone, quinidine, clarithromycin, rifampin, PPIs, atorvastatin	No monitoring required; prolongs ecarin clotting time, aPTT, PT/INR, thrombin time	No antidote available
Dalteparin	Inhibition of factor Xa and IIa	Subcutaneous	Elimination: renal Half-life (normal renal function): 2–5 h Duration of effect: 12 h	Hemorrhage, thrombocytopenia (including HIT), abnormal liver enzymes, local injection site hematoma	Concomitant anticoagulants	No routine monitoring required; anti-Xa levels may be monitored in obese patients (>190 kg); other coagulation tests not affected	Protamine sulfate (1% solution), at a dose of 1 mg protamine for every 100 units of dalteparin given

Enoxaparin	Inhibition of factor Xa and IIa	Subcutaneous, IV	Elimination: renal (40%) Half-life (normal renal function): 7 h Duration of effect: ~12 h	Hemorrhage, thrombocytopenia (including HIT), nauseam diarrhea, abnormal liver enzymes, local injection site hematoma	Concomitant anticoagulants	No routine monitoring required; anti-Xa levels may be monitored in obese patients (>190 kg); other coagulation tests not affected	Protamine sulfate (1% solution) at a dose of 1 mg of protamine for every 1 mg of enoxaparin if administered <8 h; if >8 h 0.5 mg of protamine per 1 mg of enoxaparin
Fondaparinux	Inhibition of factor Xa	Subcutaneous	Elimination: renal (77%) Half-life (normal renal function): 17–21 h	Hemorrhage, fever, nausea, anemia, abnormal liver enzymes, local injection site hematoma	Concomitant anticoagulants	No routine monitoring required; other anticoagulation tests not affected	No antidote available; intermittent dialysis

(continued on next page)

Table 4
(continued)

	Mechanism of Action	Route	Pharmacokinetics	Common Adverse Events	Common Drug Interactions	Monitoring	Reversal
Heparin	Inhibition of factor Xa and IIa by binding to antithrombin	Subcutaneous, IV	Elimination: renal Half-life (normal renal function): 1–2 h	Hemorrhage, local injection site hematoma, hyperkalemia, hypersensitive reaction, HIT abnormal liver enzymes, osteoporosis (long-term administration)	Concomitant anticoagulants	Routine monitoring of aPTT or anti-Xa when used as treatment	Protamine sulfate (1% solution), at a dose of 1 mg per 100 units of UFH if administered <1 h, 0.5 mg of protamine per 100 units of UFH if administered within 1–2 h, 0.25 mg of protamine per 100 units of UFH if administered >2 h ago
Rivaroxaban	Inhibition of factor Xa	By mouth	Elimination: renal (66%), hepatic (28%) Half-life (normal renal function): 5–9 h	Hemorrhage, abnormal liver enzymes, thrombocytopenia	Substrate for CYP 3A4 and P-gp: fluconazole, ketoconazole, itraconazole, ritonavir, conivaptan, macrolide antibiotics, diltiazem, verapamil, quinidine, amiodarone, carbamazepine, phenytoin, rifampin, St. John's wort, clopidogrel	No routine monitoring required. aPTT and PT may be increased in some	No antidote available, not dialyzable

| Warfarin | By mouth | Vitamin K antagonist, inhibition of factors II, VII, IX, and X | Elimination: renal (92%) Half-life: 20–60 h | Hemorrhage, skin necrosis (early onset, <7 d), purple toe syndrome (late onset, 7–10 wk), abnormal liver enzymes | Substrate for CYP 2C9, 3A4, and 1A2. Amiodarone, trimethoprim/sulfamethoxazole, metronidazole, azole antifungals, clarithromycin, erythromycin, diltiazem, ritonavir, ciprofloxacin, levofloxacin, cimetidine, carbamazepine, phenytoin, rifampin, St. John's wort, grapefruit juice | INR | Vitamin K depending on INR; by mouth formulation preferred See **Table 5** for specific management of supratherapeutic INR |

Abbreviations: aPTT, activated partial thromboplastin time; HIT, heparin-induced thrombocytopenia; IV, intravenous; P-gp, P-glycoprotein; PT, prothrombin time; UFH, unfractionated heparin.

[a] Currently not FDA approved for DVT prophylaxis in the United States.

Data from Refs.[47–52]

Table 5		
Management of warfarin toxicity		
INR Range	**Significant Bleeding**	**Supratherapeutic INR Management**
3–5	No	Decrease warfarin dose or omit next dose Monitor INR more frequently and resume warfarin at a lower dose when INR is in range
5–9	No	Omit 1–2 doses of warfarin or omit 1 dose and administer vitamin K by mouth 2.5 mg once only (if at high risk for bleeding) Monitor INR more frequently and resume warfarin at a lower dose when INR is in range
>9	No	Hold warfarin and administer vitamin K by mouth 2.5–5 mg immediately; administer additional vitamin K if necessary (maximum 10 mg) Monitor INR more frequently and resume warfarin at a lower dose when INR is in range
Any INR	Yes	Hold warfarin and administer vitamin K 10 mg IVPB over 30 min; supplement with fresh frozen plasma, prothrombin complex concentrate, or recombinant factor VIIa depending on urgency Monitor INR more frequently and resume warfarin at a lower dose when INR is in range

Abbreviation: IVPB, intravenous piggyback (IV short-term infusion).

anticoagulation, or who have a thromboembolus within the IVC or iliac veins,[68] concomitant with the anticoagulant therapy, or in high-risk patients who have a contraindication to, or a complication of, anticoagulation such as hemorrhage or thrombocytopenia. The filters should be removed generally within 3 to 4 months if no thromboembolism has developed.

- Patients with stroke syndrome should be treated with some form of prophylaxis for VTE according to the National Institutes of Health Consensus Conference,[69] and extensive clinical experience.[70] In patients in whom hemorrhagic stroke has been ruled out, anticoagulation prophylaxis with repeated doses of low-dose heparin or LMWH compounds have been documented to be effective and should be continued until the time of discharge. Patients with a first episode of VTE, with reversible risk factors or asymptomatic calf thrombi, should be treated for at least 3 months. Patients with idiopathic VTE need anticoagulation for 6 to 12 months. Patients with recurrent VTE, cancer, or genetic risk factors should receive anticoagulation beyond 12 months to lifetime.
- Patients with traumatic brain injury (TBI) have an estimated incidence of DVT of 40%, placing them at high risk of death caused by pulmonary embolus.[71] There is no standard of care for the initiation of DVT prophylaxis and treatment in patients with TBI. The effectiveness of routine screening for DVT at rehabilitation admission has not been proved. Either heparin or LMWH within 24 to 72 hours after severe TBI or intracranial bleed is safely used[72] after consultation with the neurosurgeon about the risk of rebleed. In patients with TBI, the risk for DVT is increased by advanced age, severe injury, significant fractures, prolonged immobilization, and presence of clotting disorder.[73] In those patients who cannot undergo pharmacologic prophylaxis because of risk of bleeding (because of behavior alteration, fall risk, agitation), mechanical compression devices can be used; however, tolerance of these devices can be low for patients with agitation or requiring restraints. The duration of DVT prophylaxis is not clearly defined

in the TBI population. In general, the prophylaxis may be discontinued if the patient is able to ambulate greater than 30 m.

Heparin-Induced Thrombocytopenia

Heparin-induced thrombocytopenia (HIT) is a rare, but serious, life-threatening complication of UFH therapy, and to a significantly lesser extent with LMWH. HIT is an immune-mediated reaction caused by antibodies formed against complexes of platelet factor (PF4) and heparin, forming heparin-PF4-antibody complexes. Activated platelets with heparin-PF4-antibody complexes bind to surfaces of other activated platelets and undergo aggregation in the circulation, leading to thrombocytopenia.[74–76] The most serious complications caused by HIT are life-threatening venous thrombosis such as PE or proximal DVT or arterial thrombosis such as limb artery occlusion leading to limb ischemia, stroke, myocardial infarction, or cerebral venous thrombosis. Other complications include skin lesions, skin necrosis, and, in rare instances, anaphylactoid reactions.

Diagnosis of hit
The following is the typical presentation of HIT[74–77]:

1. Thrombocytopenia (platelet count <150,000/mm^3) or platelet count reduction of greater than 50% from baseline
2. Thrombocytopenia onset is typically 5 to 14 days after heparin exposure (no prior exposure, or last heparin exposure more than 100 days); however, exceptions exist (listed later)
3. Platelet nadir is typically greater than or equal to 20,000/mm^3
4. Observed thrombosis (presentation listed earlier) secondary to thrombocytopenia.

HIT is rarely manifested before 5 days after heparin exposure. Thrombocytopenia before 5 days can be either an acute, benign thrombocytopenia that does not require UFH discontinuation, or it can be early-onset HIT, which occurs within hours of heparin exposure in patients who received heparin in the previous 100 days, and it requires immediate discontinuation of UFH.[74–76] Other causes of thrombocytopenia have to be excluded, such as bacterial infections, sepsis, bone marrow disease, and medications other than heparin that can cause thrombocytopenia. It is reasonable to start patients on alternative anticoagulant therapy if they have a high or intermediate probability of HIT and continue alternative anticoagulation until HIT is confirmed or ruled out by laboratory testing.

Treatment of hit
It is recommended to immediately discontinue UFH after high clinical suspicion of HIT,[74–77] and this includes all types of heparin such as subcutaneous heparin, heparin flushes, or LMWH; initiate anticoagulation with alternative nonheparin anticoagulants such as direct thrombin inhibitors (eg, lepirudin, argatroban, or bivalirudin), and factor Xa inhibitor (eg, fondaparinux) immediately after discontinuation of heparin to prevent thrombosis. In patients with HIT who experience thrombosis, oral anticoagulants, such as warfarin, should be initiated only after platelet count has recovered to more than 150,000/mm^3. Use of LMWH is not recommended for the treatment of HIT because there is a high cross-reactivity with circulating heparin antibodies. Treatment with nonheparin anticoagulants in patients with HIT should continue until the platelet count has recovered to more than 150,000/mm^3 or for at least 4 weeks considering that the risk for thrombosis remains high for 2 to 4 weeks after treatment is initiated.

Table 6
Recommended anticoagulant therapy for DVT prophylaxis

Condition	Recommended Pharmacologic Prophylaxis	Initiation of Pharmacologic Prophylaxis	Dose	Duration
Elective hip replacement	LMWH (enoxaparin or dalteparin)	12 h before surgery, or 12–24 h after surgery at usual prophylactic dose, or 4–6 h after surgery at half dose then increase to usual prophylactic dose	Enoxaparin subcutaneous 30 mg twice a day, or enoxaparin 40 mg once daily, or dalteparin[a]	At least 10 d and up to 35 d for all options
	Fondaparinux (patients ≥50 kg only)	6–24 h after surgery	2.5 mg subcutaneously once daily	
	Vitamin K antagonist (warfarin)	Before surgery or the evening of surgical day	Target INR 2.5 (range INR 2–3)	
Elective knee replacement	LMWH (enoxaparin)	12–24 h after surgery at usual prophylactic dose	30 mg subcutaneous twice a day	At least 10 d and up to 35 d for all options
	Fondaparinux (patients ≥50 kg only)	6–8 h after surgery	2.5 mg subcutaneously once daily	
	Vitamin K antagonist (warfarin)	Before surgery or the evening of surgical day	Target INR 2.5 (range INR 2–3)	
Hip fracture surgery	Fondaparinux (patients ≥50 kg only)	6–8 h after surgery	2.5 mg subcutaneously once daily	At least 10 d and up to 35 d for all options
	LMWH (enoxaparin)	12–24 h after surgery	Enoxaparin 40 mg subcutaneously once daily	
	Vitamin K antagonist (warfarin)	Before surgery or the evening of surgical day	Target INR 2.5 (range INR 2–3)	
	Low-dose UFH	After surgery	5000 units every 8–12 h	

Patients with trauma	LMWH (enoxaparin)	As soon as considered safe	Enoxaparin 30 mg subcutaneous twice a day	Up to hospital discharge; if patient with impaired mobility transferred to rehabilitation, either LMWH or warfarin (INR 2.5, range 2–3)
Acute SCI	LMWH (enoxaparin)	After clinical evidence that primary hemostasis has been achieved	Enoxaparin 30 mg subcutaneously twice a day	Continue LMWH or convert to warfarin (target 2.5, range 2–3) for duration of rehabilitation phase

This text was written before the publication of the 2012 ACCP Antithrombosis guidelines, therefore all recommendations are based on the 2008 ACCP guideline update. For the most recent version of the updated guideline please refer Ref.[104]

[a] Dalteparin prophylaxis dosing options for hip replacement surgery: (1) postoperative regimen, 2500 units 4–8 hours after surgery (may be delayed if hemostasis is not achieved) after surgery, then maintenance 5000 units once daily at least 6 hours after postsurgical dose; (2) preoperative regimen, 2500 units within 2 hours before surgery 2500 units 4–8 hours after surgery (may be delayed if hemostasis is not achieved), then maintenance 5000 units once daily at least 6 hours after postsurgical dose; (3) preoperative regimen, 5000 units 10–14 hours before surgery, 5000 units 4–8 hours after surgery (may be delayed if hemostasis is not achieved), then maintenance 5000 units once daily, allowing 24 hours between previous dose.

Data from Hirsh J, Guyatt G, Albert G, et al. Antithrombotic and thrombolytic therapy: American College of Chest Physicians evidence-based clinical practice guidelines. Chest 2008;133:715–1095.

In patients with heparin-induced thrombosis, treatment should be continued for at least 3 to 6 months after the event.

PAIN MANAGEMENT

Pain can be described in a multitude of ways and can present as an acute or chronic condition but, beyond its subjective nature, it is generally described as an unpleasant sensory and emotional experience associated with actual or potential tissue damage.[78–80] Regardless of the cause or the type of pain the patient is experiencing, efficacy and safety in the use of analgesics require knowledge of the agents available and the complications of their use.

Pain medications or analgesics consist of several drug classes based on their mechanism of action. Currently available agents include NSAIDs, opioids/opiates, and acetaminophen. Other drug classes that have a role in pain management include antidepressants and anticonvulsants.

NSAIDs are the primary class of analgesics used for the treatment of mild to moderate somatic or visceral pain.[79] There are several agents in this class and selecting which to use can be confusing but, no matter which agent is chosen, the use of NSAIDs requires some precaution, particularly with chronic therapy, because there is an increased risk for gastric ulceration and certain subclasses have been associated with increased cardiac complications, stroke, and increased mortality.[81,82] Use of PPIs or H-2 blockers, as well as limiting the duration of use, may lessen the risk of peptic ulcer disease. Other ADRs to be aware of in the use of NSAIDs are worsening asthma, dyspepsia, renal impairment, increased blood pressure, and poor control in heart failure.

Treatment of more severe pain generally requires the use of opioids as well as the conversion of the patient from oral to parenteral drug administration. Adverse reactions to opioids generally include sedation, pruritus, constipation, and, in severe cases, respiratory depression. Dose increases should be based on patient self-reported pain based using validated pain scales as well as tolerance to side effects and vital signs (particularly respiratory rate). Consideration should also be made to scheduled doses of medication versus as-needed dosing. Scheduled doses of opioids has the potential for greater pain control but the risk for overdose is greater. Just as pain syndromes are varied in their presentation, so is the response of the patient to the medications, so the switch from one agent to another is often required. When changing opioid agents, it is important to take specific precautions to prevent an overdose (**Box 2**).

Methadone is a useful agent in patients with uncontrolled severe chronic pain syndromes but its conversion is variable and is based on the morphine equivalent dose (see **Table 7**; **Table 8**). This variability in conversion rates can lead to inadvertent overdoses and potential ADEs or sentinel events (eg, death). However, if the provider is aware of this nuance, the proper dose adjustment can be made and the risk for ADEs can be reduced.[83]

Box 2
Conversion algorithm for opioids

1. Calculate 24-hour opioid requirement for pain
2. Convert 24-hour opioid requirement to an oral morphine equivalent from a dose equivalence table (see **Table 7**) and use 25% to 60% of that dose
3. Convert 24-hour morphine equivalent to the intended opioid of change
4. Divide the new 24-hour opioid dose into an appropriate dosing frequency

---

Table 7
Equianalgesic doses of narcotic medications

| Drug | Equianalgesic Dose (mg) | |
	Oral	Parenteral
Buprenorphine	—	0.4
Butorphanol	—	2
Codeine	200	—
Fentanyl	—	0.1
Hydrocodone	30	—
Hydromorphone	7.5	1.5
Meperidine	300	75
Methadone	See **Table 8**	Variable
Morphine	30	10
Oxycodone	20	—
Oxymorphone	10	1
Tapentadol	75	—

Data from Lexi-Comp Online. Available at: http://online.lexi.com/crlsql/servlet/crlonline. Accessed December 15, 2011. Opioid Analgesics; and American Pain Society (APS). Principles of analgesic use in the treatment of acute pain and cancer pain. 6th edition. Glenview (IL); 2008. p. 60025.

Although NSAIDs and opioids are useful in somatic or visceral pain, they may lack efficacy in patient complaints of neuropathic pain characterized by sensations of burning and tingling or a shooting and lightning-bolt presentation. Agents that are not typically associated with being pain medications (eg, antidepressants, particularly those that have norepinephrine reuptake inhibition) are commonly used as well as anti-convulsants, the mechanisms of which are not well elucidated. TCAs, as well as the serotonin-norepinephrine reuptake inhibitors (SNRIs), have shown benefit but SNRIs are generally preferred because of less anticholinergic activity and QTc prolongation, leading to improved tolerability and safety profile.[83] If an anticonvulsant is warranted, gabapentin may be considered as an initial choice because of its preferential side effect profile, because other anticonvulsants carry a heavy side effect burden and may require blood monitoring for assessment of toxicity. Drug selection is generally up to the provider but switching or augmenting therapy with any other agent is a valid option and may prove beneficial.

Safety in pain control is a valid concern for health care providers but it should not predispose them to undertreating patients. with an understanding of the available medications and how they should be used, physiatrists can manage a patient's pain to an appropriate degree and be comfortable with the treatment.

Clinical pearls

- Avoid chronic use of NSAIDs to prevent gastric bleeding events
- Always apply a dose reduction of 25% to 60% when converting from one opioid to another to prevent potential overdose
- Take care when converting to methadone and be aware that the conversion ratio changes based on the dose in morphine equivalents
- Medications not generally indicated for pain may be used for the treatment of neuropathic pain

Table 8
Guidelines for conversion to oral methadone in adults

Oral Morphine Dose or Equivalent (mg/d)	Oral Morphine/Oral Methadone (Conversion Ratio)
<90	4:1
90–300	8:1
>300	12:1

Data from Lexi-Comp Online. Available at: http://online.lexi.com/crlsql/servlet/crlonline. Accessed December 15, 2011. Opioid Analgesics.

SLEEP DISORDERS: INSOMNIA AND HYPERSOMNIA

Currently approximately 70 million Americans suffer from a sleep disorder, but the occurrence of sleep disorders is higher among patients who are hospitalized and in rehabilitation. Most commonly encountered sleep disorders in the rehabilitation population include insomnia, hypersomnia, sleep apnea, narcolepsy, and circadian rhythm disorders. Risk factors in the rehabilitation population that can contribute to sleep disorders, in addition to the normal risk factors, are TBI, stroke, medications, and uncontrolled pain.[84]

Sleep Neurochemistry and Sleep Cycles

The neurochemistry of sleep is complex and it involves multiple neurotransmitters in the brain that are responsible for promoting sleep as well as arousal and wakefulness. Serotonin is involved in sleep onset, so decrease of serotonin results in reduced sleep. Serotonin is also converted to melatonin, which is synthesized at night, inhibited by light, and has the same effect on sleep as serotonin. Dopamine, norepinephrine, and acetylcholine are involved in arousal and wakefulness, and decrease in these neurotransmitters promotes decreased alertness and sleepiness. The normal sleep cycle is divided into rapid eye movement (REM) and non–rapid eye movement (NREM) sleep. NREM sleep is further divided into 4 stages (1, 2, 3, and 4). During an average sleep, a person would normally alternate through REM and NREM sleep 3 to 6 times, each cycle lasting approximately 90 to 120 minutes.[85,86]

Treatment Options for Insomnia

Nonpharmacologic therapy for insomnia is as important as pharmacologic therapy.[87–91] Patients should be educated regarding normal sleep habits, sleep hygiene, and stress management. Pharmacologic treatment of insomnia is recommended after nonpharmacologic therapies fail, and the lack of sleep has a significant impact on the patient's social, occupational, or daytime functioning.

Initial recommended treatment of insomnia is a short-action or intermediate-action benzodiazepine receptor agonist (BzRA) medication or the melatonin receptor agonist, ramelteon. Insomnia medications and their common doses are presented in **Table 9**. These medications have been proved safe and effective in reducing sleep latency and nocturnal awakenings and increasing total sleep time. Alternative BzRA agents with longer half-life may be selected if a patient does not respond to the initial treatment; however, these medications with prolonged half-lives may lead to potential accumulation and prolonged sedation, leading potentially to falls, therefore they are not generally first-line treatment. Benzodiazepines not specifically approved for insomnia (lorazepam, clonazepam) may be used if patients have a comorbid condition such as anxiety that may benefit from treatment.

Table 9
Medications used for the treatment of insomnia

Medication Class	Pharmacokinetics	Recommended Dosage	Onset of Action	Indication
Benzodiazepine Receptor Antagonists (Schedule IV Controlled Substance)				
Nonbenzodiazepines				
Zolpidem tartrate	Half-life: 1.4–4.5 h Excretion: urine (48%), feces (29%)	10 mg immediately before bedtime Controlled release: 12.5 mg immediately before bedtime	30 min	Short to intermediate acting Sleep onset Controlled release Sleep onset and sleep maintenance
Eszopiclone	Half-life: 6 h Excretion: urine	2 mg immediately before bedtime (maximum 3 mg)	30 min	Intermediate acting Sleep onset and sleep maintenance
Zaleplon	Half-life: 0.5–1 h Excretion: urine (70%), feces (17%)	10 mg at bedtime (range 5–20 mg)	20 min	Short acting Sleep onset
Benzodiazepines				
Temazepam	Half-life: 4–18 h Excretion: urine	7.5 mg–30 min at bedtime	30–60 min	Short to intermediate acting Sleep maintenance
Flurazepam	Half-life: 47–100 h Excretion: urine (active metabolites)	15–30 mg at bedtime Avoid use in geriatrics if possible	15–30 min	Long acting Sleep maintenance
Melatonin Receptor Antagonist (Nonscheduled)				
Ramelteon	Half-life: 1–2.6 h Excretion: urine (86%), feces (4%)	8 mg within 30 min of bedtime	30 min	Short acting Sleep onset

Sedating low-dose antidepressants such as trazodone, mirtazapine, and doxepin or amitriptyline may be prescribed if the patient is not responding to the initial treatment or the patient has a comorbid condition such as depression that may benefit from treatment, although higher doses may be necessary for the treatment of the depression. In addition, these medications may be an option in patients with a history of substance abuse because of their low abuse potential.

Hypnotic medications can be dosed either nightly or intermittently, between 2 to 5 times per week. As-needed dosing of hypnotic medications is generally not recommended because of the potential of daytime sedation and potential arousal conditioning in anticipation of the medication. Duration of treatment should be guided based on the patient's needs and preferences.

Off-label and Over-the-Counter Medications for Treatment of Insomnia

The use of off-label prescription medications such as gabapentin, tiagabine, quetiapine, and olanzapine is not recommended because of lack of evidence for the treatment of chronic insomnia, and the potential for adverse events, unless there is a comorbid condition that is the primary indication for the medication. Over-the-counter nonprescription medications such as antihistamines are not recommended for long-term treatment of chronic insomnia because of the lack of evidence in the treatment of chronic insomnia and the potential risk of side effects such as daytime drowsiness and sleepiness, cognitive impairment, as well as anticholinergic side effects if used long term.[91]

L-Tryptophan is a dietary supplement that is available over the counter and has been used as a sleep aid, in addition to its many other potential uses. Its proposed mechanism of action is that it increases serotonin and melatonin levels in the brain, which are helpful in inducing sleep. Studies with L-tryptophan and its effectiveness are conflicting and not well controlled, but there is evidence that it may be effective in inducing sleep.[92]

Adverse Events from Insomnia Medications

Medications such as zolpidem and eszopiclone have been studied for up to 12 months and have been shown to be safe. If longer treatment periods are necessary, frequent evaluation is necessary to monitor for efficacy and side effects. Discontinuation of hypnotic medications after long-term use can cause rebound insomnia as well as physical and psychological withdrawal. When discontinuing hypnotic medications, slow tapering of the medication is necessary over several weeks or months, until the lowest effective, safe dose has been reached.[88]

Hypersomnia and Narcolepsy

Excessive daytime sleepiness and narcolepsy are rare among the general population, but they are frequently seen in patients who have experienced TBI.[84,86]

Modafinil, a psychostimulant, has been used in patients with excessive daytime sleepiness and narcolepsy to improve alertness, increase daytime alertness, improve mood, and prevent sleep, but it has no effect on cataplectic symptoms. Dextroamphetamine and methylphenidate also are FDA approved for the treatment of narcolepsy (**Table 10**). They are also classified as psychostimulants like modafinil; however, they have higher abuse potential.[93,94]

Stimulants improve alertness, increase daytime performance, improve mood, and prevent sleep; however, they can induce insomnia, hypertension, palpitations, and irritability. Modafinil, dextroamphetamine, and methylphenidate have been used in patients after TBI and they have limited evidence in their effectiveness in reducing

Table 10
Drugs used for the treatment of narcolepsy

Medication Class	Pharmacokinetics	Recommended Dosage	Onset of Action
Medications for Treatment of Excessive Daytime Sleepiness			
Dextroamphetamine	Half-life: 10–13 h Excretion: urine	10 mg once daily May increase dose by 10 mg in weekly interval (max: 60 mg/d)	1–1.5 h
Methylphenidate	Half-life: 3–4 h Excretion: urine	10 mg 2–3 times/d (max: 60 mg/d)	2 h
Modafinil	Half-life: 15 h Excretion: urine	200 mg once daily in the morning	2–4 h
Sodium oxybate[a]	Half-life: 0.5–1 h Excretion: pulmonary	4.5 g per day (divided in 2 equal doses) Increase dose in 2 week intervals Average dose 6–9 g/d (max: 9 g/d)	30–75 min
Medications for Treatment of Cataplexy			
Fluoxetine	Half-life (days) 4–16 h (active metabolites) Excretion: urine	20–80 mg per day	—
Imipramine	Half-life: 6–18 h Excretion: urine (as metabolites)	50–250 mg daily May be in divided dose	—
Nortriptyline	Half-life: 28–31 h Excretion: urine, feces	50–200 mg once daily Can be given in single or divided doses	—
Venlafaxine	Half-life: 5–7 h Excretion: urine	75–375 mg daily IR formulation: 2–3 divided doses ER formulation: once daily	—

[a] Also effective in treating cataplexy.

daytime fatigue and daytime sleepiness.[95] Sodium oxybate, a derivative of GABA, is the only medication that is effective in treating daytime sleepiness as well as the cataplexy, hallucinations, and sleep paralysis associated with narcolepsy. The most common side effects from this medication include nausea, somnolence, confusion, dizziness, and incontinence. Other medications that can be used for the treatment of cataplexy, paralysis, and hallucinations are TCAs, SSRIs, and venlafaxine (see **Table 10**).[94,95]

NONSTEROIDAL ANTIINFLAMMATORY DRUG-INDUCED GASTROPATHY

NSAIDs are commonly used in the treatment of patients with musculoskeletal pain because of their antiinflammatory and analgesic properties. In addition, low-dose aspirin is commonly used for prevention of CV diseases and ischemic stroke because of its antiplatelet activity. NSAIDs and aspirin reduce the synthesis of mucosal-protective prostaglandins (PGs) from arachidonic acid by inhibiting the cyclooxygenase-1 (COX-1) enzyme. Most NSAIDs available on the market are nonselective and block COX-1 and COX-2 enzymes, whereas celecoxib is the only selective COX-2 inhibitor NSAID and it is associated with less GI hemorrhage because of the lack of inhibition of COX-1.[96–98] Commonly used NSAID medications used in the rehabilitation population are listed in **Box 3** in order of decreasing GI toxicity.

Risk Factors and Prevention of NSAID-Induced Gastropathy

The American College of Gastroenterology has classified patients in 3 groups (high, moderate, and low risk) according to the number of risk factors present for developing NSAID-related gastropathy.[96] They include history of complicated peptic ulcer disease and the presence of multiple risk factors such as (1) age more than 65 years, (2) high-dose NSAID therapy, (3) previous history of uncomplicated ulcer, and (4) concurrent use of aspirin (including low dose), corticosteroids, or anticoagulants. The current guidelines by the American College of Gastroenterology recommend designing prevention strategies by considering the patient's risk factors for developing NSAID-induced gastropathy as well as balancing CV risks because most NSAIDs, especially COX-2 selective inhibitors, have been associated with increased CV risks. Most evidence for the prevention of NSAID-induced gastropathy is with PPIs and misoprostol (**Table 11**). H_2-receptor agonists are not recommended for prevention of NSAID-induced gastropathy because they are only effective in high doses. Details of these recommendations are listed in **Table 12**.

DRUG-INDUCED COGNITION ADVERSE EFFECTS

Cognition is the process by which our minds use information and apply knowledge. This process is responsible for maintaining attention, understanding language, problem solving, and making decisions. Several medications have been noted to impair cognition, particularly the anticonvulsants. A review of previous studies found that phenytoin has a high association with cognitive impairment, whereas phenobarbital and valproic

---

Box 3
NSAIDs

Nonselective NSAIDs in decreasing order of GI toxicity

1. Indomethacin
2. Naproxen
3. Diclofenac
4. Ketorolac
5. Sulindac
6. Piroxicam
7. Ibuprofen
8. Meloxicam
9. Nabumetone
10. Etodolac

Selective NSAIDs

1. Celecoxib

Data from Cook DJ, Fuller HD, Guyatt GH, et al. Risk factors for gastrointestinal bleeding in critically ill patients. N Engl J Med 1994;330:337–81; and Schalansky B, Hwang JH. Prevention of nonsteroidal anti-inflammatory drug-induced gastropathy. J Gastroenterol 2009;44:44–52.

Table 11
Agents for prevention of NSAIDs-induced gastropathy

Medication Class	Mechanism of Action	Dosage and Route	Adverse Events	Drug Interactions
PPIs				
Dexlansoprazole	Suppresses gastric acid secretion by inhibition of the H$^+$/K$^+$ ATPase in the gastric parietal cells	30–60 mg daily, by mouth	Diarrhea, nausea, vomiting, abdominal pain, headaches, rash, acute interstitial nephritis, hip fractures, *Clostridium difficile* infections	CYP 2C19, 3A4 Lansoprazole ⋙ rabeprazole ⋙ omeprazole ⋙ esomeprazole > pantoprazole Clopidogrel, delavirdine, erlotinib, posaconazole, dabigatran, St. John's wort, rifampin
Esomeprazole		20–40 mg daily, by mouth, IV		
Lansoprazole		30 mg daily, by mouth		
Omeprazole		40 mg daily, by mouth		
Pantoprazole		40 mg daily, by mouth, IV		
Rabeprazole		20 mg daily, by mouth		
Misoprostol	Synthetic prostaglandin E1 analogue that replaces the protective prostaglandin consumed with NSAIDs	200 μg 4 times daily with food, by mouth	Diarrhea, abdominal pain, dyspepsia, flatulence	Antacids

acid derivatives have a more moderate effect, and carbamazepine is free or has minimal impairment.[99] Another drug class of concern is the antipsychotics, particularly the first-generation antipsychotics that cause dopamine blockade in the mesocortical dopaminergic tract, which is thought to regulate cognition and executive function.[100] Atypical or second-generation antipsychotics have less activity in this region of the brain and are theorized to have less impact, or even improvement in cognition, particularly in schizophrenic patients.[99,101] These medications should be used in patients with cognitive impairments only after consideration of the risks versus benefits of treatment.

Table 12
Recommendations for prevention of NSAIDs-induced gastropathy

	Low GI Risk	Moderate GI Risk	High GI Risk
Low CV risk	NSAID alone (the least GI-toxic NSAID at the lowest dose possible)	NSAID + PPI or misoprostol	Alternative therapy if possible or COX-2 inhibitor + PPI or misoprostol
High CV risk (low-dose aspirin required)	Naproxen + PPI or misoprostol	Naproxen + PPI or misoprostol	Avoid all NSAIDs or COX-2 inhibitors. Use alternative therapy

Data from Lanza FL, Chan FK, Quigley EM, et al. Practice Parameters Committee of the American College of Gastroenterology. Guidelines for prevention of NSAID-related ulcer complications. Am J Gastroenterol 2009;104:728–38.

Table 13
Medication classes associated with neuropsychiatric reactions

Drug Class	Common Medications in Class	Neuropsychiatric Complication
Anticonvulsants	Levetiracetam, topiramate	Aggression, psychosis
Antiretrovirals	Efavirenz, didanosine, lamivudine	Depression, psychosis, aggression, sleep disturbances, delirium
Antihypertensives	Propranolol, clonidine	Depression, mania
Hormone modulators	Luprolide, estrogen	Depression, aggression, agitation
Parkinson medication	Ropinirole, bromocriptine	Psychosis, hypomania, sleep disturbances, delirium, anxiety
Antibiotics	Cycloserine, nitrofurantoin	Depression, anxiety, delirium, fatigue, irritability
Opioids	Propoxyphene, meperidine	Dysphoria, delirium, mood changes, psychosis

Data from Turjanski N, Lloyd GG. Psychiatric side-effects of medications: recent developments. Adv Psychiatr Treat 2005;11:58–70.

DRUG-INDUCED NEUROPSYCHIATRIC DISTURBANCES

Understanding that side effects associated with commonly used medication are not limited to purely physical consequences is important. Several medications can be responsible for psychiatric and neurologic complications such as depression, mood alterations, psychosis, anxiety, and sleep disturbances. **Table 13** gives a general overview of drug classes and their associated psychiatric complications. The degree to which the medications can cause these symptoms depends on the specific medications as well as their ability to cross the blood-brain barrier.[102,103]

REFERENCES

1. Reducing and preventing adverse drug events to decrease hospital costs. Available at: http://www.ahrq.gov/qual/aderia/aderia.htm. Accessed December 15, 2011.
2. Nebeker JR, Barach P, Samore MH. Clarifying adverse drug events: a clinician's guide to terminology, documentation, and reporting. Ann Intern Med 2004;140: 795–801.
3. World Alliance for Patient Safety Forward Programme 2005. Geneva (Switzerland): World Health Organization; 2004.
4. Institute of Medicine. To err is human: building a safer health system. Washington, DC: National Academy Press; 1999.
5. Leape LL, Bates DW, Cullen DJ, et al. Systems analysis of adverse drug events. JAMA 1995;274:35–43.
6. Budnitz DS, Shehab N, Kegler SR, et al. Medication use leading to emergency department visits for adverse drug events in older adults. Ann Intern Med 2007; 125:755–65.
7. Cornish PL, Knowles SR, Marchesano R, et al. Unintended medication discrepancies at the time of hospital admission. Arch Intern Med 2005;165:424–9.
8. Agency for Healthcare Research and Quality (AHRQ). Medication reconciliation. Available at: http://psnet.ahrq.gov/primer.aspx?primerID=1. Accessed December 15, 2011.

9. The case for medication reconciliation—adapted from the Institute for Healthcare Improvement's Getting Started kit: prevent adverse drug events (medication reconciliation) how-to-guide. Nurs Manage 2005;22. Available at: http://www.ihi.org/IHI/Programs/Campaign. Accessed December 15, 2011.

10. Schnipper JL, Kirwin JL, Cotugno MC, et al. Role of pharmacist counseling in preventing adverse drug events after hospitalization. Arch Intern Med 2006; 166(5):565–71.

11. Schnipper JL, Hamann C, Ndumele CD, et al. Effect of an electronic medication reconciliation application and process redesign on potential adverse drug events: a cluster-randomized trial. Arch Intern Med 2009;169(8):771–80.

12. Adherence to long-term therapies: evidence for action. Geneva (Switzerland): World Health Organization; 2003.

13. National Council of Health Information and Education. Enhancing prescription medicine adherence. Rockville (MD): 2007.

14. Marinker M, Blenkinsopp A, Bond C, et al. From compliance to concordance: achieving shared goals in medicine taking. London: Royal Pharmaceutical Society of Great Britain; 1997.

15. Kramer JM, Hammill B, Anstrom K, et al. National evaluation of adherence to [beta] blocker therapy for 1 year after acute myocardial infarction in patients with commercial health insurance. Am Heart J 2006;152(3):454, e1–8.

16. Beckles GL, Engelgau MM, Narayan KM, et al. Population-based assessment of the level of care among adults with diabetes in the U.S. Diabetes Care 1998;21: 1432–8.

17. To err is human; building a safer health system. Institute of Medicine. Washington (DC): National Academies Press; 2000.

18. Feldman JA, DeTullio PL. Medication noncompliance: an issue to consider in the drug selection process. Hosp Formul 1994;29:204–11.

19. Medication compliance-adherence-persistence digest. Washington (DC): American Pharmacists Association; 2003.

20. Ziegler DK, Mosier MC, Buenaver M, et al. How much information about adverse effects of medication do patients want from physicians? Arch Intern Med 2001; 161:706–13.

21. Cramer JA. Overview of methods to measure and enhance patient compliance. In: Cramer JA, Spilker B, editors. Patient compliance in medical practice and clinical trials. New York: Raven Press; 1991. p. 3–10.

22. Krueger KP, Felkey BG, Berger BA. Improving adherence and persistence: a review and assessment of interventions and description of steps toward a national adherence initiative. J Am Pharm Assoc (2003) 2003;43(6):668–78.

23. Cramer JA, Mattson RH, Prevey ML, et al. How often is medication taken as prescribed? JAMA 1989;261:3273–7.

24. Guidance for medication assessment in patients with swallowing (dysphagia) or feeding disorders. Pharmacy Benefits Management-Strategic Healthcare Group (PBM), June 2006. Available at: http://www.pbm.va.gov. Accessed December 21, 2011.

25. AGS/BGS Clinical practice guideline: prevention of falls in older persons (2010). American Geriatrics Society. Available at: http://www.americangeriatrics.org/health_care_professionals/clinical_practice/clinical_guidelines_recommendations/2010/. Accessed December 21, 2011.

26. Deeg DJ, Comijs HC, Thomése GC, et al. [The Longitudinal Ageing Study Amsterdam: a survey of 17 years of research into changes in daily functioning]. Tijdschr Gerontol Geriatr 2009;40(6):217–27 [in Dutch].

27. Campbell AJ, Borrie MJ, Spears GF. Risk factors for falls in a community-based prospective study of people 70 years of age and older. J Gerontol 1989;44(4): M112–7.

28. Buchner DM, Larson EB. Falls on fractures in patients with Alzheimer's-type dementia. JAMA 1987;257:1492–5.

29. Leipzig RM, Cumming RG, Tinetti ME. Drugs and falls in older people: a systematic review and meta-analysis, Part I. Psychotropic drugs. J Am Geriatr Soc 1999;47:30–9.

30. Leipzig RM, Cumming RG, Tinetti ME. Drugs and falls in older people: a systematic review and meta-analysis, Part II. Cardiac and analgesic drugs. J Am Geriatr Soc 1999;47:40–50.

31. Woolcott JC, Richardson KF, Wiens MO, et al. Meta-analysis of the impact of 9 medication classes on falls in elderly persons. Arch Intern Med 2009;169(21): 1952–60.

32. Medow MS, Stewart JM, Sanyal S, et al. Pathophysiology, diagnosis, and treatment of orthostatic hypotension and vasovagal syncope. Cardiol Rev 2008; 16(1):4–20.

33. Riefkohl EZ, Bieber HL, Burlingame MB, et al. Medications and falls in the elderly: a review of the evidence and practical considerations. P T 2003; 28(11):724–6, 733.

34. Zermansky AG, Alldred DP, Petty DR, et al. Clinical medication review by a pharmacist of elderly people living in care homes- randomized controlled trial. Age Ageing 2006;35(6):586–91.

35. Haumschild MJ, Karfonta TL, Haumschild MS, et al. Clinical and economic outcomes of a fall-focused pharmaceutical intervention program. Am J Health Syst Pharm 2003;60(10):1029–32.

36. Hutchison LC, O'Brien CE. Changes in pharmacokinetics and pharmacodynamics in the elderly patient. J Pharm Pract 2007;20(1):4–12.

37. Hutchinson LC. Biomedical principles of aging. In: Hutchinson LC, Sleeper RB, editors. Fundamentals of geriatric pharmacotherapy. Bethesda (MD): American Society of Health System Pharmacists; 2010. p. 53–70.

38. Delafuente JC. Pharmacokinetic and pharmacodynamic alterations in the geriatric patient. Consult Pharm 2008;23:324–34.

39. Starner CI, Gray SI, Guay DR, et al. Geriatrics. In: DiPiro JT, Talbert RL, editors. Pharmacotherapy: a pathophysiologic approach. 6th edition. New York: McGraw-Hill; 2008. p. 57–67.

40. Woosley RL. Drugs that prolong the QT interval and/or induce torsades de pointes. Arizona Center for Education and Research for Therapeutics. Available at: http://www.azcert.org/medical-pros/drug-lists/printable-drug-list.cfm. Accessed December 29, 2011.

41. Quaranta LA. Seizures. In: Tisdale JE, Miller DA, editors. Drug-induced diseases. Bethesda (MD): ASHP Publications Production Center; 2005. p. 111–23.

42. Dallenbach FM, Bovier PA, Desmeules J, et al. Detecting drug interactions using personal digital assistants in an out-patient clinic. QJM 2007;100:691–7.

43. Larson AM, Kaplan MM. Drugs and the liver: metabolism and mechanisms of injury. February 3, 2011, Uptodate Web site. Available at: http://www.uptodate.com/contents/drugs-and-the-liver-metabolism-and-mechanisms-of-injury. Accessed December 28, 2011.

44. Flockhart DA. Drug interactions: cytochrome P450 drug interaction table. Indiana University School of Medicine; 2007. Available at: http://medicine.iupui.edu/clinpharm/ddis/table.aspx. Accessed December 28, 2011.

45. Ansell J, Hirsh J, Hylek E, et al. Pharmacology and management of vitamin K antagonists: American College of Chest Physicians evidence-based clinical practice guidelines. Chest 2008;133:160S–98S.
46. Lexi-Comp Web site. Available at: http://online.lexi.com/crlsql/servlet/crlonline. Accessed December 29, 2011.
47. Hirsh J, Guyatt G, Albert G, et al. Antithrombotic and thrombolytic therapy: American College of Chest Physicians evidence-based clinical practice guidelines. Chest 2008;133:71S–109S.
48. Product information: LOVENOX(®) injection, enoxaparin sodium injection. Bridgewater (NJ): Aventis Pharmaceuticals; 2005.
49. Product information: FRAGMIN(®) subcutaneous injection, dalteparin sodium subcutaneous injection. Woodcliff Lake (NJ): Eisai; 2009.
50. Product information: ARIXTRA (®) subcutaneous injection, fondaparinux sodium subcutaneous injection. Research Triangle Park (NC): GlaxoSmithKline; 2008.
51. Product information: PRADAXA (®) oral capsules, dabigatran etexilate mesylate oral capsules, Boehringer Ingelheim Pharmaceuticals. (per FDA), Ridgefield (CT), 2011.
52. Product information: XARELTO(®) oral tablets, rivaroxaban oral tablets. Titusville (NJ): Janssen Pharmaceuticals; 2011.
53. Partsch H. Ambulation and compression after deep vein thrombosis: dispelling myths. Semin Vasc Surg 2005;18(3):148–52.
54. Trujillo-Santos J, Perea-Milla E, Jimenez-Puente A, et al. Bed rest or ambulation in the initial treatment of patients with acute deep vein thrombosis or pulmonary embolism: findings from the Riete registry. Chest 2005;127(5):1631–6.
55. Prandoni P, Lensing AW, Prins MH, et al. Below-knee elastic compression stockings to prevent the post-thrombotic syndrome: a randomized, controlled trial. Ann Intern Med 2004;141(4):249–56.
56. Merli GJ, Crabbe S, Paluzzi RG, et al. Etiology, incidence, and prevention of deep vein thrombosis in acute spinal cord injury. Arch Phys Med Rehabil 1993;74:1199–205.
57. Merli GJ, Herbison GJ, Ditunno JF, et al. Deep vein thrombosis: prophylaxis in acute spinal cord injured patients. Arch Phys Med Rehabil 1988;69:661–4.
58. Jensen MP. The validity and reliability of pain measures in adults with cancer. J Pain 2003;4:2–21.
59. Price DD, Harkins SW, Baker C. Sensory-affective relationships among different types of clinical and experimental pain. Pain 1987;28:297–307.
60. Price DD, McGrath PA, Rafii A, et al. The validation of visual analogue scales as ratio scale measures for chronic and experimental pain. Pain 1983;17:45–56.
61. Paciaroni M, Ageno W, Agnelli G. Prevention of venous thromboembolism after acute spinal cord injury with low-dose heparin or low-molecular-weight heparin. Thromb Haemost 2008;99:978–80.
62. Spinal Cord Injury Thromboprophylaxis Investigators. Prevention of venous thromboembolism in the rehabilitation phase after spinal cord injury: prophylaxis with low-dose heparin or enoxaparin. J Trauma 2003;54:1111–5.
63. Teasell RW, Hsieh JT, Aubut JA, et al. Venous thromboembolism after spinal cord injury. Arch Phys Med Rehabil 2009;90:232–45.
64. Hebbeler SL, Marciniak CM, Crandall S, et al. Daily vs twice daily enoxaparin in the prevention of venous thromboembolic disorders during rehabilitation following acute spinal cord injury. J Spinal Cord Med 2004;27:236–40.
65. [Anonymous]: Prevention of thromboembolism in spinal cord injury. Consortium for Spinal Cord Medicine. J Spinal Cord Med 1997;20:259–83.

66. Price DD, Bush FM, Long S, et al. A comparison of pain measurement characteristics of mechanical visual analogue and simple numerical rating scales. Pain 1994;56:217–26.
67. Green D. Diagnosis: prevalence, and management of thromboembolism in patients with spinal cord injury. J Spinal Cord Med 2003;26:329–34.
68. Farrar JT, Portenoy RK, Berlin JA, et al. Defining the clinically important difference in pain outcome measures. Pain 2000;88:287–94.
69. Office of Medical Applications of Research National Institutes of Health. Consensus Conference: prevention of venous thrombosis and pulmonary embolism. JAMA 1986;256:744–9.
70. Brandstater ME, Roth EJ, Siebens HC. Venous thromboembolism in stroke: literature review and implications for clinical practice. Arch Phys Med Rehabil 1992; 73(Suppl):S379–91.
71. Cifu DX, Kaelin DL, Wall BE. Deep venous thrombosis: incidence on admission to a brain injury rehabilitation program. Arch Phys Med Rehabil 1996;77:1182–5.
72. Geerts WH, Bergqvist D, Pineo GF, et al. Prevention of venous thromboembolism: American College of Chest Physicians evidence-based clinical practice guidelines. Chest 2008;133:381S–453S.
73. Rogers F, Cipolle M, Velmahos G, et al. Practice management for the prevention of venous thromboembolism in trauma patients: the EAST Practice Management Guidelines Work Group. J Trauma 2002;53:142–64.
74. Arepally GM, Ortel TL. Heparin-induced thrombocytopenia. N Engl J Med 2006; 355:809–17.
75. Selleng K, Warkentin TE, Greinacher A. Heparin-induced thrombocytopenia in intensive care patients. Crit Care Med 2007;35:1165–76.
76. Haines ST, Witt DM, Nutescu EA. Venous thromboembolism. In: Dipiro JT, Talbert RL, Yee GC, et al, editors. Pharmacotherapy: a pathophysiologic approach. 7th edition. New York: McGraw-Hill; 2008. p. 331.
77. Warkentin TE, Greinacher A, Koster A, et al. Treatment and prevention of heparin-induced thrombocytopenia: American College of Chest Physicians evidence-based clinical practice guidelines (8th edition). Chest 2008;133:340S–80S.
78. International Association for the Study of Pain (IASP). Available at: http://www.iasp-pain.org. Accessed December 2011.
79. Grond S, Radbruch L, Meuser T, et al. Assessment and treatment of neuropathic cancer pain following WHO guidelines. Pain 1999;79:15–20.
80. Grabois M, Monga T. Pain management in rehabilitation. New York (NY): Demos Medical Publishing; 2002. p. 352.
81. Vergara M, Catalán M, Gisbert JP, et al. Meta-analysis: role of *Helicobacter pylori* eradication in the prevention of peptic ulcer in NSAID users. Aliment Pharmacol Ther 2005;21(12):1411–8.
82. Gislason GH, Jacobsen S, Rasmussen JN, et al. Risk of death or reinfarction associated with the use of selective cyclooxygenase-2 inhibitors and nonselective nonsteroidal antiinflammatory drugs after acute myocardial infarction. Circulation 2006;113:2906–13.
83. Strickland JM. Palliative pharmacy care. 1st edition. Bethesda (MD): American Society of Health-System Pharmacists; 2009. p. 153–68.
84. Ouellet M, Beaulieu-Bonneau S. Sleep disorders in rehabilitation patients. In: Stone JH, Blouin M, editors. International encyclopedia of rehabilitation. 2012. Available at: http://cirrie.buffalo.edu/encyclopedia/en/article/43/. Accessed December 26, 2011.
85. Siegel JM. The neurotransmitters of sleep. J Clin Psychiatry 2004;65(Suppl 16): 4–7.

86. Roth T. Characteristics and determinants of normal sleep. J Clin Psychiatry 2004;65(Suppl 16):8–11.
87. Kamel NS, Gammack JK. Insomnia in the elderly: cause, approach, and treatment. Am J Med 2006;119:463–9.
88. Ramakrishnan K, Scheid DC. Treatment options for insomnia. Am Fam Physician 2007;76:517–26.
89. Larive LL. Sleep disorders. In: Tisdale JE, Douglas DA, editors. Drug-induced diseases: prevention, detection, and management. 1st edition. Bethesda (MD): ASHP; 2005. p. 185.
90. Singer CM, Applebee GA. Sleep disorders. In: Feldman MD, Christensen JF, editors. Behavioral medicine: a guide for clinical practice. 3rd edition. New York: McGraw-Hill; 2008. Chapter 28. Available at: http://www.accessmedicine.com. Accessed December 19, 2011.
91. Schuttle-Rodin S, Broch L, Buysse D, et al. Clinical guideline for the evaluation and management of chronic insomnia in adults. J Clin Sleep Med 2008;4(5):487–504.
92. Schneider-Helmert D, Spinweber CL. Evaluation of L-tryptophan for treatment of insomnia: a review. Psychopharmacology 1986;89:1–7.
93. Morgenthaler TI, Kapur VK, Brown T, et al. Practice parameters for the treatment of narcolepsy and other hypersomnias of central origin. Sleep 2007;30(12):1705–11.
94. Roth T. Narcolepsy: treatment issues. J Clin Psychiatry 2007;68(Suppl 13):16–9.
95. Kaiser PR, Valko PO, Werth E, et al. Modafinil ameliorates excessive daytime sleepiness after traumatic brain injury. Neurology 2010;75:1780–5.
96. Cook DJ, Fuller HD, Guyatt GH, et al. Risk factors for gastrointestinal bleeding in critically ill patients. N Engl J Med 1994;330:337–81.
97. Lanza FL, Chan FK, Quigley EM, et al. Practice Parameters Committee of the American College of Gastroenterology. Guidelines for prevention of NSAID-related ulcer complications. Am J Gastroenterol 2009;104:728–38.
98. Schalansky B, Hwang JH. Prevention of nonsteroidal anti-inflammatory drug-induced gastropathy. J Gastroenterol 2009;44:44–52.
99. Trimble MR. Anticonvulsant drugs and cognitive function: a review of the literature. Epilepsia 1987;28:S37–45.
100. Stahl SM. Stahl's essential psychopharmacology: neuroscientific basis and practical applications. 3rd edition. New York: Cambridge University Press; 2008. p. 273–5.
101. Keefe RS, Silva SG, Perkins DO, et al. The effects of atypical antipsychotic drugs on neurocognitive impairment in schizophrenia: a review and meta-analysis. Schizophr Bull 1999;25(2):201–22.
102. Cespedes MS, Aberg JA. Neuropsychiatric complications of antiretroviral therapy. Drug Saf 2006;29(10):865–74.
103. Turjanski N, Lloyd GG. Psychiatric side-effects of medications: recent developments. Adv Psychiatr Treat 2005;11:58–70.
104. Antithrombotic Therapy and Prevention of Thrombosis, 9th ed: American College of Chest Physicians Evidence-Based Clinical Practice Guidelines. Chest 2012;141(2 Suppl).

Falls in the Inpatient Rehabilitation Facility

Marc K. Ross, MD*, Ethan Egan, MD, Mohammed Zaman, MD, Besem Aziz, MD, Tad Dewald, BA, MPH, Salem Mohammed

KEYWORDS

• Falls • Acute rehabilitation • Inpatient rehabilitation facilities

Older adults are rehabilitated for a variety of conditions in an inpatient rehabilitation facility (IRF) and they are often at an increased risk for falling during their stay. This article (1) provides an overview of the incidence, prevalence, and impact of falls in facilities that provide inpatient rehabilitation; (2) provides some key factors to be considered in the assessment of the patient admitted to the IRF for risk factors associated with falling; and (3) identifies strategies that can help reduce the risk of falling in patients admitted to an IRF.

EPIDEMIOLOGY OF FALLS IN HOSPITALS, IRFs, AND LONG-TERM HEALTH CARE SETTINGS

Falls occur frequently in older persons. Approximately 30% of persons older than 65 years fall at least once a year and 15% fall at least twice.[1–5] Patient falls are a leading cause of adverse events and injury in hospitals.[6] Among older adults, falls are the leading cause of death due to injury and are also the most common cause of nonfatal injuries and hospital admissions for trauma. In 2008, more than 19,700 older adults died of unintentional fall injuries. In 2009, 2.2 million nonfatal fall injuries among older adults were treated in emergency departments and more than 581,000 of these patients were hospitalized.[7]

Falls are the commonest safety incident among hospitalized patients and account for 32% of incident reports at hospitals in the United Kingdom.[8] Rates from 5 to 18 falls per 1000 bed days have been described in intervention and observational studies.[9] Falls are the most common type of inpatient accident, accounting for up to 70% of inpatient accidents.[6] Patients often fall more than once, and the average is 2.6 falls per person per year.[10] Rates from 2.9 to 13 falls per 1000 bed days have been reported. Up to 30% of such falls may result in injury, including fracture, head and

Department of Rehabilitation Medicine, Kingsbrook Rehabilitation Institute, 585 Schenectady Avenue, Brooklyn, NY, USA
* Corresponding author.
E-mail address: mross@kingsbrook.org

Phys Med Rehabil Clin N Am 23 (2012) 305–314
doi:10.1016/j.pmr.2012.02.006
1047-9651/12/$ – see front matter © 2012 Elsevier Inc. All rights reserved.

soft tissue trauma, all of which may in turn lead to impaired rehabilitation and comorbidity.[11,12]

In 2003, 1.5 million people aged 65 years and older lived in nursing homes.[13] Approximately 5% of adults aged 65 years and older live in nursing homes, but nursing home residents account for approximately 20% of deaths from falls in this age group. Each year, a typical nursing home with 100 beds reports 100 to 200 falls, with many also unreported.[14] Falls among nursing home residents occur frequently and repeatedly. Approximately 1800 older adults living in nursing homes die each year from fall-related injuries, and those who survive falls frequently sustain hip fractures and head injuries that result in permanent disability and reduced quality of life. Approximately 10% to 20% of falls in nursing home cause serious injuries and 2% to 6% cause fractures.[15] Between half and three-quarters of nursing home residents fall each year, which is twice the rate of falls for older adults living in the community. Falls result in disability, functional decline, and reduced quality of life. Fear of falling can cause further loss of function, depression, feelings of helplessness, and social isolation.[16]

IMPACT OF FALLS: COST TO SOCIETY

In 2000, the total direct medical costs of all fall injuries for people aged 65 years and older exceeded $19 billion: $0.2 billion for falls that are fatal and $19 billion for falls that are nonfatal. The costs involved in the treatment of fall injuries increase rapidly with age. In 2000, medical costs for women, who comprised 58% of older adults, were 2 to 3 times higher than the costs for men. In 2000, the direct medical cost of fatal fall injuries totaled $179 million. Traumatic brain injuries and injuries to the lower extremities cause approximately 78% of deaths due to fall and account for 79% of total costs. Injuries to internal organs were responsible for 28% of deaths due to fall and accounted for 29% of costs. Fractures were the most common and most costly nonfatal injuries. Just more than one-third of nonfatal injuries were fractures, but these accounted for 61% of total nonfatal costs, or $12 billion. Hospitalizations accounted for nearly two-thirds of the costs of nonfatal fall injuries and emergency department treatment accounted for 20%.[17] Falls can result in increased length of hospital stay, discharge to a long-term care facility, and increased costs. Patients with serious fall-related injury had charges that were $4233 higher than those for patients who did not fall.[12,18] Among community-dwelling older adults, fall-related injury is one of the 20 most expensive medical conditions. In 2002, approximately 22% of community-dwelling seniors reported falling in the previous year. Medicare costs per fall averaged between $9113 and $13,507. Among community-dwelling seniors treated for fall injuries, 65% of direct medical costs were for inpatient hospitalizations; 10% each for medical office visits and home health care, 8% for hospital outpatient visits, 7% for emergency department visits, and 1% each for prescription drugs and dental visits. Approximately 78% of these costs were reimbursed by Medicare.[19] Approximately 30% of patient falls in hospitals result in physical injury, with 4% to 6% resulting in serious injury.[20,21] Traumatic brain injury (TBI) accounts for 46% of fatal falls among older adults.[22] Falls in hospital may lead to injury, in up to 30% of cases, and associated mortality and morbidity.[23] The death rates from falls among older men and women have increased over the past decade.[22,24] Of those who fall, 20% to 30% suffer moderate-to-severe injuries that make it hard for them recover or live independently and increase their risk of early death. Older adults are hospitalized for fall-related injuries 5 times more often than they are for injuries from other causes.[2]

IMPACT OF FALLS ON PATIENTS

Falls can result in serious physical and emotional injury, poor quality of life, increased length of stay in the hospital, admission to a long-term care facility, and increased cost.[12,25–29] Falls are also associated with higher anxiety and depression scores, loss of confidence, and increased fear of the consequences of falling, such as physical injuries, activity curtailment, loss of functional ability, need for institutionalization, and death.

Falls are associated with increased length of hospital stay and higher rates of discharge to long-term institutional care,[30–32] both of which can significantly affect the life of an older adult. Twenty to thirty percent of people who fall suffer moderate to severe injuries, such as lacerations, hip fractures, or head traumas. These injuries make it hard to recover or live independently and increase the risk of early death.[24,33] Approximately 42% of falls result in some form of injury and 8% in serious injury.[18] 5% of falls lead to a fracture and 5% lead to other serious injuries. Approximately 1 in 4 people who fall consults a hospital emergency department or primary care physician after the fall. Other consequences are loss of function and mobility, fear of falling, and increased institutionalization.[34] Falls cause 90% of the fractures of the forearm, hip, and pelvis in the elderly.[35] Falls are strong predictors of mortality in elderly female patients who sustain a hip fracture. For both men and women, previous falls is a risk factor for future falls.

FALLS IN THE IRF: GENERAL CONSIDERATIONS

Falls in an IRF setting brings on a different challenge for patients who have preexisting risk factors for falls (ie, neurologic diseases, amputations, poly-pharmacy, advanced age, multiple health care providers). In IRF, patients are challenged to achieve a higher level of function than they had before admission through intensive rehabilitation (3 h/d and 5 to 7 d/wk). In the IRF, between 2.92 and 15.9 falls per 1000 days occur compared with the general hospital rates that range between 2.45 and 3.73 per 1000 days[36] Patients with stroke and brain injury have a high incidence of falls on IRF units.[36]

The common denominators that contribute to falls in the IRF setting must be understood to identify patients at high risk and target interventions that can be useful in reducing their risk for falling.

Risk factors for falls in patients admitted to the IRF include advanced age, medical complexity, physical impairments (ie, muscle weakness, loss of sensation, visual-spatial deficits, and cognitive impairments), which result in a decreased level of function as documented by standardized outcome measures, such as the function of independence measure. Additional factors to consider include

1. Timing of fall: (daytime vs evening vs night). Although there are limited studies that report the impact of timing on falls, in one study, it was reported that 85% of falls occur during the day.[36]
2. Number of days from time of admission to fall: A study on patients with stroke found that falls occur within the first 4 weeks of admission, with the first week having the highest prevalence.[37] In the authors' institution, patients admitted to the IRF unit have the highest incidence of falls in the first week of their admission.
3. Location of falls: In the IRF setting most falls occur in the patient's room[36]
4. Altered sleep-wake cycles can also be a contributing factor to falls in patients with impairments related to neurologic conditions (ie, patients with brain injury fall at night, compared with patients with stroke who fall during the day).[36] Sleep medication may also contribute to falls.[38]

5. Mobility devices: In a previous study that deals with falls in patients with physical disabilities, mobility devices were associated with falling[38]
6. Environmental risk factors: A patient's space in a room in the IRF is small and that space can be compromised by items near the patient's bed, such as nightstand, table, intravenous (IV) poles, wheelchairs, walkers, and chairs. The bed may be positioned at a higher level and brakes not set in the locked position. Liquid spills, telephone lines, and electrical cords can all compromise the patient's safety and contribute to falls.[36]
7. Multiple transition points and multiple caregivers can contribute to patient disorientation: Patients admitted to IRF might have had received care in multiple different settings before their hospitalization, which include medical and surgical wards as well as intensive care units. In each of these settings, there are multiple different providers: physicians, nurses, therapists, and nutritionists. The complexity of the patient's movement throughout an institution is continued in the IRF where the patient may be moved several times while in the rehabilitation setting for a variety of reasons.

ASSESSMENT OF THE OLDER ADULTS AT RISK FOR FALLING IN AN IRF

Patients are usually admitted to an IRF from either a medical or surgical ward in the same hospital or from another institution. The admitted patients usually have a combination of factors that increase their risk for falling as described earlier. Common reasons for admission include neurologic injuries or diseases (stroke, spinal cord injury, multiple sclerosis, and TBI), major limb amputations, fractures, joint replacements, myocardial infarction, and pulmonary disease exacerbations.

In addition to their underlying disease-specific impairment, the patient may also have generalized weakness secondary to prolonged bed rest and disuse-related muscle atrophy. Muscle strength reduces by 10% to 20% per week or 1% to 3% per day from complete immobility.[39] A study showed that 60 days of bed rest lead to 75% of volume loss in the calf muscle. Another study showed that 5-week bed rest reduced muscle strength by 8% in knee extension and 12% in hip extension.[40] Three to 5 weeks of complete bed rest may lead to up to 50% decrease in muscle strength.

Presence of contractures, pain, malnutrition, incontinence, and multiple comorbidities can further compound the clinical picture.

Medical History

A careful review of the medical history can provide significant information on the risk factors of falling in the IRF. This can be obtained from the review of the medical records with the patients and their family. Important information to obtain in addition to a thorough history of hospital course to date includes, (1) history of prior functional level, cognitive and physical abilities for performing activities of daily living, and instrumental activities of daily living; (2) history of prior falls or near falls at home or on the medical/surgical ward before transfer to IRF. If falls had occurred, it is important to inquire about the factors that contributed to the falls as well as the number of falls; (3) review of medications before hospitalization and from referring institution for polypharmacy; (4) if available, reports on the most recent functional level from physical and occupational therapist; (5) review of systems for patient reports of weakness, dizziness, impaired balance, pain, vision, and hearing difficulties.

Physical Examination

The physical examination of all patients admitted to an IRF should include elements that evaluate the potential for falls. Some key elements of this evaluation include (1) blood pressure and heart rate taken in the supine, sitting, and, whenever possible, standing positions, to assess for orthostatic changes; (2) vision assessment, peripheral vision and evaluation for visual-spatial deficits; (3) cognitive evaluation: level of alertness, orientation, and immediate and delayed recall. Cognitive impairment and misperception of functional ability is an important risk factor for falls and an important part of the evaluation process[41]; (4) neurologic evaluation: motor strength, sensation to light touch, pinprick, proprioception, sitting and standing balance, and presence of spasticity; (5) orthopedic evaluation: range of motion restrictions and presence of contractures, pain, and tenderness in bones, joints, and spine; and (6) functional evaluation: ability to transfer from bed to wheelchair, ambulation with appropriate assistive device (identify the type of device), and functional reach.

There are multiple tools to assess fall, which have been used in long-term care settings[41] and many of them share common elements, such as (1) history of falling; (2) observations of impaired judgment, agitation, impaired gait; (3) self-reports of dizziness; (4) incontinence; (5) use of high–fall risk medications (ie, tranquilizers, diuretics, antihypertensives, antiparkinsonian drugs, antidepressants); (6) sensory deficits; (7) motor weakness; and (8) gait abnormalities.[42–46]

INTERVENTIONS TO MINIMIZE THE RISK OF FALLS IN AN IRF

There are several potentially helpful interventions to minimize the risk of falls in the IRF setting. Some examples are described below as well as in Appendix A:

1. Prompted toileting before bedtime.
2. Family education on causes of falls in the patient's room and strategies to minimize the risks of fall in the IRF. This is especially important in patients with cognitive impairments. Having a family member at the patient's bedside is not a guarantee to prevent patient fall. Family members should be educated to inform the nursing staff if the patient is exhibiting high fall-risk behavior.
3. Multidisciplinary rounds several times a week by a team that consists of a physician, nurse, and therapist should occur at times when there is a high risk for falls. This team can evaluate the environmental risk factors, review patient's medical record for high-risk medications and educate patient and family.
4. Expanded activities in common areas.
5. Medication review of high–fall risk medications.
6. Check for orthostatic changes in blood pressure and heart rate.
7. Environmental modifications: (1) check that bed is in the lowest position and with brakes on (2) switch on the night light (3) clean up liquid spills (4) remove wheelchairs and footrests, chairs, table from frequently traveled pathway around the patient's bed; (5) remove electrical wires, IV poles, telephone wires, from the area commonly traveled by the patient; (6) keep call bell, glasses, dentures within reach.
8. Ensure adequate levels of nursing staff at times of day when fall risk is highest.
9. Use slip-resistant socks or footwear.
10. Limit ability to prescribe medications in the patient's medical record to the primary rehabilitation physician to minimize confusion raised when there are several consultants involved in the patient's care.
11. Limit the use of restraints: Limiting the use of physical restraints has been shown to decrease the rate of falls in patients after -stroke or patients admitted to a brain injury unit.[47] Analyses of the effectiveness of physical restraints for 263,068 residents of nursing home included full bed rails on all open sides of the bed, half-rail

on one side, trunk restraints, limb restraints, or chairs to prevent rising. All outcomes examined, including behavior issues, cognitive performance, falls, walking dependence, activities of daily living, pressure ulcers, and contractures, were significantly worse for restrained residents compared with matched residents who were not restrained.

12. Alarms: The implementation of alarms reduces the duration of time the patient lies on the floor after a fall, and also monitors patients who may be attempting dangerous bed or chair transfers. Pressure sensitive pads can be placed on a bed or a chair, which activates an alarm alerting the staff and reminding the patient that they require assistance to mobilize.

13. Visual cues: Visual cues can help communicate the level of fall risk of a patient among the health care professionals and other personnel on the wards. Patient can be placed on a 3-color system indicating the risk of fall: red = high risk, yellow = medium risk, and green = low risk. The fall risk can be assessed using the Morse fall scale, and individual interventions can be placed for the different risk categories. Patients at high risk can be placed on an alarm system and hip protectors along with every 2-hour check by the staff.[48]

14. Orthostatic hypotension: Treatment of orthostatic hypotension help in reducing the incidence of falls. Treatment options include reducing the dose of hypotensive medications, optimizing fluid intake, use elastic stocking, and consider medications, such as fludrocortisones or midodrine.

15. Hip protectors: Hip fracture is one of the morbidities associated with falls. Hip protectors shunt impact energy away from the greater trochanter toward softer tissues anterior, posterior, and inferior to the proximal femur, preventing fracture. Trials conducted to evaluate the effectiveness of placement of hip protectors have yielded mixed results. Some have found hip protectors to protect and reduce the risk of fractures, such as for patients in nursing home.[49] Others, however, have found no significant difference.[50,51] It is possible that the main discrepancy between these 2 findings is the low compliance rate with hip protectors because patients may complain of discomfort caused by the bulkiness of the hip protectors and the difficulty in getting dressed with them. However, hip protectors have been shown to be efficacious in patients with good compliance and who are at a high risk for hip fractures.[52]

Rehabilitation Interventions in the IRF to Minimize the Risk of Falling

The IRF facility is an ideal place to address the various factors that contribute to falls using the expertise of various team members and consultants. Some interventions include (1) exercising key muscle groups to improve strength and endurance for ambulation and activities of daily living as well as maximizing the range of motion in major joints of the limbs, (2) gait training with appropriate assistive devices on different terrains and stairs, (3) progressive balance training, (4) evaluation of prosthetic and orthotic devices for proper fit, (5) training in activities of daily living and evaluation for appropriate assistive devices to minimize the risk of falling, (6) educating patient and family members about the risk of falling and strategies that can be used to minimize the risk, (7) counseling on minimizing alcohol intake because that can also contribute to falls, (8) home evaluation for environmental risk factors, (9) appropriate discharge planning to minimize the risk of falls at home, and (10) consider supplementation of Vitamin D because there is some literature linking a higher rate of falls with low serum 25-hydroxyvitamin D concentration (<19 ng/mL (25 nmol/L).[53]

REFERENCES

1. Hausdorff JM, Rios DA, Edelber HK. Gait variability and fall risk in community–living older adults: a 1–year prospective study. Arch Phys Med Rehabil 2001; 82(8):1050–6.
2. Hornbrook MC, Stevens VJ, Wingfield DJ, et al. Preventing falls among community–dwelling older persons: results from a randomized trial. Gerontologist 1994; 34(1):16–23.
3. Nevitt MC, Cummings SR, Kidd S, et al. Risk factors for recurrent nonsyncopal falls: a prospective study. JAMA 1989;261(18):2663–8.
4. Tinetti ME, Doucette J, Claus E, et al. Risk factors for serious injury during falls by older persons in the community. J Am Geriatr Soc 1995;43(11):1214–21.
5. Tromp AM, Pluijm SM, Smit JH, et al. Fall-risk screening test: a prospective study on predictors for falls in community-dwelling elderly. J Clin Epidemiol 2001;54(8): 837–44.
6. Sutton JC, Standen PJ, Wallace WA. Patient accidents in-hospital: incidence, documentation and significance. Br J Clin Pract 1994;48:63–6.
7. Centers for Disease Control and Prevention, National Center for Injury Prevention and Control. Web–based Injury Statistics Query and Reporting System (WIS-QARS) [online]. Accessed January 20, 2012.
8. National Patient Safety Agency. Slips trips and falls in hospital. London: NPSA; 2007. Available at: http://www.npsa.nhs.uk. Accessed February 22, 2012.
9. Oliver D, Connelly J, Victor C, et al. Strategies to prevent falls and fractures in hospitals and care homes and effect of cognitive impairment. Systematic review and meta-analyses. BMJ 2007;334:82–7.
10. Rubenstein LZ, Robbins AS, Josephson KR, et al. The value of assessing falls in an elderly population. A randomized clinical trial. Ann Intern Med 1990;113(4):308–16.
11. Rhymes J, Jaeger R. Falls–prevention and management in the institutional setting. Clin Geriatr Med 1988;4:613–22.
12. Bates D, Pruess K, Souney P, et al. Serious falls in hospitalised patients; correlates and resource utilisation. Am J Med 1995;99:137–43.
13. National Center for Health Statistics. Health, United States, 2005. With chartbook on trends in the Health of Americans. Hyattsville (MD): National Center for Health Statistics; 2005.
14. Rubenstein LZ, Josephson KR, Robbins AS. Falls in the nursing home. Ann Intern Med 1994;121:442–51.
15. Rubenstein LZ, Robbins AS, Schulman BL, et al. Falls and instability in the elderly. J Am Geriatr Soc 1988;36:266–78.
16. Rubenstein LZ. Preventing falls in the nursing home. JAMA 1997;278(7):595–6.
17. Stevens JA, Corso PS, Finkelstein EA, et al. The costs of fatal and nonfatal falls among older adults. Inj Prev 2006;12:290–5.
18. Hitcho EB, Krauss MJ, Birge S, et al. Characteristics and circumstances of falls in a hospital setting. J Gen Intern Med 2004;19:732–9.
19. Carroll NV, Slattum PW, Cox FM. The cost of falls among the community-dwelling elderly. J Manag Care Pharm 2005;11(4):307–16.
20. Morse JM, Prowse MD, Morrow N, et al. A retrospective analysis of patient falls. Can J Public Health 1985;76:116–8.
21. Ash KL, MacLeod P, Clark L. A case control study of falls in the hospital setting. J Gerontol Nurs 1998;24:7–15.
22. Stevens JA. Fatalities and injuries from falls among older adults–United States, 1993–2003 and 2001–2005. MMWR Morb Mortal Wkly Rep 2006;55(45):1221–4.

23. Australian Council on Safety. Falls prevention in hospitals and residential aged care facilities. Best practice guidelines. Brisbane (Australia): Australian Council on Safety; 2005.

24. Alexander BH, Rivara FP, Wolf ME. The cost and frequency of hospitalization for fall-related injuries in older adults. Am J Public Health 1992;82(7):1020–3.

25. Kempen GI, Sanderman R, Scaf-Klomp W, et al. The role of depressive symptoms in recovery from injuries to the extremities in older persons. A prospective study. Int J Geriatr Psychiatry 2003;18:14–22.

26. Kong KS, Lee FK, Mackenzie AE, et al. Psychosocial consequences of falling: the perspective of older Hong Kong Chinese who had experienced recent falls. J Adv Nurs 2002;37:234–42.

27. Scaf-Klomp W, Sanderman R, Ormel J, et al. Depression in older people after fall-related injuries: a prospective study. Age Ageing 2003;32:88–94.

28. Kosorok MR, Omenn GS, Diehr P, et al. Restricted activity days among older adults. Am J Public Health 1992;82:1263–7.

29. Tinetti ME, Williams CS. The effect of falls and fall injuries on functioning in community-dwelling older persons. J Gerontol A Biol Sci Med Sci 1998;53: M112–9.

30. Vetter N, Ford D. Anxiety and depression scores in elderly fallers. Int J Geriatr Psychiatry 1989;4:168–73.

31. Murphy J, Isaacs B. The post fall syndrome. A study of 36 elderly inpatients. Gerontology 1982;28:265–70.

32. Oliver D. Bed falls and bedrails–what should we do? Age Ageing 2002;31:415–8.

33. Sterling DA, O'Connor JA, Bonadies J. Geriatric falls: injury severity is high and disproportionate to mechanism. J Trauma 2001;50(1):116–9.

34. Stel VS, Smit JH, Pluijm SM, et al. Consequences of falling in older men and women and risk factors for health service use and functional decline. Age Ageing 2004;33(1):58–65.

35. Koval KJ, Meek R, Schemitsch E, et al. Geriatric trauma: young ideas. J Bone Joint Surg Am 2003;85:1380–8.

36. Frisina PG, Guellnitz R, Alverzo J. A time series analysis of falls and injury in the inpatient rehabilitation setting. Rehabil Nurs 2010;35(4):141–6.

37. Lee IE, Stokic DS. Risk factors for falls during inpatient rehabilitation. Am J Phys Med Rehabil 2008;87:341–50.

38. Lin JT, Lane JM. Falls in the elderly population. Phys Med Rehabil Clin N Am 2005;16:109–28.

39. Trappe TA, Burd NA, Louis ES, et al. Influence of concurrent exercise or nutrition countermeasures on thigh and calf muscle size and function during 60 days of bed rest in women. Acta Physiol (Oxf) 2007;191(2):147–59.

40. Berg HE, Eiken O, Miklavcic L, et al. Hip, thigh and calf muscle atrophy and bone loss after 5-week bedrest inactivity. Eur J Appl Physiol 2007;99(3):283–9.

41. Shimada H, Suzukawa M, Ishizaki T, et al. Relationship between subjective fall risk assessment and falls and fall-related fractures in frail elderly people. BMC Geriatr 2011;11:40.

42. Brians LK, Alexander K, Grota P, et al. The development of the RISK tool for fall prevention. Rehabil Nurs 1991;16(2):67.

43. Oliver D, Britton M, Seed P, et al. Development and evaluation of evidence-based risk assessment tool (STRATIFY) to predict which elderly patients will fall. BMJ 1997;315:1049–53.

44. Conley D, Schultz AA, Selvin R. The challenge of predicting patients at risk for falling: development of the Conley Scale. Medsurg Nurs 1999;8(6):348.

45. Vassallo M, Poynter L, Sharma JC, et al. Fall risk-assessment tools compared with clinical judgment: an evaluation in a rehabilitation ward. Age Ageing 2008;37: 277–81.
46. Nyberg L, Gustafson Y. Using the downton index to predict those prone to falls in stroke rehabilitation. Stroke 1996;27:1821–4.
47. Castle NG, Engberg J. The health consequences of using physical restraints in nursing homes. Med Care 2009;47:1164.
48. Barnett K. Reducing patient falls project: January 2001-March 2002. Mid Yorkshire Hospitals NHS Trust; 2012. Available at: http://www.premierinc.com/safety/topics/falls/downloads/E-14-falls-project-uk.pdf. Accessed February 22, 2012.
49. Sawka AM, Boulos P, Beattie K, et al. Hip protectors decrease hip fracture risk in elderly nursing home residents: a Bayesian meta-analysis. J Clin Epidemiol 2007; 60:336.
50. Parker MJ, Gillespie WJ, Gillespie LD. Effectiveness of hip protectors for preventing hip fractures in elderly people: systematic review. BMJ 2006;332:571.
51. Kannus P, Parkkari J, Niemi S, et al. Prevention of hip fracture in elderly people with use of a hip protector. N Engl J Med 2000;343:1506.
52. Cameron ID, Cumming RG, Kurrle SE, et al. A randomised trial of hip protector use by frail older women living in their own homes. Inj Prev 2003;9(2):138–41.
53. Bischoff HA, Stähelin HB, Dick W, et al. Effects of vitamin D and calcium supplementation on falls: a randomized controlled trial. J Bone Miner Res 2003;18:343.

APPENDIX A: IRF ENVIRONMENTAL FALL PREVENTION CHECKLIST

• Orientating the patient to the ward area, placing a call light within reach, instructing the patient on when and how to call for assistance, and teaching patients how to transfer and to safely use assistive devices.	• Exit signs exist and are visible
• Keeping the bed low when not performing physical care; locking wheels into position on beds, lockers, wheelchairs, and commodes; and wiping up fluids	• Hallways and corridors clear of obstacles
• Reduce the usage of bed rails because increased use has been shown to correlate with increased risk of falling	• Furniture and equipment are sturdy and wheels are locked
• Implementation of sensor alarms, bedside commodes, and hip protectors	• Furniture and equipment are suitable for the specific needs of the unit
• Proper lighting and cluster-free environment with nonobstructed pathway for the patient to ambulate	• Chairs, geri chairs, and wheelchairs are suitable
• Floor is clean and dry	• Commode/seat lifts are properly installed (not loose)
• Consider the use of sitters for cognitively impaired or keep them near visual sight for the staff	• Door handles are secure
• Provide physically safe environment (ie, eliminate spills, clutter, electrical cords, and unnecessary equipment)	• Handrails in halls are present, accessible and properly secured to walls
• Call bell/light within reach	• Patients' clothing fit well and do not drag on the floor

• Bed in low position	• Slippers have nonslip soles
• Bedside table within reach	• Grab bars next to the toilet
	• Toilet seat at a height that allows easy transfer
• Room furniture arranged to allow patient space when walking and grab bars/hand rails are accessible	• Night light in the bathroom
• Identify patient with a colored wrist band for patients at risk of falls	• Flooring is level and free of tripping hazards, such as broken tiles or thresholds that are above the level of the floor

Patient Safety Considerations in the Rehabilitation of the Individual with Cognitive Impairment

Brad T. Tyson, MA, Martha T. Pham, MS, Natashia T. Brown, PhD, Thomas R. Mayer, PsyD*

KEYWORDS

- Cognitive impairment • Patient safety • Rehabilitation
- Activities of daily living • Executive functioning

Deficits in cognitive functioning are associated with myriad safety concerns, including greater difficulties performing activities of daily living (ADLs) in a safe manner, medication errors, motor vehicle accidents, impaired awareness of deficits, decision-making capacity, falls, and travel away from home. The purpose of this article is to give rehabilitation clinicians quick reference information about cognitive functioning, safety considerations in patients with cognitive impairment, and methods to enhance patient safety. The information is divided into two sections. The first section provides a brief overview of the primary cognitive domains assessed in rehabilitation patients. The second section addresses the most relevant safety concerns in rehabilitation patients and recommendations that may be helpful in limiting adverse outcomes in the continuity of care.

ASSESSMENT OF COGNITIVE IMPAIRMENT IN REHABILITATION PATIENTS

Cognitive impairment is apparent in rehabilitation patients with traumatic brain injury, stroke, dementia, and other neurologic conditions. Furthermore, it is well established

Disclosures: No commercial party having a direct financial interest in the results of this article has or will confer a benefit on the authors or any organization with which the authors are associated.

Traumatic Brain Injury and Coma Recovery Unit, Department of Physical Medicine and Rehabilitation, Kingsbrook Jewish Medical Center, Kingsbrook Rehabilitation Institute, 585 Schenectady Avenue, Brooklyn, NY 11203, USA

* Corresponding author. Department of Physical Medicine and Rehabilitation, Kingsbrook Jewish Medical Center, 585 Schenectady Avenue, Brooklyn, NY 11203.

E-mail address: tmayer@kingsbrook.org

Phys Med Rehabil Clin N Am 23 (2012) 315–334
doi:10.1016/j.pmr.2012.02.007
1047-9651/12/$ – see front matter © 2012 Elsevier Inc. All rights reserved.

that cognitive impairment is a prominent feature in many psychiatric disorders, such as depression and schizophrenia. Perhaps less well known is that cognitive impairment is documented in many diseases systemically, including cardiovascular disease without obvious cerebrovascular involvement,[1] obesity,[2] diabetes,[3] cancer,[4] and many chronic pain populations.[5–7] Although the term, *cognition*, is used to denote countless processes, the domains typically assessed in rehabilitation patients include attention, visual spatial functioning, language, memory, and executive functioning.

Brevity and depth are essential features of an inpatient cognitive assessment. Because patients may not be accurate historians, linking patient and family information is important. Clinical interviews should inquire about recent changes in cognitive, emotional, and behavioral functioning. There are several validated cognitive measures available for brief screening purposes. Perhaps the most widely used is the Mini-Mental State Examination (MMSE). Newer variations of the MMSE, such as the Saint Louis University Mental Status examination and the Montreal Cognitive Assessment, are equally brief and more comprehensive. Longer screening measures with more breadth and depth include the Brief Neurocognitive Examination, Neurobehavioral Cognitive Status Examination, Repeatable Battery for the Assessment of Neuropsychological Status, and Dementia Rating Scale. Comprehensive neuropsychological testing can be conducted on an outpatient basis and is most commonly completed approximately 6 months after brain injury. A full review of neuropsychological tests is beyond the scope of this article. For a complete review, the reader is referred to more detailed resources.[8]

Attention and Related Functions

Attention is a widely distributed cerebral process that encompasses many interrelated cognitive functions and serves as the gateway of sensory information flow into the brain. At the most basic level, attention requires arousal and alertness. The reticular activating system and associated thalamic nuclei are primarily responsible for this basic level of arousal and alertness. The anterior cingulate gyrus is heavily involved in initiating attention, focusing attentional resources, and developing control. The dorsolateral prefrontal cortex works together with the anterior cingulate in performing the most complex and highest order attentional processes.

After arousal, the hierarchical nature of attention skills that are hypothesized to be successively more complex include sustained, selective, alternating, and divided attention. The ability to sustain attention for increasing lengths of time becomes the first gauge of attentional sophistication. Selective attention is the ability to attend to relevant information while ignoring irrelevant stimuli. Distractibility, a common feature of prefrontal injury, suggests an inability to selectively attend effectively. Alternating attention entails the ability to disengage, switch, and re-engage attention. Divided attention involves simultaneous awareness of 2 or more activities and the ability to switch or alternate attention between those activities. Many neuropsychological tests of attention are multifactorial, requiring aspects, such as motor speed, reaction times, visual and auditory tracking, selective responding, and other capacities. Accurate identification of deficit areas requires careful evaluation of the constituent components of each task.

Orientation, working memory, and processing speed are closely related features of attention. Orientation, the awareness of self in relation to surroundings, requires successful integration of attention, perception, and memory. Questions related to orientation are featured on most mental status examinations. Patients may be asked to state their name, the location, the date, and their circumstance. Orientation is extremely vulnerable to the effects of brain dysfunction. Impaired awareness for time and place is the most common disorientation and typically occurs with widespread cortical involvement, lesions to limbic structures, or damage to the reticular activating system. Impaired orientation is, therefore, strongly suggestive of cerebral dysfunction. Working memory involves immediate awareness of sensory information and the ability to store and manipulate that information temporarily. During working memory processes, information is attended to, organized, manipulated, highlighted, and discarded. Repeating digits forward and backward is the classic test of working memory. Processing speed refers to the rate at which information is perceived and processed and is typically assessed with timed visual motor attentional tasks. It relies heavily on the integrity of cerebral white matter. Working memory and speed of information processing tend to peak in young adulthood and are among the first cognitive abilities to decline with age.[9] Furthermore, measures of working memory and processing speed are 2 of the most sensitive neuropsychological tasks for brain injury of any kind.

In sum, attention is one of the most important cognitive abilities to assess because it serves as a good measure of overall brain functioning. Impaired attention is related to poor safety outcomes in ADLs, driving behavior, medication management, awareness of limitations, decision-making capacity, mobility, and travel away from home. Patients with moderate to severe attentional impairments have difficulty functioning independently and likely require intensive supervision.

Visual Spatial Functioning

Visual spatial functioning is largely a task of the nondominant hemisphere and is interdependent with attentional mechanisms. Visual spatial ability is an integrated perceptual ability that includes visual attention, form recognition, localization of objects in space, visual construction, visual synthesis, and visual organization. Lesions to the right parietal lobe have been associated with impaired understanding of spatial relationships, impaired spatial conceptualization and imagery, visual inattention, tactile inattention, and impaired body awareness.[10] Lesions overlapping into the occipital cortex may give rise to various visual agnosias.

In evaluating visual spatial functioning, it is important to distinguish nondominant hemisphere visual spatial impairment from deficits due to disorders of the eye, oculomotor deficits, and lesions along the primary visual pathway. Neuropsychological measures of visual spatial functioning commonly involve replicating a figure, identifying a spatial relationship, reconfiguring the pieces of an object, locating a hidden object, or recreating a design out of blocks.

Visual attention deficits are among the most commonly impaired aspects of visual spatial functioning and are highly amenable to cognitive rehabilitation. Visual inattention or neglect involves impaired awareness of visual information, almost always to the left side of space, reflecting its common association with right hemisphere lesions. Patients may neglect the left side of their body, disregard people to the left side of space, or even ignore food on the left side of their plate. Visual inattention is tested with line bisection tasks, cancellation tasks, and clock drawing. An impaired clock drawing, with all the numbers lined up on the right side, is a classic sign of visual inattention. Visual inattention is commonly seen in the acute stages of traumatic brain injury or stroke and tends to dissipate quickly. Later neuropsychological testing, however, may reveal residual signs of inattention long after brain injury.

Visual inattention represents one extreme of visual spatial dysfunction, but other, more subtle deficits also have an impact on patient safety. Even mild visual attention deficits are related to accident-prone behavior.[11] For instance, driving and navigation of any kind is heavily dependent on visual attention, depth perception, form recognition, and localization of objects in space. Accidents, falls, getting lost, and taking the wrong medications may also result from poor visual spatial functioning.

Language

Language is a means of processing and transmitting information, organizing sensory perceptions, codifying thoughts, and expressing emotions. The development of language does not require speech or even audition as evidenced by deaf and/or mute individuals who communicate with sign language. Perhaps more than any other cognitive ability, the acquisition of language is influenced by sensitive and critical periods of development. Individuals who do not acquire language during these periods have marked impairments in cognition. The left hemisphere is dominant for language in approximately 95% of right handers and 70% of left handers. Overall, approximately 96% of the population is left hemisphere dominant for language. Therefore, patients with damage to the left hemisphere should always be closely evaluated for language deficits.

Clinical evaluation of language commonly includes observation of spontaneous speech, verbal comprehension, repetition, confrontation naming, verbal fluency, reading, and writing. Assessment includes open-ended questions to evaluate aspects of speech and content, accuracy of command following, repetition of simple phrases, naming of common objects, reading a magazine or newspaper, and writing one's name. Bedside language examination can detect obvious aphasias but may fail to identify more subtle deficits because many tasks are routine or overlearned. More detailed language testing and aphasia examinations can be done in collaboration with neuropsychologists and speech therapists.

There are many safety concerns related to deficits in language expression and comprehension. Expressive aphasias preclude patients from communicating medical history and current symptoms, making their needs known, and calling for help in emergency situations. Receptive aphasias limit a patient's ability to understand medical results, care instructions, and medication regimens. Language is a core cognitive ability that is responsible for all verbally mediated information processing. Inner self-talk is central to many attention and executive functions, such as evaluating, planning, organizing, self-awareness, and decision making. When language is impaired, patient safety and independence is compromised in many ADLs.

Memory

Memory is a multifaceted process that requires encoding, storage, and retrieval of sensory information. At its most basic level, memory requires attention to the environment. Working memory represents the initial processing stage of memory as attentional information is transferred to a more immediate storage in the hippocampus. Working memory and immediate memory are commonly referred to as short-term memory. The left hemispheric hippocampus is primarily responsible for immediate verbal memory. Damage may lead to deficits in learning new semantic information. The right hemispheric hippocampus is more responsible for the immediate visual and perceptual components of memory, such as episodic and emotional features. Damage may lead to impaired recall of complex visual and auditory patterns that cannot be easily verbalized. Long-term memories are not stored in the hippocampus but rather distributed throughout the cortex, especially the temporal lobes.

Long-term memory consists of 2 broad aspects of memory, declarative (explicit) and nondeclarative (implicit) memory. Declarative memory is conscious learning and recall of events and facts, of which episodic memory and semantic memory are 2 subtypes. Declarative memory depends on intact functioning of the temporal limbic structures and interconnected cortical regions. Episodic (autobiographic) memory involves recall of verbal and visual information, details of when and where, and information associated with personal experiences and events. Semantic memory is recall of verbally stored facts and knowledge. Well-learned semantic facts are stored in a diffuse cerebral network and tend to be more resistant to aging, damage, and disease. Conversely, episodic memory is more likely to decline with age. Nondeclarative (implicit) memory is memory for skills and habits and unconscious learning and recall more generally. Procedural memory, priming, classical conditioning, and operant conditioning represent nondeclarative memory abilities. Most nondeclarative memory abilities remain intact in normal aging and even the early stages of Alzheimer disease.[12]

Assessment of verbal memory typically involves recalling varying amounts of words or a story both immediately and after a delay of 5 to 30 minutes. Visual memory tasks require immediate or delayed recall of a picture, spatial arrangement, or design. Early assessment of memory impairment is important because it serves as a baseline from which to compare future findings. Serial assessment is particularly relevant in identifying and staging mild cognitive impairment and dementia. Because memory is so vital to everyday functioning, memory impairment has a significant impact on safety in ADLs, medication adherence, driving, decision-making capacity, and travel away from home.

Executive Functioning

Executive functioning is variously defined, but is generally thought to include the ability to plan, organize, sequence, shift, strategize, execute, inhibit responses, form goals, reason abstractly, monitor thought processes and behavior, perform searches, and allocate resources. Because of the heterogeneity of these functions, many dislike the umbrella term, *executive functioning*; however, the term prevails in the common nomenclature. The prefrontal cortex initiates and coordinates cognition and acts as an executive or supervisory system overseeing cognitive processes and operations. Prefrontal systems become very active when a person performs a novel task by integrating information from its 3 main divisions: the dorsolateral, orbitofrontal, and anterior cingulate cortices. The prefrontal cortex is susceptible to injury from head trauma and vascular damage. Damage to the prefrontal cortex does not necessarily lead to executive dysfunction. Furthermore, lesions to areas outside of the prefrontal cortex and the cerebellum can also cause executive-type impairments.

Blumenfeld[13] identifies order, restraint, and initiative as the 3 higher cognitive functions of the prefrontal cortex. Order is processed in the dorsolateral prefrontal cortex and includes abstract reasoning, working memory, perspective taking, planning, insight, sequencing, and temporal organization. Restraint is an orbitofrontal function that entails judgment, foresight, perseverance, delaying gratification, inhibiting socially inappropriate behavior, self-monitoring, and decision making. Initiative involves curiosity, spontaneity, motivation, drive, creativity, shifting cognitive set, mental flexibility, and aspects of personality. Initiative is a function of the anterior cingulate gyrus and interaction of the anterior cingulate and dorsolateral prefrontal cortices. Mateer's[14] model of executive functioning includes 6 key components, including initiation and drive (starting behavior), response inhibition (stopping behavior), task persistence (maintaining behavior), organization (organizing actions and thoughts), generative thinking (creativity, fluency, and cognitive flexibility), and awareness (monitoring and modifying one's own behavior).

The executive functions are the most complex and difficult cognitive domain to evaluate and identify. Many individuals with executive impairments perform well on structured tasks, such as IQ tests, but have difficulty with unstructured real world activities. It is, therefore, useful to interview friends or family members regarding executive-type changes in cognition and behavior. Neuropsychological tests of executive functioning measure features, such as complex attention, fluency, novel problem solving, and decision-making ability. No single test, however, effectively captures the broad spectrum of executive disturbance.

Executive functioning may be the strongest of all cognitive domains in the prediction of everyday independent functioning. Executive impairment does more to determine the extent of community reintegration than does damage to any other cognitive system.[15] Many patients with executive impairments demonstrate problems with organization and execution of everyday action, such as errors performing a sequence of action, with the potential for poor safety outcomes.[16] Executive disruption is associated with impairments in ADLs, difficulty organizing medication regimens, motor vehicle accidents, impaired awareness of deficit, decision-making capacity, and decreased independent functioning necessitating supervision.

SAFETY CONCERNS IN THE PATIENT WITH COGNITIVE IMPAIRMENT AND RECOMMENDATIONS TO LIMIT ADVERSE OUTCOMES

The second section of this article focuses on the most common safety concerns faced by rehabilitation clinicians in the assessment and treatment of patients with cognitive impairment. These concerns include safety related to ADLs, medication adherence, driving an automobile, impaired awareness of deficit, decision-making capacity, substance abuse, suicide, falls, and wandering. This section discusses the most relevant safety issues guiding clinical decision making (**Table 1**), related impairments, assessment procedures, referral sources, and recommendations to limit adverse outcomes (**Table 2**).

Instrumental Activities of Daily Living

ADLs are typically divided into 2 types, basic ADLs (BADLs) and instrumental ADLs (IADLs). BADLs include things related to basic self-care, such as grooming, dressing, feeding, toileting, and bathing. IADLs involve more complex tasks instrumental to successful day-to-day functioning, such as shopping, cooking, money management, medication management, communication skills, handling transportation needs, and community activities. Although physical and cognitive deficits interact to decrease effectiveness in performing ADLs in general, BADLs tend to be more significantly impacted by physical factors and IADLs more significantly affected by cognitive impairments. Furthermore, IADLs are necessary to maintain a household as well as safety and independence and tend to precede impairment in ADLs. The capacity to execute ADLs is typically assessed by physical and occupational therapists, whereas neuropsychologists are commonly asked to collaborate in the prediction of IADL functioning. There is a significant association between neuropsychological test performance and the ability to carry out IADLs. Neuropsychological performance has been associated with IADLs in multiple rehabilitation groups, including individuals with traumatic brain injury,[17] heart transplantation,[18] vascular dementia,[19] Alzheimer disease,[20] HIV,[21] and schizophrenia[22] as well as community-dwelling older adults.[23] There are safety issues inherent in many IADLs related to cooking and leaving appliances on; leaving the house and getting lost or injured; taking medication properly; driving or coordinating transportation; organizing important activities, such as doctor's appointments or pharmacy visits; and dealing with emergencies.

Executive functioning is often at the core of impairments in IADLs. Patients with brain injury typically fare better when performing routine tasks in familiar environments, without distraction, and in the presence of overlearned situational cues. New environments and novel tasks present safety hazards to those with cognitive impairments.[24] Increased frustration and psychological distress can be disorganizing for patients with brain injury and limiting exposure to stressful environments may reduce potential dangers. Functional impairment and safety concerns increase with degree of cognitive impairment necessitating supervision.

Patient and family educational support is central to reducing safety risks in IADLs. Patients and families must be made aware of IADL limitations to make necessary adjustments in supervision needs or find strategies to compensate for IADL deficits. Cognitive rehabilitation has shown effective in improving executive dysfunction and IADL performance, thereby reducing safety risks. There is substantial evidence to support interventions for attention, memory, social communication skills, executive function, and comprehensive-holistic neuropsychologic rehabilitation after traumatic brain injury.[25] Compensatory strategies, such as memory books, calendars, smart phones, and alarming devices, assist in increasing independence in IADLs. These strategies have greater use with low-risk activities, such as keeping appointments, going shopping, and paying bills. IADLs of higher risk (ie, medication adherence and driving) deserve greater scrutiny in ensuring safety and are discussed in the following sections.

Medication Adherence

Medication adherence is broadly defined as the accurate use of medication. This includes proper administration of medicine in the correct dosage, at the appropriate time, and in agreement with any special instructions.[26] Rates of medication compliance are lower than 50% in most studies and tend to decline over time in almost all chronic diseases.[27] Medication nonadherence is associated with declines in overall health and increased risk of hospitalization,[28] increased morbidity and mortality,[29] and higher health care costs.[30] Approximately 10% of hospital admissions are directly attributable to nonadherence with prescription drug regimens, and 23% of nursing home admissions are seen secondary to poor compliance with medical regimens.[31] Medication nonadherence is particularly prevalent in patients who require compliance, such as those with complex medical problems and geriatric patients. Approximately 90% of patients over age 65 regularly take some form of medication, and inappropriate drug discontinuation occurs in up to 40% of this population.[32] As many as 20% of older adults commit medication errors that potentially have serious health consequences.[33] Nonadherence increases with number of drugs prescribed, number of side effects, and overall complexity of instructions and medication regimen.

A prominent cause of medication nonadherence among older adults is related to memory difficulty. Patients with dementia may have difficulty remembering which medications they are taking, when to take the medications, the names of the medications, and even the reasons for their use. Executive functioning deficits contribute to difficulty in adhering to demanding or complex medication regimens, such as those seen in older adults and in patients with multiple medical problems, HIV/AIDS, and cancer. Patients with executive functioning deficits may even perseverate on medication taking and unintentionally overdose. Poor comprehension of medication instructions and medication regimens may play a role in medication nonadherence. Visual impairments and presentation of written instructions can also affect adherence.

Medication adherence is vital to patient health and safety. Increasing adherence involves many factors and application of multiple methods. Factors associated

Table 1
Checklist of key safety concerns guiding clinical decision making

Safety Issue	Key Areas of Inquiry
Instrumental activities of daily living	What level of supervision is necessary to ensure the patient's safety? How does the patient function in new or novel environments? What are the obstacles impeding patient independence? How can these obstacles be overcome?
Medication adherence	Can the patient name the medications he/she is taking, the doses, when he/she is supposed to take the medications, and the reason for their use? How complex is the patient's medication regimen? Are there any unnecessary medications that can be eliminated? Are there any cultural or motivational factors influencing the use of any prescribed medications?
Driving a motor vehicle	Does the patient have a visual impairment? Is it corrected? When was the last time the patient passed a state driver licensing examination? Are there observable deficits in attention, visual spatial functioning or executive functioning, or neuropsychological test results that warrant a driving evaluation?
Awareness of deficit	What is the patient's understanding of his/her condition and limitations? Does the patient use compensatory strategies, conscious or unconscious, suggesting accommodation to changes in functioning? What are the relative contributions of psychological denial and neurologically based injury to the patient's impaired awareness? Is the impaired awareness generalized or specific and does it accompany other cognitive impairments? What are consequences of the patient's impaired awareness and how likely is he/she to engage in dangerous activities?

Decision-making capacity	Can the patient communicate a choice, appreciate the consequences of the choice, reason about the choice, provide a rational explanation of the choice, understand the context in which the choice was made, and know the inherent risks, benefits, and alternatives?
	Can the patient describe the medical condition accurately?
	Can the patient understand the significant benefits, risks, and alternatives to the proposed medical care?
	Can the patient make and communicate a health care decision?
Substance abuse	Does the patient have a history of substance abuse?
	Is the patient currently abusing substances?
Suicide	Does the patient have a personal or family history of suicide attempts?
	Does the patient have past or present suicidal ideation?
	Does the patient have a plan or intent?
	Does the patient have access to a lethal means?
	Is the patient using alcohol or drugs in excess?
	Is the patient grieving a recent loss or separation?
Falls	Is the patient's medical condition associated with an increased risk of falls?
	What environmental barriers increase the risk for falls at home?
	Are there any sedating medications in the patient's regimen that can be replaced or eliminated?
	Does the patient have any significant cognitive impairments that increase the risk of falls?
Wandering	Does the patient experience periods of confusion, disorientation, or memory impairment?
	What is the patient's level of supervision?
	Has the patient wandered in the past and how did he/she get away?
	Is the caregiver aware and in control of all the exits points in the environment?
	What are the boundaries at which point the patient would be considered lost?

Table 2
Safety concerns and recommendations to limit adverse outcomes

Safety Issue	Specific Concerns	Related Impairments	Assessment and Referral Sources	Strategies and Recommendations
Instrumental activities of daily living	Operating appliances, travel away from the home, new or novel environments, organizing important activities, dealing with emergencies	Executive functioning	Patient and caregiver report; medical records; assessment by physical therapists, occupational therapists, neuropsychologists, and/or speech therapists	Caregiver and patient education, increasing the level of supervision, cognitive rehabilitation, low stress environments, routine daily schedule and avoiding changes
Medication adherence	Missing medications, not reaching therapeutic dose, unintentional overdose, inappropriate discontinuation	Memory, executive functioning, language comprehension	Patient and caregiver report, medical records, assessment by occupational therapists and neuropsychologists, home health aid assessment and monitoring	Explanation of use and side effects at appropriate cognitive level, check for understanding, printed instructions, limiting prescriptions, cost-benefit analyses, external memory aids
Driving a motor vehicle	Motor vehicle accidents, getting lost	Vision, visual spatial functioning, attention, executive functioning	Neuropsychological assessment, driving simulators, driving evaluations, state driving tests for licensure	Completion of a driving evaluation, cognitive rehabilitation
Awareness of deficit	Engaging in risky activities beyond an individual's cognitive or physical limitations	Executive functioning	Medical history, comparing patient and caregiver report, behavioral observation, response to performance, errors and feedback	Education, therapeutic alliance, reviewing medical records, activities designed to highlight limitations with direct feedback

Decision-making capacity	Noncompliance with necessary medical treatments, independent living	Attention, executive functioning	Informal observation, neuropsychological testing, capacity evaluation	Completion of a capacity evaluation
Substance abuse	Delayed neurologic recovery, further neurologic damage, overdose	Executive functioning, personality characteristics	Patient and caregiver report/history, toxicology screening	Outpatient/inpatient substance abuse treatment, mobilization of social support
Suicide	Suicidal ideation, gestures, attempts	Depression, substance abuse	Suicide risk assessment evaluating level of depression, ideation, intent, a plan, and means	Psychotherapy, medication, inpatient psychiatric hospitalization
Falls	Physical trauma, head injury	Attention, memory, visual spatial functioning, executive functioning	Review of medical records (gait, hypotension, polypharmacy, sedative use) neuropsychological assessment, environmental obstacles at home	Education, cognitive rehabilitation, physical conditioning, gripping shoes, environmental modifications
Wandering	Getting lost, injury, death	Confusion, disorientation, memory	History of wandering, neuropsychological assessment	Supervision, environmental modifications

with increased medication adherence include intact cognitive functioning, greater psychological stability, less drug or alcohol abuse, greater familiarity with medication, beliefs about medication effectiveness, few side effects, health literacy, the establishment of routines and regimens, and social support.[34] There are several methods to help increase medication adherence in patients with cognitive impairment. Physicians should provide a thorough explanation of medication instructions at an appropriate cognitive level to patients, inform and bring together a patient's family and social supports, discuss cost/benefit analyses when appropriate, review side effects, encourage and provide detailed responses to patient questions, have patients repeat verbal instructions, and provide written instructions. They can develop a simplistic medication schedule that matches a patient's daily routine or specific times of the day that become associated with taking the medication. Pillboxes are an effective external memory aid for patients with impaired memory. These should be kept in the same routinely accessed location, such as by the sink in the bathroom or kitchen. Calendars, erasable boards, and notepads located on a refrigerator with written instructions and daily plans are effective if routinely used. Daily planners, medication charts, pill alarms, and alarms programmed into phones or watches help improve planning, organization, and memory. Limiting the number of medications may increase compliance and reduce medication regimen complexity. Cognitive rehabilitation techniques improve cognitive impairments, and providing education about adherence techniques may be particularly helpful. Discharge education groups for rehabilitation inpatients are effective when medication adherence is discussed and informational materials are distributed. Written instructions in large fonts and simple language may improve comprehension and visual impairments. Medication nonadherence is complex and results from a unique combination of cognitive, emotional, and behavioral factors that dictates subtle tailoring of treatment recommendations to each patient. Therefore, it is important to identify cognitive risk factors associated with nonadherence and recommend multiple methods that are known to increase adherence.

Driving a Motor Vehicle

Cognitive abilities determine driving behavior and safety errors, which in turn predict accidents. Cognitively impaired individuals as a group perform significantly worse than controls on driving measures and the risk of crashes and injury increases with degree of cognitive impairment. Safe driving requires the coordination of motor responsivity, attention, visual perceptual ability, executive functioning, and memory. These abilities are impaired by physical and mental fatigue, drugs and alcohol, advancing age, medical complications, neurologic disorders, and psychiatric disorders. Any disorder affecting vision or perception can have a negative impact on or preclude driving. A certain level of muscular strength and psychomotor reactivity is necessary for safe driving. Patients with sleep disturbances, drowsiness, and fatigue are at increased risk for crashes. Alcohol and drug use increase the risk of automobile accidents exponentially. Furthermore, prescription drugs, such as opiates, anticonvulsants, antidepressants, antihypertensives, antilipemics, hypoglycemic agents, and sedatives, have all been associated with an increased risk of car accidents. To safely operate a motor vehicle requires a higher level of functional ability and integration than any other activity of daily living.

Attention and executive functioning are often cited as the most important cognitive abilities related to driving. Safety issues relate not only to vigilance in rapidly shifting environmental conditions but also to whether or not an individual has the cognitive capacity to recognize slowly changing environmental conditions, such as knowing to watch out for children in a school zone or taking an alternative route if a road is blocked.[35] More specifically, performances on measures of tasks of processing speed, working memory, selective attention, shifting attention, and divided attention have shown a strong relationship to driving performance in patients.[36-38] Distractibility by electronic devices, competing stimuli, and rapidly shifting environments is particularly treacherous. As attentional complexity and environmental demands increase, the risks for dangerous driver errors and crashes increase. Impaired decision making is another critical factor in driver errors that lead to vehicular crashes. Poor impulse control, such as thrill seeking and aggression, is closely related to decision making and influences driving outcomes. Other emotional and behavioral problems, such as increased stress, depression, anxiety, and psychosis, can have a negative impact on driver performance. Driving safety declines in all forms of memory impairment. Although global positioning system devices assist with navigation, they easily divert attention and are not always accurate. Therefore, routine and alternative routes home should be memorized to prevent getting lost.

Physical capabilities, cognitive ability, and personality characteristics all contribute to safe driving and are highly individualized. Patients with physical impairments that prevent safe driving should be given assistive devices or discontinue driving. The research literature indicates that patients with moderate to severe cognitive impairment should not drive. It is more common, however, to be faced with decisions about patients with milder cognitive deficits that are more difficult to predict. Cognitive rehabilitation may improve cognitive ability related to driving, particularly if safe driving is one of the goals of the therapy. Specifically, speed of processing training has been associated with reductions in dangerous driving maneuvers.[39] Patients may be referred for more intensive driving testing, such as drive simulators, and/or asked to pass state driving tests for licensure. Although it is prudent to recommend discontinuation of driving when there is any concern for patient safety, allowing a patient with cognitive deficits the opportunity to demonstrate capacity and safety in driving through specialized occupational therapy evaluations and/or behind the wheel evaluations conducted by authorized driving schools allows greater levels of independence.

Impaired Awareness of Deficit

Impaired awareness of deficit is a common result of acquired brain injury, which produces significant barriers to patient recovery and presents unique challenges to rehabilitation clinicians attempting to maximize patient safety. Up to 45% of patients with moderate to severe traumatic brain injury demonstrate awareness deficits.[40] At the most extreme, impaired awareness of deficit manifests as anosognosia, literally translated to "no knowledge of disease." Anosognosia is a surprisingly frequent feature of brain injury. Up to 18% of acute hemiparetic stroke patients show unawareness of their paretic limb.[41] Patients with a limited understanding of the nature, degree, and impact of their impairments may be resistant to therapy and engage in dangerous activities because they do not appreciate their limitations. A generalized impaired awareness is often observed in rehabilitation patients with traumatic brain injury, schizophrenia, and dementia. Focal lesions cause specific types of impaired awareness for motor, sensory, visual, and linguistic deficits. Examples include impaired awareness of hemiparesis and hemiplegia, left inattention, impaired awareness of partial or complete blindness, and impaired awareness of disordered speech.

Impaired awareness is most closely related to executive dysfunction, specifically working memory and self-monitoring deficits. Episodic memory deficits may also be related. Some individuals accurately assess their physical status but are much less reliable in their assessment of their cognitive, emotional, and behavioral skills. Individuals with traumatic brain injury are much less likely to complain of changes in personality, such as impaired judgment, reduced insight, irritability, impulsivity, affective instability, and problems with interpersonal functioning in general.[42]

Impaired awareness of deficit may be attributable to psychological denial, neurologic damage, or some combination of the two. Behavioral signs related to defensive or nondefensive methods of coping help distinguish these patients. Denial is defined here as an adaptive psychological defense mechanism that spares an individual from the emotional pain of acknowledging deficits. When evidence for limitations is brought to the attention of an individual with denial, it is not uncommon for the individual to give momentary recognition followed by an explanation that discounts the feedback. Sentences that begin with "Yes, but…" are common in patients who use denial.[43] When pressed, these individuals may become irritated and agitated. Unawareness due to neurologic injury is usually found with damage to the nondominant prefrontal, insular, and/or parietal cortices. In contrast to individuals with psychological denial, patients with a neurologic basis for their impaired awareness may seem puzzled or show indifference when given feedback about their impairments. In cases of pure anosagnosia, by definition, there is no defensive reaction.[44]

In assessment of awareness deficits, the most common strategies include a patient's self-report of abilities and disabilities, comparison of a patient's self-report and other observers' reports, observing a patient's response to deficits and limitations, observing a patient's use of compensatory strategies, and comparing a patient's prediction of performance with the performance on physical examination and cognitive testing.[45]

Many different approaches have been attempted to increase the level of awareness in individuals with brain injury. These include patient and caregiver education regarding unawareness in the context of brain injury, activities designed to highlight limitations and deficits, exploring discrepancies between patient and observer reports, reviewing medical records, and videotaping individuals with brain injury to provide feedback regarding their behavior. The most important early intervention is development of a therapeutic alliance. In the presence of a trusting therapeutic relationship, an individualized treatment plan that moves from simple awareness tasks to more complex awareness tasks can be developed and implemented. These hierarchically ordered exercises help patients experience errors and changes in their ability to increase their awareness about the nature and degree of these changes. This helps initiate patient discussion integrated with clinician education. The rehabilitation plan is more likely to be successful if it is engaging and interesting to patients. In patients with denial or a combination of denial and organically based impaired awareness, an educational approach may be most appropriate. Coordination of a multidisciplinary team of physical therapists, occupational therapists, neuropsychologists, and speech therapists is necessary in more complex cases, such as anosagnosia for hemiparesis and hemiplegia, blindness, or aphasia. Patients whose beliefs are less rigid may be more responsive to feedback and therefore have a better prognostic profile.

Decision-Making Capacity

Capacity is a clinical term used in evaluation of an individual's ability to make decisions in specific areas, including managing financial affairs, entering into contracts, making a will or advanced directive, consenting to medical treatment, participating in research, driving, and living independently or selecting a living situation. A capacity assessment may be performed by any licensed physician but is usually performed by a psychiatrist or psychologist. Capacity is often confused with the term, competency. Competency refers to a legal determination, made by a judge, of an individual's ability to retain decision-making power regarding a particular activity or set of activities.

Capacity relates to safety in several areas of patient functioning and along the spectrum of treatment continuum. For example, during acute hospital care or acute rehabilitation, capacity may need to be assessed when a patient is asked to consent to medical procedures or agree to take a prescribed medication. At this level of care, capacity may be questioned at time of discharge when making plans about a living situation, the ability to live alone, or the level of supervision needed. Once a patient is living in the community, the ability to drive, manage finances, and enter into contracts is of greater concern.

Outcomes of capacity evaluations can have serious consequences in a patient's life, especially if it is determined that an individual does not have capacity. For example, patients may be placed in a nursing home against their will. No one wants to restrict individual freedoms, yet there are potential safety consequences when someone who does not have capacity is allowed to go home without adequate supervision.

Capacity is rarely a dichotomous, static clinical finding. It can change over time as a person's status improves or deteriorates. For example, medical decision-making capacity was found to improve in patients with traumatic brain injury over a period of 6 months.[46] In some situations, capacity is enhanced by compensating for a patient's sensory impairments (visual or auditory), communication barriers (aphasia, dysarthria, foreign language, and others), or fatigue limitations. The presence of cognitive impairment in itself does not constitute proof of impaired capacity. Capacity is most closely associated, however, with memory, comprehension, and executive functioning.

Decision-making capacity involves assessment of a patient's ability to understand and appreciate a given decision. Several interrelated factors evaluated in decision making include the ability to communicate a choice, appreciate the consequences of the choice, reason about the choice, provide a rational explanation of the choice, understand the context in which the choice was made, and know the inherent risks, benefits, and alternatives.[47] Capacity to consent to medical care involves assessment of an individual's ability to understand the significant benefits, risks, and alternatives to proposed care and to make and communicate a health care decision.[48]

The framework for capacity evaluations involves the following: legal standards, functional elements (BADLs and IADLs), diagnosis (temporary vs permanent and prognosis), cognitive underpinnings, psychiatric or emotional factors, values (race, ethnicity, culture, gender, sexual orientation, and religion), risk considerations, and steps to enhance capacity. Capacity is assessed through informal means, such as observing an individual and/or clinical interview with the individual, family, and treatment staff, and by using cognitive tests and functional assessment instruments. Some of the more commonly used capacity instruments include the Adaptive Behavior Assessment System, Aid to Capacity Evaluation, Capacity Assessment Tool, Financial Capacity Instrument, and Independent Living Scale. Formal testing has the advantage of greater inter-rater reliability, but capacity evaluations are best conducted using a combination of informal and formal testing procedures.

Substance Abuse

It is not yet known whether traumatic brain injury itself increases the risk for substance abuse. Research suggests that a younger age, male gender, substance abuse history and psychiatric history are significant factors in determining risk for substance misuse following brain injury.[49,50] For individuals with a history of substance abuse, there is likely a decline in use for the first year, but many return to their preinjury level of use 28 months after the injury, a factor that can increase the risk for future head injuries.[51] Limited consistent support systems, poor access to health care, difficulty adjusting to functional changes, avoidant coping strategies, and deficits in executive functioning also increase the risk for substance use.

Premorbid substance abuse history is linked to aggressive behaviors up to 6 months after a traumatic brain injury.[52] Alcohol or drug use at any point postinjury can be harmful and compound the effects of a traumatic brain injury, especially during the first several years when the brain is recovering.[53] Individuals with brain injury may have a lower tolerance to substances due to the presence of fewer neurons to absorb the alcohol or drug and postinjury prescription medications interfering with alcohol/drug absorption. Substance use inhibits new connections between neurons, complicates existing medical conditions, and interacts with prescription medications to create new medical problems. Drug use can exacerbate problems with cognition and increase the risk for seizures and falls that can lead to a subsequent trauma and additional brain damage. It is, therefore, important to recommend abstinence from alcohol and illicit drugs after any acquired brain injury. It is also essential for all clinical staff to inquire about alcohol and drug use, past and present, for several years after a brain injury. Those who are abusing substances or at risk for substance abuse may benefit from support groups and psychotherapeutic interventions. Inpatient treatment may be necessary in more extreme cases.

Suicide

The experience of traumatic brain injury and the related cause often precipitates a complex series of medical, cognitive, and emotional experiences leading to an impaired ability to cope. Persons with traumatic brain injury carry a 4-fold greater risk of committing suicide than the general population.[54] Individuals with brain damage frequently have co-occurring conditions that increase the risk of attempted or completed suicide, such as chronic disease, chronic pain, substance abuse, and psychiatric disorders.[55] Curry[56] outlined several critical suicide risk factors in depression, including a history of suicide attempts, acute suicidal ideation, severe hopelessness, attraction to death, family history of suicide, acute overuse of alcohol, and loss/separations. The highest risk group was found to have suicidal ideation, intent, a plan, a means to lethality, and the fewest inhibitors (reasons not to complete the act). It is, therefore, imperative to assess the risk level of suicidality/homicidality by asking a patient about thoughts of suicidality/homicidality, any potential plans of action, and access to lethal means. Patients with increased risk for suicide may need to be treated in an inpatient psychiatric setting to ensure safety.

Falls

Falls are the second most common source of traumatic brain injury in any age group, behind motor vehicle accidents, and the most common cause of traumatic brain injury in the elderly.[57] Up to three-quarters of older adults with cognitive impairments or dementia fall each year and the number of falls increases with degree of dementia severity.[58] Fatalities as a result of fall-related traumatic brain injury are most common in those over age 75. Disorders affecting the frontal lobe, subcortical structures, and cerebellum are associated with an increased risk of falls.

Falls occur because of an interaction of environmental factors, medical problems, and cognitive impairment. Miller and colleagues[59] describe 4 common issues that have been implicated in increased risk for falls in the elderly. These include postural hypotension, gait and balance instability, polypharmacy, and the use of sedative medications. Sedative use impairs attention and is a major risk factor for falls. Hyperactive symptoms are an additional risk factor associated with falls.[60] The role of visual perceptual disturbances is apparent in falls. Impairments in attention, memory, and executive functioning have also been linked to falls. Processing speed is linked to various indices of mobility as well as falls in older adults.[61] Depression also increases the risk for falls in older adults.[62]

Interventions to improve cognitive function may be helpful in reducing falls among older adults. Educational efforts can be beneficial in preventing falls. The Brain Injury Association of America suggests that physical conditioning, review of medications, use of comfortable and gripping shoes, and modification of the environment reduce falls in older adults. Modification examples include reducing waxed or slippery floors, decreasing potential hazards in the bathtub or shower, removing loose rugs, removing or altering sharp furniture and potential snags, and increasing the amount of light in and outside the house. One study showed that modification of the environment decreased falls by 60% annually.[63]

Wandering

Individuals with cognitive impairment are at a higher risk for harm due to wandering, which occurs as a result of disorientation, confusion, and memory dysfunction. The Alzheimer's Association estimates that 60% of individuals with Alzheimer disease wander and become lost at some point. These incidents may result in injury or death due to hyperthermia, drowning, and dehydration.[64] Wandering can be reduced using behavioral measures and environmental modifications. Behavioral measures include supervision, keeping a person oriented, and avoiding complicated tasks and changes in routine. Environmental modifications include keeping the house layout consistent and familiar, setting boundaries of travel, and controlling exits.

SUMMARY

Preventable injury is one of the most significant health care issues in the United States. Preventing adverse safety outcomes is particularly relevant in rehabilitation patients. Integration of information and recommendations stemming from allied disciplines, such as rehabilitation medicine, physical therapy, occupational therapy, speech therapy, and neuropsychology, is the most effective way to limit potential adverse outcomes in patients with cognitive impairment. Consensus of what the cognitive issues are, how they are managed, and what precautions need to be taken is the ultimate goal. With dedication to prevention and treatment along with education and resources provided to patients and caregivers, a substantial drop in adverse safety outcomes can be achieved. Education and prevention counseling by health care professionals in the clinical setting as well as at the community level (senior centers, media, and so forth) is the most effective generalized approach in limiting adverse safety outcomes in patients with cognitive impairment.

REFERENCES

1. Cohen RA, Gunstad J. The neuropsychology of cardiovascular disease. New York: Oxford University Press; 2009.
2. Farr SA, Yamada KA, Butterfield DA, et al. Obesity and hypertriglyceridemia produce cognitive impairment. Endocrinology 2008;149(5):2628–36.
3. Brands A, Biessels GJ, de Haan EH, et al. The effects of type 1 diabetes on cognitive performance: a metanalysis. Diabetes Care 2005;28(3):726–35.
4. Pereira J, Hanson J, Bruera E. The frequency and clinical course of cognitive impairment in patients with terminal cancer. Cancer 1997;79(4):835–42.
5. Kewman DG, Vaishampayan N, Zald D, et al. Cognitive impairment in musculo-skeletal pain patients. Int J Psychiatry Med 1991;21(3):253–62.

6. Schuler M, Njoo N, Hestermann M, et al. Acute and chronic pain in geriatrics: clinical characteristics of pain and the influence of cognition. Pain Med 2004;5(3): 253–62.

7. O'Bryant SE, Marcus DA, Rains JC. The neuropsychology of recurrent headache. Headache 2006;46(9):1364–76.

8. Strauss E, Sherman EM, Spreen O. A compendium of neuropsychological tests. New York: Oxford University Press; 2006.

9. Schaie K. The course of adult intellectual development. Am Psychol 1994;49(4): 304–13.

10. Lezak MD, Howieson DB, Loring DW. Perception. In: Neuropsychological assessment. 4th edition. New York: Oxford University Press; 2004. p. 611–46.

11. Diller L, Weinberg J. Evidence for accident prone behavior in hemiplegic patients. Arch Phys Med Rehabil 1970;51:358–63.

12. Kuzis G, Sabe L, Tiberti C, et al. Explicit and implicit learning in patients with Alzheimer's disease and Parkinson's disease with dementia. Neuropsychiatry Neuropsychol Behav Neurol 1999;12(4):265–9.

13. Blumenfeld H. Higher order cerebral function. In: Neuroanatomy through clinical cases. Sunderland (MA): Sinauer and Associates; 2003. p. 821–909.

14. Mateer CA. The rehabilitation of executive disorders. In: Stuss DT, Winocur G, Robertson I, editors. Cognitive neurorehabilitation. New York: Guilford; 1999. p. 314–32.

15. Solhberg MM, Mateer CA. Management of dysexecutive symptoms. Cognitive rehabilitation: an integrative neuropsychological approach. New York: Guilford; 2001. p. 230–68.

16. Marcotte TD, Scott JC, Kamat R, et al. Neuropsychology and the prediction of everyday functioning. In: Marcotte TD, Grant I, editors. Neuropsychology of everyday functioning. New York: Guilford; 2010. p. 5–38.

17. Farmer JE, Eakman AM. The relationship between neuropsychological functioning and instrumental activities of daily living following acquired brain injury. Appl Neuropsychol 1995;2(3–4):107–15.

18. Putzke JD, Williams MA, Daniel JF, et al. Activities of daily living among heart transplant candidates: neuropsychological and cardiac function predictors. J Heart Lung Transplant 2000;19:995–1006.

19. Boyle PA, Paul R, Moser D, et al. Executive impairments predict functional declines in vascular dementia. Clin Neuropsychol 2004;18(1):75–82.

20. Cahn-Weiner DA, Ready RE, Malloy PF. Neuropsychological predictors of everyday memory and everyday functioning in patients with mild Alzheimer's disease. J Geriatr Psychiatry Neurol 2003;16(2):84–9.

21. Heaton RK, Marcotte TD, Minte MR, et al. The impact of HIV-associated neuropsychological impairment on everyday functioning. J Int Neuropsychol Soc 2004;10(3):317–31.

22. Jeste SD, Patterson TL, Palmer BW, et al. Cognitive predictors of medication adherence among middle aged and older outpatients with schizophrenia. Schizophr Res 2003;63(1–2):49–58.

23. Royall DR, Palmer R, Chiodo LK, et al. Normal rates of cognitive change in successful aging: the freedom house study. J Int Neuropsychol Soc 2005;7:899–909.

24. Lowenstein D, Acevedo A. The relationship between instrumental activities of daily living and neuropsychological performance. In: Marcotte TD, Grant I, editors. Neuropsychology of everyday functioning. New York: Guilford; 2010. p. 93–112.

25. Cicerone KD, Langenbahn DM, Braden C, et al. Evidence based cognitive rehabilitation: updated review of literature from 2003 through 2008. Arch Phys Med Rehabil 2011;92:519–30.

26. Gould ON, McDonald-Miszczak L, Gregory J. Prediction accuracy and medication instructions: will you remember tomorrow? Aging Neuropsychol C 1999;6: 141–54.
27. Dunbar-Jacob J, Erlen JA, Schlenk EA, et al. Adherence in chronic disease. Annu Rev Nurs Res 2000;18:48–90.
28. Col N, Fanale JE, Kronholm P. The role of medication compliance and adverse drug reactions in hospitalizations of the elderly. Arch Intern Med 1990;150:841–5.
29. Ganguli M, Dodge HH, Mulsant BH. Rates and predictors of mortality in an aging, rural, community-based cohort: the role of depression. Arch Gen Psychiatry 2002;59:1046–52.
30. Gryfe CI, Gryfe BM. Drug therapy of the aged: the problem of compliance and roles of physicians and pharmacists. J Am Geriatr Soc 1984;32:301–7.
31. Herzog L, Dufresne J, Greene V. Medication regimens: causes of noncompliance. Washington, DC: The U.S. Department of Health and Human Services; 1990.
32. Jackson JE, Ramsdell JW, Renvall M, et al. Reliability of drug histories in a specialized geriatric outpatient clinic. J Gen Intern Med 1984;4:39–43.
33. Lamy PP, Salzman C, Nevis-Oleson J. Drug prescribing patterns, risks, and compliance guidelines. In: Salzman C, editor. Clinical geriatric psychopharmacology. 2nd edition. Philadelphia: Williams and Wilkins; 1992. p. 15–37.
34. Barclay TR, Wright MJ, Hinkin CH. Medication management. In: Marcotte TD, Grant I, editors. Neuropsychology of everyday functioning. New York: Guilford; 2010. p. 136–67.
35. Rizzo M, Kellison IL. The brain on the road. In: Marcotte TD, Grant I, editors. Neuropsychology of everyday functioning. New York: Guilford; 2010. p. 168–208.
36. Legenfelder J, Schultheis MT, Al-Shihabi T, et al. Divided attention and driving: a pilot study using virtual reality technology. J Head Trauma Rehabil 2002; 17(1):26–37.
37. Whelihan WM, DiCarlo M, Paul RH. The relationship of neuropsychological functioning to driving competence in older persons with early cognitive decline. Arch Clin Neuropsychol 2005;20(2):217–28.
38. Worringham C, Wood JM, Kerr G, et al. Predictors of driving outcome in Parkinson's disease. Mov Disord 2003;21(2):230–5.
39. Roenker DL, Cissell GM, Ball KK, et al. Speed of processing training and driver simulator training result in improved driving performance. Hum Factors 2003; 45(2):218–33.
40. Freeland J. Awareness of deficits: a complex interplay of neurological, personality, social and rehabilitation factors. Magazine 1996;4:32–4.
41. Baier B, Karnath HO. Incidence and diagnosis of anosagnosia for hemiparesis revisited. J Neurol Neurosurg Psychiatry 2005;76(3):358–61.
42. Flashman L, Amador X, McAllister TW. Awareness of deficit. In: Silver JM, McAllister TW, Yudofsky SC, editors. Textbook of traumatic brain injury. Washington, DC: American Psychiatric Publishing, Inc; 2005. p. 353–67.
43. Prigatano GP, Klonoff PS. A clinician's rating scale for evaluating impaired self-awareness and denial of disability after brain injury. Clin Neuropsychol 1998; 12(1):56–67.
44. Prigatano GP, Morrone-Strupinsky J. Management and rehabilitation of persons with anosagnosia and impaired self-awareness. In: Prigatano GP, editor. The study of anosagnosia. New York: Oxford University Press; 2009. p. 495–516.
45. Solhberg MM, Mateer CA. The assessment and management of unawareness. In: Cognitive rehabilitation: an integrative neuropsychological approach. New York: Guilford Press; 2001. p. 296–305.

46. Marson DC, Herbert K. Assessing civil competencies in older adults with dementia: consent capacity, financial capacity, and testamentary capacity. In: Larabee G, editor. Forensic neuropsychology: a scientific approach. New York: Oxford; 2005. p. 334–77.

47. Novak TA, Sherer M, Penna S. Neuropsychological practice in rehabilitation. In: Frank RG, Caplan B, editors. Handbook of rehabilitation psychology. 2nd edition. Washington, DC: American Psychological Association; 2010. p. 165–78.

48. American Psychological Association and American Bar Association. Assessment of older adults with diminished capacity. Washington, DC: American Psychological Association; 2008.

49. Center for Substance Abuse Treatment. Treating clients with traumatic brain injury. Substance abuse treatment advisory 2010;9(2):1–8.

50. Horner MD, Ferguson PL, Selassie AW, et al. Patterns of alcohol use 1 year after traumatic brain injury: a population-based, epidemiological study. J Int Neuropsychol Soc 2005;11:322–30.

51. Kreutzer JS, Witol AD, Marwitz JH. Alcohol and drug use among young persons with traumatic brain injury. J Learn Disabil 1996;29:643–51.

52. Tateno A, Jorge RE, Robinson RG. Clinical correlates of aggressive behavior after traumatic brain injury. J Neuropsychiatry Clin Neurosci 2003;15:155–60.

53. Corrigan JD. Substance abuse. In: High WM, Sander AM, Struchen MA, et al, editors. Rehabilitation for traumatic brain injury. New York: Oxford University Press; 2005. p. 133–55.

54. Teasdale TW, Engberg AW. Suicide after traumatic brain injury: a population study. J Neurol Neurosurg Psychiatry 2001;71(4):436–70.

55. Mainio A, Kyllonen T, Viilo K, et al. Traumatic brain injury, psychiatric disorders and suicide: a population-based study of suicide victims during the years 1988-2004 in northern Finland. Brain Inj 2007;21(8):851–5.

56. Curry ML. Eight factors found critical in assessing suicide risk. Mon Psychol 2000;31:2.

57. Elovic E, Zafonte R. Prevention. In: Silver JM, McAllister TW, Yudofsky SC, editors. The textbook of traumatic brain injury. Washington, DC: American Psychiatric Publishing Inc; 2005. p. 727–47.

58. Shaw F, Bond J, Richardson D, et al. Multifactorial intervention after a fall in older people with cognitive impairment and dementia presenting to the accident and emergency department: randomised controlled trial. BMJ 2003;326:73.

59. Miller KE, Zylstra RG, Standridge JB. The geriatric patient: a systematic approach to maintaining health. Am Fam Physician 2000;61:1089–104.

60. Kattin K, Gustafason Y, Sandman P. Factors associated with falls among older cognitively impaired people in geriatric settings. Am J Geriatr Psychiatry 2005; 13(6):501–9.

61. Vance DE, Ball K, Roenker DL, et al. Predictors of falling in older Maryland drivers: a structural equation model. J Aging Phys Act 2006;14:254–69.

62. Seeman TE. Social ties and health: the benefits of social integration. Ann Epidemiol 1996;6(5):442–51.

63. Plautz B, Beck DE, Selmar C, et al. Modifying the environment: a community-based injury reduction program for elderly residents. Am J Prev Med 1996;12: 33–6.

64. Rowe MA, Bennett V. A look at deaths occurring in persons with dementia lost in the community. Am J Alzheimers Dis Other Demen 2003;18(6):343–8.

Safety Concerns and Multidisciplinary Management of the Dysphagic Patient

Claudia Giammarino, MS, CCC-SLP[a],*,
Elizabeth Adams, MA, CCC-SLP[a], Christina Moriarty, MS[a],
Adrian Cristian, MD, MHCM[b]

KEYWORDS

- Comprehensive and integrated speech pathology approach
- Swallowing • Dysphagia • Medical errors • Patient safety

"To err is human; to forgive, divine."
—Alexander Pope

The father of Western medicine, Hippocrates, introduced the concept of patient safety. The modernized version of this oath, for contemporary medicine, "primum non nocere," (first do no harm),[1] must be upheld, not only by physicians, but also by the entire interdisciplinary health care team. The interdisciplinary team is responsible for providing medical care based on a patient-centered model while maintaining professional and ethical standards. However, an emerging body of research suggests that ineffective, inappropriate care, or fatal error, arises from the lack of productive communication between patients, families, and medical caregivers.[2] This has prompted the evolution of a new health care discipline, patient safety, which became increasingly prominent in the 1990s. The World Health Organization (WHO) reported that heath care errors collide with 1 in every 10 patients around the world.[3] The Joint Commission's Annual Report on Quality and Safety, 2007, identified the root causes of more than 50% medical errors are attributable to poor interdisciplinary communication and inadequate and incomplete education to patients and their families.[4] The purpose of this article is to bridge the gap between the discipline of patient safety and its relationship to the diagnosis of dysphagia.

[a] Department of Speech-Language Pathology and Audiology, The Kingsbrook Jewish Rehabilitation Institute, Kingsbrook Jewish Medical Center, 585 Schenectady Avenue, Brooklyn, NY 11203, USA
[b] Department of Rehabilitation Medicine, Kingsbrook Jewish Rehabilitation Institute, Kingsbrook Jewish Medical Center, 585 Schenectady Avenue, Brooklyn, NY 11203, USA
* Corresponding author.
E-mail address: cgiammarino@kingsbrook.org

Phys Med Rehabil Clin N Am 23 (2012) 335–342
doi:10.1016/j.pmr.2012.02.008
1047-9651/12/$ – see front matter © 2012 Elsevier Inc. All rights reserved.

pmr.theclinics.com

DYSPHAGIA ACROSS HEALTH CARE SETTINGS

Dysphagia is a widespread term in any medical institution, yet it has various perceived definitions by members of the hospital and rehabilitation team. The definition, being complex and involving many physiologic components and neuromuscular interactions, may result in varying levels of understanding by the interdisciplinary team. Deglutition entails simultaneous and interactive movements involving the oral, pharyngeal ,and esophageal stages of swallowing. As discussed in an article from Becker and colleagues,[5] dysphagia clinically manifests itself with complications arising during eating, drinking, and reduced secretion management. In addition to the physical consequences, dysphagia is also a disorder involving psychosocial and emotional complications for patients and families.[6] Dysphagia may lead to several complications, such as dehydration, malnutrition and weight loss, pulmonary complications, and pneumonia.[5]

The incidence and prevalence of dysphagia across health care settings varies. The American Speech-Language and Hearing Association reports that the epidemiologic studies indicate that the prevalence may be as high as 22% for individuals over age 50.[7] Reports indicate that 61% of adults with dysphagia are admitted to acute trauma centers; 41% are admitted to rehabilitation settings Thirty percent to 75% of patients reside in skilled nursing facilities, and 25% to 30% are admitted to hospitals.[7] The likelihood of dysphagia is more common in certain patient populations. In total, between 300,000 to 600,000 patients across the United States are afflicted with dysphagia yearly.[7] The prevalence of dysphagia in patients who have been diagnosed with stroke is 25% to 70%, with 10% to 30% of this population identified as having dysphagia with aspiration.[7] Other disorders with a high prevalence of dysphagia include traumatic brain injury, amyotrophic lateral sclerosis, Parkinson disease, and head and neck cancer.[7]

Within the last 2 decades, the health care industry has undergone a pivotal change in medical and technological advances. This progression has increased the number of dysphagic patients with medically complex diagnoses, such as pulmonary, circulatory, gastrointestinal, and neurologic involvement,[8] who are treated by the speech–language pathologist (SLP). The management of dysphagia in this population requires specialized training by the SLP, as well as a sophisticated understanding of diagnostic and treatment methods. As such, SLP treatment protocols and recommendations are a medically essential aspect of patient care.

IDENTIFICATION OF DYSPHAGIA

Approximately 10 million Americans are referred to SLPs yearly for evaluations of swallowing.[7] Evaluations to rule dysphagia can be conducted along the entire continuum of care: acute, rehabilitation unit, subacute rehabilitation, and the home setting. Early identification of dysphagia signs in the medical and rehabilitation settings is the responsibility of all members of the medical team. The speech pathologist within each clinical setting should educate the medical team on the early signs that would raise suspicion of a dysphagia diagnosis. The following clinical pearls can be incorporated into a patient's history and physical examination, upon admission, to any clinical setting. An answer of "yes" to one or more of the following questions may indicate that a patient is at high risk for a swallowing impairment; therefore, a referral to the SLP is strongly recommended (**Box 1**).

COMPERHENSIVE AND INTEGRATED SPEECH PATHOLOGY APPROACH

As a member of the health care team, the SLP serves a myriad of roles during the diagnosis of dysphagia. Routine dysphagia screening by the SLP may not always be possible. Therefore, the SLP needs to rely on the medical team for referrals when dysphagia is suspected. However, failure or incomplete screening of the patient's swallowing by the medical team may delay or prevent the initial referral to the SLP, placing the patient at risk for dysphagia related complications. To expedite this referral process, the SLP should also assume the role of educating the medical team on the clinical indicators as listed in **Box 1**. Once the initial referral is received, the SLP may begin using the comprehensive and integrated speech pathology approach, (CISPA), focusing on the patient as the nucleus of this model. The SLP's implementation of this approach will ensure effective dysphagia management, contributing to the safety of the patient. **Fig. 1** outlines the components of the CISPA, summarizing the process of evaluation, treatment, and education for patients, families, and the medical team, implemented by the SLP.

In settings where an SLP may not be readily available, not all CISPA components may be implemented. Therefore, it becomes the responsibility of the medical team to monitor the patient's safety with the prescribed diet, as well as document clinical indicators of the swallowing impairment. Dysphagia monitoring recommendations may include close monitoring of pulmonary status, laboratory tests, patient's weight, food intake, anecdotal reports of dysphagia-related complications.

Implementation of the CISPA encourages broad interdisciplinary communication between the SLP, the medical team, the patient, and the patient's family. When there is a breakdown of communication by the interdisciplinary team, medical errors may result. This breakdown may occur at any stage along the critical pathway detailed in **Fig. 2**, directly affecting the dysphagic patient's safety. It is essential that SLPs implement, encourage, and maintain a continuity of care and involvement with the patient after dysphagia has been diagnosed.

CRITICAL PATHWAYS LEADING TO MEDICAL ERRORS IMPACTING SAFETY FOR PATIENTS WITH DYSPHAGIA

Medical errors should be defined as failed processes that are linked to adverse outcomes.[9] The epidemiology of medical errors can be vast; however, human error was attributed to be the root cause according to the 2007 Joint Commission Report on Quality and Safety.[3] These findings led to the development of patient safety programs across medical institutions and settings. The acute rehabilitation setting should be considered the bond between the patient's hospital stay and the patient's

---

Box 1
Clinical indicators of a possible swallowing impairment

Does the patient have a previously documented dysphagia?

Does the patient have difficulty maintaining alertness during a meal?

Is the patient breathing with difficulty?

Does the patient have difficulty swallowing his or her secretions?

Does the patient have an open mouth posture with drooling?

Does the patient have difficulty swallowing and coughing on command?

Is the patient's voice wet–gurgly and congested?

Is the patient's speech slurred?

Does the patient report difficulty during a meal?

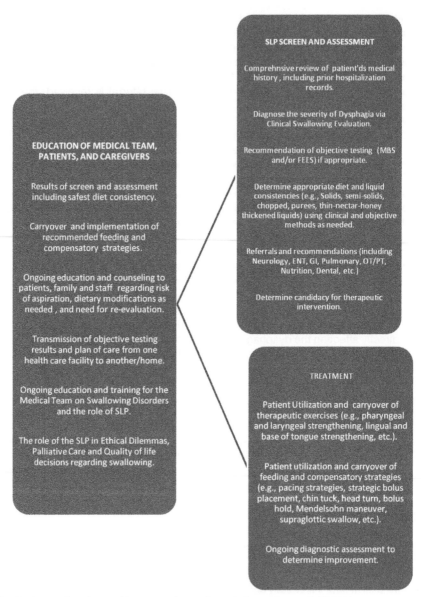

Fig. 1. Comprehensive and integrated speech pathology approach (CISPA).

recovery. However, the missing link for providing quality care may be the transition of patient care information from 1 institution to another. **Fig. 2** illustrates the sequence of patient events that may occur during the assessment and treatment phase, from admission to discharge. Additionally, **Fig. 2** illustrates medical errors that may arise when there is a breakdown in this cycle. As team members review the patient's hospital discharge and transfer information, they should not only focus on information that has been provided, but also on information that may have been omitted, such as previously conducted modified barium swallows (MBS) and fiberoptic endoscopic

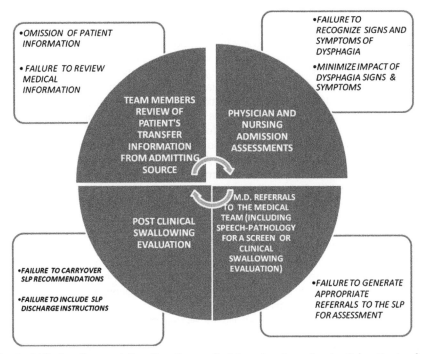

Fig. 2. Critical pathways delineating the medical team's role and potential patient safety risks for patients with dysphagia.

evaluation of swallowing (FEES). Omission of information regarding the patient's swallowing status will interfere with continuity of care and delay referrals to the SLP. In addition, this may also greatly impact patient safety. The following medical errors, including incorrectly prescribed diets, failure to continue dysphagia rehabilitation, and failure to use compensatory strategies as directed, may result in pulmonary compromise, choking, dehydration, weight loss, and the need for costly rehospitalization. The need for thorough reporting is essential, since the Joint Commission Standard (2009) states that the hospital discharge summary is the sole document mandated to report the patient's plan of care upon discharge to a posthospital setting.[7]

A retrospective study conducted by Kind and colleagues[10] examined omission of dysphagia recommendations from hospital discharge summaries from a large academic medical center from 2003 to 2005. The sample size consisted of 187 adult stroke, hip and/or pelvis, or hip–femur fractures. All final dysphagia recommendations from SLPs were abstracted, coded, and compared for each inpatient who received a dysphagia evaluation and was subsequently discharged to a subacute setting. Results illustrated that, in general, physicians completely omitted 45% of all SLP dysphagia recommendations. Physician omissions of SLP recommendations may have been attributed to concentration on physician-prescribed therapies rather than SLP recommendations.[10] Frequently omitted recommendations included postural and compensatory techniques, rehabilitative techniques, meal pacing, sizing and procedural techniques, medication and pill recommendations, care provider and communication recommendations, and environmental/other, in the final discharge patient summary. These omissions may increase the dysphagic patient's risk of dysphagia-related complications. Therefore, a multidisciplinary model revolving around a patient-centered care approach is recommended for patients from admission to discharge.

SLP's use of the CISPA may reduce the number of errors that occur in the critical pathway, resulting in improved safety for the dysphagic patient. Improving patient safety with implementation of CISPA components provides a guide for improved communication between SLPs, the physician, the medical staff, the patient, and the patient's caregivers. Improved communication between the physician and the speech pathologist may result in timelier evaluations for the patients, prescription of the safest diet consistency, and implementation of referrals and recommendations derived from the evaluation. Recommendations may also include the decision to maintain nonoral feeding for patients with severe dysphagia. When dysphagia is not readily remediated through alteration of diet and/or use of compensatory feeding strategies, alternative means of nutrition/hydration/medication are needed to maintain the highest level of patient safety. The expertise and immediate intervention of the SLP may aid in reducing the pulmonary complications that can arise from dysphagia and other related complications. Family and caregivers have an integral role in maintaining patient safety by implementing the compensatory feeding and swallow strategies as learned through interaction with the SLP. The recommendation for diet consistency should follow the patient as he or she transitions from 1 setting to another. The ultimate goal is a patient-centered approach, with the multidisciplinary team ensuring that accurate information is disseminated.

The study by Kind and colleagues[10] illustrates that important information is deleted from discharge summaries that accompany the patient from the acute care facility to the subacute setting. As previously discussed, the loss of this information interferes with a patient-centered, multidisciplinary approach. The discharge summary is the essential link between the acute care and rehabilitation settings. It should provide all of the essential information needed to ensure a safe transition from 1 facility to another. However, Kind noted, "Despite the critical communication role discharge summaries play, they are not standardized and often lack important components that experts recognize as crucial to insuring patient safety." Based on these findings, a movement away from a physician-driven discharge summary may be needed. To improve patient safety and interdisciplinary communication, a multidisciplinary discharge summary should be implemented. Every discipline involved in the patient's care would be responsible for outlining patient-specific recommendations, thereby optimizing patient safety. A transitional medical record can be created, which can travel with the patient as he or she is transferred from 1 setting to another. It can be accessed by the primary care physician as well as by the patient and his or her caregivers. In view of the fact that the discharge summary is the sole item mandated by the Joint Commission, it stands to reason that this document should be a more complex, descriptive record of the plan of care suggested by the medical team. In the care of the dysphagic patient, this document may reduce errors that occur when recommendations for specific diet consistency, compensatory feeding strategies, and caregiver modifications are omitted.

Errors of omission, as discussed by Kind and colleagues,[10] reveal that physicians are more likely to include physician-prescribed therapies rather than SLP recommendations in the discharge summary. In addition to the SLP's role of assessment and treatment planning for dysphagia patients, a further role in education of the medical team is critical. SLP's recommendations made for dysphagic patients are based on extensive knowledge and training. Furthering the knowledge of the medical team becomes a key component, ensuring that patient safety is addressed at all professional levels. Using the multidisciplinary model when formulating discharge summaries reduces the need for physicians to make choices regarding which patient care recommendations are most crucial. The ultimate goal of the multidisciplinary model will allow for all disciplines to report recommendations on the patient's transitional record.

SUMMARY

In the United States, 300,000 to 600,000 people are diagnosed with dysphagia.[7] Management of dysphagia requires a multidisciplinary team approach. Increasing interdisciplinary communication may provide the groundwork for decreasing medical errors and improving patient safety. The Institute for Healthcare Improvement reports increasing evidence that lack of communication between patients and caregivers may result in decreased quality of care and increased frequency of medical and fatal errors.[2] The health care industry has undergone important medical and technological advances over the past 2 decades. These changes have increased the number of dysphagic patients with medically complex diagnoses. This has prompted a transformation in the SLP's role in assessment, intervention, and education of patients, caregivers, and the medical team. Education of the medical team by the SLP is a key component. This may improve early identification of a swallowing impairment and may generate more timely referrals to the SLP. Discussed in this article is integrating a swallow screen in the medical team's initial assessment, which includes clinical indicators of a possible swallowing impairment.

This paper details the CISPA, providing a method for effectively evaluating and treating the dysphagia patient in an integrated format, involving the entire medical team. The CISPA may contribute to a reduction in communication breakdown between the multidisciplinary team. Inclusion of the patient, caregiver, and multidisciplinary team in the plan of care and discharge plan will foster a more holistic approach to patient care. As a result, a reduction of medical errors along the critical pathways may emerge, with improvement in patient safety. Further research is recommended investigating the benefits of a multidisciplinary approach to patient care, implementation of CISPA, and use of a standardized transitional patient discharge plans to determine improvement of patient safety for dysphagic patients.

REFERENCES

1. Geraghty K. Why do freshly minted doctors still recite the Hippocratic oath? 2000. Available at: http://www.ama-assn.org/amednews/2000/05/01/prca0501.htm. Accessed November 30, 2012.
2. Botwinick L, Bisognano M, Haraden C. Leadership guide to patient safety. IHI innovation series white paper. Camabridge (MA): Institute for Health Care Improvement; 2006.
3. Who Health Organization. WHO launches nine patient safety solutions. World Health Orangization-Media Centre; 2007. Available at: www.who.int/mediacentre/news/releases/2007/pr22/en/index.html. Accessed November 30, 2012.
4. The Joint Commission. Improving America's hospitals; Annual report of patient quality and safety. TJC Annual report 2007. Available at: www.jointcommission.org/assets/1/6/2007_Annual_Report.pdf. Accessed October 24, 2012.
5. Becker R, Nieczaj R, Egge K. Functional dysphagia therapy and PEG treatment in a clinical geriatric setting. Dysphagia 2011;28:108–16.
6. Bennett JW, Steele CM. Food for thought: The impact of dysphagia on quality of life. Perspectives on Swallowing and Swallowing Disorders (dysphagia) 2005;14:24–7.

7. Castrogiovanni A. Communication facts: Special populations: Dysphagia-2008 edition. ASHA. Available at: www.asha.org/Research/reports/dysphagia/. Accessed January 30, 2012.

8. Puntil-Sheltman J. Medically fragile patients: Fitting dysphagia into the bigger clinical picture. The ASHA Leader 2002. Available at: http://www.asha.org/Publications/leader/2002/021008/021008.htm. Accessed October 24, 2012.

9. Hofer TP, Kerr EA, Hayward RA. What is an error? Eff Clin Pract 2000;3:261–9.

10. Kind A, Anderson P, Hind J. Omission of dysphagia therapies in hospital discharge communications. Dysphagia 2011;26:49–61.

Safety Considerations for Patients with Communication Disorders in Rehabilitation Medicine Settings

Adrian Cristian, MD, MHCM[a],*, Claudia Giammarino, MS, CCC-SLP[b],
Michael Olds, MD[a], Elizabeth Adams, MA, CCC-SLP[b],
Christina Moriarty, MS[b], Sabina Ratner, BS[a],
Shruti Mural, BSc[a], Eric C. Stobart, BS[a]

KEYWORDS

• Communication • Patient safety • Rehabilitation medicine

More than 2 million people in the United States have a communication disorder that prevents them from communicating effectively. Communication disorders can be caused by congenital (cerebral palsy), acquired (stroke, brain injury, spinal cord injury, or cancer), or degenerative (amyotrophic lateral sclerosis or muscular dystrophy) conditions.[1]

People with complex communication needs are often seen in rehabilitation settings. They can present with (1) speech that is difficult to understand, (2) problems with comprehension of what is being said to them, and (3) problems making their needs known.[2] Other etiologies may include language barriers and hearing and vision impairments. This "communication-vulnerable state" can result in feelings of frustration, distress, misdiagnosis, and unrecognized pain.[3] In a 6-year study (1997–2002), the Joint Commission on Accreditation in Health Care Organizations attributed "communication" as the root cause of "sentinel events" in hospitals that were associated with unnecessary extended hospital stays and death.[4]

[a] Department of Rehabilitation Medicine, Kingsbrook Rehabilitation Institute, Kingsbrook Jewish Medical Center, 585 Schenectady Avenue, Brooklyn, NY 11203, USA
[b] Department of Speech-Language Pathology and Audiology, The Kingsbrook Jewish Rehabilitation Institute, Kingsbrook Jewish Medical Center, 585 Schenectady Avenue, Brooklyn, NY 11203, USA
* Corresponding author.
E-mail address: acristian@kingsbrook.org

Phys Med Rehabil Clin N Am 23 (2012) 343–347
doi:10.1016/j.pmr.2012.02.017
1047-9651/12/$ – see front matter © 2012 Elsevier Inc. All rights reserved.

pmr.theclinics.com

Effective communication skills are vital to a successful life for all individuals. Communication disorders can have a significant impact on the affected person's school, work, and social relationships.[5]

TYPES OF COMMUNICATION DISORDERS

There are several varieties of communication disorders that one may encounter in the practice of rehabilitation medicine, including (1) language disorders, (2) motor speech disorders, (3) cognitive-communication disorders, (4) deafness or hearing impaired, and (5) language barriers.[5] The first two are briefly described next.

Language disorders are characterized by impaired comprehension or use of spoken and written language. The most common type of language-based communication disorders are classified as aphasias. Aphasia is a communication disorder that is acquired following brain insult. The primary cause of aphasia is a cerebral vascular accident (CVA). Aphasia hinders a person's ability to comprehend and express language. It may also affect areas of the nervous system that are involved with information processing, memory, thinking, and other higher level language functions (eg, problem solving and abstract reasoning).[6] The physiology of cortical function and its specialization is poorly understood. The exact differences between the right and left hemispheres are entirely understood. Language and fine motor function (eg, writing) are controlled by the language dominant hemisphere, the left hemisphere in 95% of right-handed individuals and 70% of left-handed individuals.[7] Aphasias are common in stroke patients and those with brain injuries. It is estimated that approximately 1 million people in the United States are living with an aphasia[5,8] and approximately 80,000 individuals acquire aphasia each year.[5,8] Language disorders can also be seen in adults who failed to develop normal language because of impaired hearing or developmental disorders.[5]

Motor speech disorders may result from neurologic diagnoses, including stroke, neuromuscular disease, developmental neurologic disorders, and obstructive neurologic lesions. Motor speech disorders can affect articulatory precision, voice, fluency, and resonance. Motor speech disorders can also differ in severity. Depending on the level of severity, motor speech disorders can significantly impact communication between the patient and the entire medical staff. Conditions that can lead to hindered communication include Parkinson disease, Huntington disease, and amyotrophic lateral sclerosis. In certain neuromuscular diseases, communication may progressively deteriorate until speech is no longer an available mode of communication.

IMPACT OF IMPAIRED COMMUNICATION ON PATIENT SAFETY

There are several characteristics and challenges common to hospitalized adult patients with communication disorders, which may have a major impact on their safety. These patients are faced with the challenge of effectively communicating personal needs and medical information to medical staff. After an acute stroke or traumatic brain injury, patients with associated cognitive impairment or aphasia are at risk for further preventable injuries. This is especially important in patients who show clinical signs of functional and cognitive impairment, but are unaware of their own physical limitations. They may not be able to adequately understand when physicians and nurses instruct them to ask for assistance with feeding, dressing needs, transfers, or toileting. This in turn can potentially lead to a fall within the room when the patient is alone.

Patients may also find it difficult to verbally express their symptoms to clinical staff. This presents a challenge for symptom management, such as pain. Obtaining an accurate medical history can be a challenge if the patient cannot provide key information. Healthcare professionals have to rely on close family members or charted documents from other facilities to obtain an accurate medical history.[9] If this information is not correct, pertinent items may be missing, which in turn can affect the patient's safety (ie, medication errors, allergic reactions, and inaccurate diagnosis).

Monitoring effectiveness of treatment for a disease can also be limited by the communication barrier. There may be situations in which patients with impaired communication have questions or concerns about a particular medical treatment. If the patient cannot communicate the concern, he or she may not be able to effectively participate in their plan of care. Patients may not understand the reason for taking a medication and therefore choose not to take it, or alternatively not take it in a safe manner. Without proper communication and expressed understanding between patient and physician, preventative or prophylactic treatment can become difficult, ineffective, and unsafe.

Patient care transition points, such as transfers between hospitals, services, attending physicians, and nurses, rely on discharge summaries and medical records for safety protection.[9,10] Patients with communication disorders can have a difficult time describing their concerns and symptoms as they move through the healthcare system.

ASSESSMENT OF THE PATIENT WITH COMMUNICATION DISORDER

It is important that the clinician evaluating a patient in a communication-vulnerable state obtain information from the patient's family, caregiver, or other clinicians whom have cared for that patient in the past. Key information includes (1) appropriate communication strategies that they have used to communicate with the patient, (2) the patient's daily routine, (3) sources of agitation for the patient, and (4) calming influences when the patient is upset.

The physical examination of the patient with a communication disorder should be performed in a quiet area. The clinician should use a calm tone of voice, face the patient, and make good eye contact. Appropriate communication aids used by the patient should be available (ie, hearing aids or prior augmentative communication systems). In many healthcare facilities, a Language Line may be available to facilitate translation to the patient's native language if a personal translator is not available.

Key elements of the physical examination (focusing on communication, cognitive-communication, and swallowing) include (1) mini mental status examination; (2) cognition level of orientation and alertness, immediate and delayed recall, and executive function; (3) hearing and vision testing (including the use of eyeglasses and hearing aids); (4) speech–language communication of basic activities of daily living wants and needs; (5) swallow screen determining risk of dysphagia (described elsewhere in this issue); and (6) upper airway assessment.

The communication screen is very useful. This screen identifies the communicative status of the patient. If the patient can verbally communicate, key questions to consider include the following: (1) Is the patient's speech intelligible? (2) Is the patient's voice strained, hoarse, or hypophonic? (3) Can the patient follow one- or two-step commands? (4) Can the patient answer yes/no questions accurately?

If the patient cannot verbally communicate, key questions to consider include the following: (1) Can the patient follow one- and two-step commands? (2) Can the patient respond to yes/no questions accurately by gesturing or eye-blink tracking? (3) Is the patient able to write? (4) Is the patient able to see without restrictions? (5) Does the patient have volitional movement of fingers, head, and eyes?

If the patient is noted to be at high risk, he or she should be referred to a speech language pathologist for further evaluation and treatment interventions. Ideally, treatment strategies are individualized for each patient. Timely identification of communication impairments permits effective environmental modifications to be implemented by the medical team. This minimizes the risk of medical errors. Speech pathologists can also evaluate the patient for augmentative and alternative communication devices and training. The evaluation may include whether the patient can use facial expressions, body language, gestures, pointing to words or photographs, line drawing, picture or word communication boards, electronic communication systems, and integrated computer software that facilitates word processing and communication.[2]

STRATEGIES TO MINIMIZE SAFETY RISKS IN INDIVIDUALS WITH COMMUNICATION DISORDERS

Strategies to minimize safety risk in this patient population have been described in the literature. An "On the Spot Communication" tool kit developed by Pearson and McBride outlines some key components: (1) use of word and picture boards; (2) modified call bells; (3) pocket amplifier of speech (for people who do not have their hearing aids with them); (4) writing boards and pen; and (5) a magnifying glass for people who do not have their eyeglasses.[11]

Iacono and Johnson[2] described additional strategies that can be used when clinicians communicate with patients who are in a communication-vulnerable state:

1. Allow ample time for the patient to express and address any and all concerns they may have about their condition or treatment.
2. Allow ample time the patient to comprehend and process information delivered by the medical team.
3. Provide the patient with written information to support verbal discussion.
4. Speak slowly, in short sentences, and avoid the use of jargon.
5. When a language barrier is present between the patient and medical team, use of in-hospital interpreters or interpreting services can be helpful.
6. Corroborate the patient's medical history, disease or hospital course, comorbid conditions, medications, and treatments provided with clinicians who know the patient well.
7. Notify all treating staff about the patient's communication disorder.
8. Identify nonverbal communication that the patient is trying to use. These may include facial and body expressions. For example, pointing to the mouth can indicate hunger or thirst, and agitated behavior can signal an internal complaint, such as distended bladder.
9. Ask short simple questions or closed-ended questions that can be answered by "yes/no" responses. Limit the choices offered to a patient to minimize confusion, and check for comprehension.
10. Clinicians should use their own body language and gestures to instruct the patient.
11. Patients using hearing aids should have these devices checked for proper function and continued effectiveness of the device in correcting the hearing deficit.
12. Clinicians should validate the patient's frustration.
13. Clinical staff should try to anticipate the patient's needs (ie, thirst or hunger).
14. Clinicians should repeat back what the patient stated to make sure that the clinician understands what the patient is trying to communicate.
15. Clinicians should understand how patients with augmentative and alternative communication devices are using these devices to communicate.

16. Clinicians should become comfortable with long periods of silence during the communication. The patient may require more time to process information and formulate responses.

SUMMARY

The accurate transmission of information from the patient to the medical team is essential for patient safety. However, many patients admitted to a healthcare facility may be in a communication-vulnerable state. This vulnerability can be the result of a variety of different impairments, including speech, language, hearing, and cognition. It becomes the responsibility of the medical team to modify the environment to obtain the most successful communication between staff and patient. The speech pathologist plays an essential role in assisting with these patients by implementing treatment strategies, environmental modifications, and staff education directed at understanding this population. The investment of time and energy by the medical staff may improve the emotional and physical comfort of these patients, and ultimately the safety of these vulnerable patients.

REFERENCES

1. American Speech-Language-Hearing Association. Information for AAC Users. 2012. Available at: http://www.asha.org/public/speech/disorders/InfoAACUsers. htm. Accessed February 15, 2012.
2. Iacono T, Johnson H. Patients with disabilities and complex communication needs: the GP consultation. Aust Fam Physician 2004;33(8):585–9.
3. Patak L, Wilson-Stronks A, Costello J, et al. Communication access within healthcare environments: a call to action. Improving patient-provider communication: a call to action 2009;39(9):372–6.
4. Pressman H, Emily N. Communication access within healthcare environments. A call for action. Patient provider communication, 1997-2012. 2012. Available at: http://www.patientprovidercommunication.org/index.cfm/article_3.htm. Accessed February 15, 2012.
5. Castrogiovanni A. Incidence and prevalence of speech, voice, and language disorders in adults in the United States: 2008 edition. Rockville (MD): American Speech-Language-Hearing Association; 2008.
6. LaPointe L. Aphasia and related neurogenic language disorders. 3rd edition. New York: Thieme; 2005.
7. Davis L, King M, Schultz J. Fundamentals of neurologic disease. New York: Demos Medical Publishing, Inc; 2005.
8. The National Institute on Deafness and other Communication Disorders. Aphasia. NIH; 2008. Available at: http://www.nidcd.nih.gov/health/voice/pages/aphasia. aspx. Accessed February 18, 2012.
9. Giammarino C, Adams E, Moriarty C. Safety concerns and multi-disciplinary management of the dysphagic patient. Phys Med Rehabil Clin N Am 2012.
10. Kind A, Anderson P, Hind J. Omission of dysphagia therapies in hospital discharge communications. Dysphagia 2011;26:49–61.
11. Available at: www.aactechconnect.com. Accessed February 15, 2012.

Patient Safety in Rehabilitation Medicine: Traumatic Brain Injury

Ajit B. Pai, MD[a,b,*], Yevgeny Zadov, DO[a], Allison Hickman, DO[b]

KEYWORDS

- Patient safety • Rehabilitation • Traumatic brain injury • Military
- Medical error • Communication • Medication reconciliation

Traumatic brain injury (TBI) contributes to a substantial number of deaths and cases of permanent disability. TBI is a contributing factor for close to a third (30.5%) of all injury-related deaths in the United States.[1] It is estimated that, on average, approximately 1.7 million people sustain a TBI annually; of these, 52,000 die, 275,000 are hospitalized, and 1.365 million (nearly 80%) are treated and released from an emergency department.[1] Adults aged 75 years and older have the highest rates of TBI-related hospitalization and death.[1] In every age group, TBI rates are higher for men than for women. In addition, boys aged 0 to 4 years have the highest rates of TBI-related emergency department visits, hospitalizations, and deaths. Within the civilian population about one-third of all TBI is caused by falls and 26.5% are caused by assault or other sources of impact other than motor vehicle accidents. Motor vehicle accidents account for another 17% of TBI, leaving 21% without an identified cause.[1]

In the general population, direct and indirect costs of TBI, such as lost productivity, totaled an estimated $55 billion to $60 billion in the United States in 2000.[1,2] However, the true cost of caring for patients with TBI is difficult to estimate because mild TBI (mTBI) in the context of other life or limb threatening injuries is thought to be under-reported.[3] The Centers for Disease Control and Prevention estimates the average

Funding sources: None.
Conflict of interest: None.
[a] Polytrauma, Hunter Holmes McGuire VA Medical Center, 1201 Broad Rock Boulevard, Richmond, VA 23249, USA
[b] Department of Physical Medicine and Rehabilitation, Virginia Commonwealth University, PO Box 980661, Richmond, VA 23298, USA
* Corresponding author. Polytrauma, Hunter Holmes McGuire VA Medical Center, 1201 Broad Rock Boulevard, Richmond, VA 23249.
E-mail address: ajit.pai@va.gov

Phys Med Rehabil Clin N Am 23 (2012) 349–370
doi:10.1016/j.pmr.2012.02.009   pmr.theclinics.com
1047-9651/12/$ – see front matter Published by Elsevier Inc.

lifetime cost of caring for a severely injured patient with TBI to be between $600,000 and $1.875 million.[4] A recent prospective cohort study of patients in a large managed care organization found that the average cost of care for patients who suffered an mTBI to be 76% higher over 3 years after injury than the costs incurred by an age-matched and sex-matched cohort of injured patients without brain injury. For moderate to severe TBI, this cost was reported at 5.75 times greater than that of non–brain-injured patients. Moreover, they noted that concomitant presence of psychiatric illness further increases the cost of care to greater than 3 times the cost of treating brain-injured patients without psychiatric illness.[5] This additional cost can be significant; research has shown that both mild and moderate to severe TBI are associated with an increased risk of subsequent psychiatric disease.[6,7]

Management of patient safety issues with regard to TBI are divided into phases of treatment and also by the types of error that can occur. The phases include the acute medical setting, including the emergency room and field evaluation, intensive care units (ICU), and general medical floors, inpatient rehabilitation facilities (IRF), transitional rehabilitation units, skilled nursing facilities (SNF) and posthospitalization follow-up. Within each of those settings, errors affecting patient safety can stem from patient assessment, medical and procedure errors, errors related to communication, and system-related issues. Each dimension can use general and specific methods to minimize patient risk and reduce errors, which will ideally lead to improved overall patient safety (**Box 1**).

[Tags: Traumatic brain injury, rehabilitation, epidemiology, prevalence, incidence, economic costs, p safety].

PATIENT SAFETY AFTER BRAIN INJURY: ACUTE MEDICAL CENTERS

In the acute trauma setting, several elements must be considered. First, emergency medical service technicians require adequate training in trauma assessment and evaluation with specific consideration for brain injury. For instance, their ability to appropriately document specific medical information related to TBI, such as the Glasgow Coma Scale and loss of consciousness, ultimately assists brain injury specialists to more accurately prognosticate patient recovery.[8] Communication between emergency response staff and emergency department personnel is important in the safe treatment of a patient with TBI. This communication is vital in preparing the team for management of expected injuries, as well as enabling primary trauma teams to have appropriate specialists available at the time of initial hospital evaluation.[9] Effective communication is an overriding theme in the successful implementation of safety culture throughout the health care continuum. According to the Joint Commission on Accreditation of Healthcare Organizations (JCAHO), almost 70% of all sentinel events

---

Box 1
Types of medical errors

- Communication
- Medication use/delivery
- Failure to escalate care
- Management of lines/tubes
- Skin assessment
- Environmental controls

are caused by breakdown in communication.[10] It is well documented that effective communication between team members is associated with lessened workloads, improved clinical outcomes, reduced adverse drug events, reduced patient morbidity, and improved job satisfaction and retention, all of which ultimately translate into improved patient safety and satisfaction (**Box 2**).[11–13]

Errors leading to a compromise of patient safety may begin in the field and thus alter emergency room evaluation and management. Such errors may include missed or inadequately managed injuries, inadequate or inappropriate use of field medications or stabilization techniques/devices, delay in transport, or transport to a facility not equipped to manage a specific level of injury. In the context of traumatic injury, when multiple systems may be affected and in need of urgent treatment, the ability to effectively triage the injuries is integral to timely and appropriate management. For this purpose, algorithms and clinical care pathways have been established, both in the United States and abroad,[14,15] to standardize prehospital and in-hospital emergent treatment of traumatic injuries including TBI. Likewise, in an effort to improve patient safety in the emergency room setting, the American College of Emergency Physicians and Centers for Disease Control and Prevention[16] have published specific recommendations for neuroimaging and decision making in individuals with mTBI. Prehospital and in-hospital clinicians rely on accurate history in the diagnosis and management of all patients; unclear histories provided by witnesses, emergency responders, or an obtunded patient can be a cause of medical error. Because of the chaotic environment in which traumatic injuries occur, protocols that outline specific triage and management of these patients can be integral to patient safety by ensuring not only appropriate medical management but also adequate documentation and communication during the course of the trauma evaluation and care delivery. These protocols are unique to each emergency management and hospital system based on available resources but should include, at a minimum, information recommended by national guidelines to effectively manage patients throughout their emergent course and across care continuums.

In addition to establishing hospital-specific protocols, other sources for improvement in patient safety have to be considered. It has been shown that neuroradiologists and neurosurgeons have good inter-rater reliability with regard to diagnosis of brain disorders.[17] However, when these vital personnel are not available for urgent evaluation of clinical imaging, there may be a decline in correct diagnosis of brain disorders. We recommend that institutions providing emergency care have neuroradiologists and neurosurgeons available in the critical first few hours after patient arrival. Misreading of radiological imaging leads to missed disorders, which produces complications such as vasospasm or herniation. Chang and colleagues[18] (2006) showed

---

Box 2
Key points of history and physical examination

- Documentation of wounds
- Medication reconciliation
- Allergy assessment
- Injury inventory
- Cognitive and physical function
- Previous level of function
- Review of radiologic and laboratory data

progression of intracranial lesion within the first 24 hours; therefore, the head computed tomography (CT) should be repeated approximately 24 hours after injury. In the interim, serial neurologic assessment should be used to evaluate for changes.

In the acute medical center, medication reconciliation is paramount in the traumatically brain-injured patient. Medications used in the acute care setting often cause slowing of cognitive recovery. Sedating medications such as opiates, anticholinergics, dopamine blockers, H_2 blockers and central-acting α-1 antagonists should be avoided, unless there is no other option. In addition, patients with TBI in the ICU setting are often sedated and on ventilators. For these patients, it is important to minimize the risk of pressure wounds by implementing hospital policies that address this specific concern (ie, daily skin evaluation, turning patients every 2 hours, protective dressings). Positioning of patients is also important, because spasticity can start early after injury. Treatment options such as range-of-motion exercises, specialty boots, or bracing can help reduce the development of contractures caused by spasticity. In addition, these patients are at risk for infection, namely pneumonia, urinary tract infection, and intravenous (IV) line infection. Routine evaluation and timely removal of indwelling urinary catheters or IV lines reduce the rate of urinary tract infection and IV line infection. In addition, occult surveillance for fracture, deep vein thrombosis, peripheral nerve injuries, or entrapments should be undertaken because they can be missed on the initial screen when lifesaving treatment is initiated (**Box 3**).

Patients with TBI often undergo neurosurgical intervention. As part of that intervention, a critical safety factor is the role of anticoagulation. Perioperative anticoagulation has not been studied in a rigorous and prospective fashion.[19] General contraindications to the use of heparin and heparinlike products include recent severe head injury, recent craniotomy, coagulopathic patients, intracranial hemorrhage, bleeding ulcer or other inaccessible bleeding sites, uncontrolled hypertension, severe hepatic or renal disease, and use less than 4 to 6 hours before an invasive procedure. The management of

---

Box 3
Key patient safety risk factors

- Communication deficits
- Medications
- Cognitive and functional deficits
- Mobility aids
- Bacterial infection/colonization
- Agitation/combativeness
- Bowel and bladder management
- Skin monitoring
- Nutritional needs
- Medications to avoid:
  - Opiates
  - Anticholinergics
  - Dopamine blockers
  - H_2 blockers
  - Central-acting α-1 antagonists

anticoagulation after cranial surgery also does not have specific recommendations; however, our institution uses the following guidelines: (1) no treatment or prophylactic dosing for venous thromboembolism (VTE) on postoperative day (POD) zero; (2) initiation of prophylactic dose, subcutaneous unfractionated heparin on POD 1 to 2, if postoperative head CT is without hemorrhage; (3) repeat head CT to evaluate progress; (4) initiation of therapeutic-dose anticoagulation on day 10 to 14 for known VTE, if no contraindication.

Intracranial hypertension is a common neurologic complication in patients with traumatic head injury. Rangel-Castillo and Robertson[20] detailed the management of intracranial pressure (ICP) in a 2006 review article. Although literature surrounding optimal methods for control of increased cerebral pressure is constantly evolving, it remains one of the most important factors in maintaining patient safety in the acute phase of patient care. Appropriate management of blood glucose can also play a significant role in maintenance of patient safety. Clinical trials support the correlation between hyperglycemia and poor overall outcome in patients with head injuries.[21] Therefore, every effort should be made to maintain euglycemia in individuals with TBI. Fevers, hypotension, and other metabolic abnormalities should be carefully managed in patients with TBI, because these are known to decrease cerebral healing and increase morbidity and mortality in patients with brain injury.[22]

ICUs are places of increased stimulus because of the number of staff, equipment, sounds, and so forth. It is well documented that agitation and delirium can increase in these settings because of the intensity of stimulation.[23–25] Agitation in the ICU setting can often lead to the use of restraints. One study found restraints were used in more than 48% of patients in the ICU.[26] Because individuals with TBI are often unable to communicate and are at high risk for agitation, there is risk of overuse of mechanical restraints. However, in patients with TBI, the use of restraints can increase agitation, which can lead to a cyclical treatment paradigm. Thus it is best to create guidelines for the use of restraints in each medical setting. Lombard and Zafonte[23] (2005) described mechanisms to reduce agitation in the patient with brain injury in the ICU setting. These mechanisms can be referenced when implementing agitation management plans to reduce the use of restraints.

Medical facilities providing acute patient care for the brain-injured patient should implement educational, multidisciplinary and interdisciplinary committees to establish best practices as appropriate for all staff involved in the management of these patients. Such action aids in increasing and maintaining patient safety and serves to provide open lines of communication should acute medical issues and complications arise.

[Tags: patient safety, acute medical center, emergency department, intensive care unit (ICU), neuroimaging, anticoagulation, intracranial pressure (ICP), agitation].

PATIENT SAFETY AFTER BRAIN INJURY: IRF

Just as in the ICU setting, there are many challenges to creating and maintaining an effective and efficient environment of safety on an inpatient rehabilitation unit. Successful patient care and progression through the rehabilitation process requires close coordination and participation by all members of the rehabilitation team, medical and ancillary consultants, as well as family and caregivers. However, the synchronization and mobilization of the large number of interdependent processes and resources needed to sustain an environment of safety on a busy rehabilitation unit are rarely optimal. As such, evolving systems of patient care and care coordination must have a core of patient safety standards and provider accountability to which all members of the rehabilitation team not only adhere but contribute. This unique team approach, although integral to patient recovery, brings with it multiple challenges and increases the probability for error if not closely monitored and actively managed.

The variety of diagnoses present in patients on the inpatient brain injury rehabilitation unit also creates unique challenges. Likewise, constructing a culture of safety in this environment is increasingly difficult because of higher populations of medically complex patients, increasing nurse/patient ratios, and the impetus for shorter rehabilitation stays and cost containment with implementation of prospective reimbursement by diagnosis-related groups. Furthermore, management of life-threatening and limb-threatening medical comorbidities must occur in the context of progressive physical challenges with the ultimate goal of maximizing functional recovery to benefit both medical and financial efficiency. Because of this, therapeutic goals must be closely coordinated to account for medical, functional, and nutritional needs that mandate flexibility during therapeutic progression. This attention and coordination must be in place from admission to discharge, and often well after, to ensure patients successfully transition their recovery to the outpatient setting. An overview of maintaining an environment of safety while addressing the medical and therapeutic challenges involved in the care of inpatient rehabilitation patients with brain injury is presented later.

As mentioned earlier, effective communication as described by the JCAHO is of utmost importance. The IRF is a unique setting that differs from acute and long-term care in the types of clinical issues faced, team composition and interaction, the higher involvement of rehabilitation professionals, and the greater involvement of patients and family members within a patient-centered care model.[27] Communication in this context must effectively flow bidirectionally from clinical therapy staff to patients and family to create a culture of safety that minimizes medical error and maximizes functional recovery. The IRF is often the last step before transitioning home, which builds a need for thorough education of patients and family members in the nuances of TBI rehabilitation and recovery. For example, the level of supervision a patient requires is of utmost importance in early discussion with family members. This discussion facilitates timely disposition and allows preparation of family and caregivers regarding the needs of the patient on return home or other discharge facility.

Inpatients in rehabilitation and their families/caregivers expect that they will not only receive quality health care during their recovery but also that they will not be harmed in the process. However, unavoidable complications do occur, and patients may also be injured because of preventable medical errors. A primary goal of ongoing patient safety is the recognition and timely management of medical errors so that they do not progress to medical injury. Many studies have documented that most morbidity and mortality from medical error is related to the use or misuse of medications and adverse drug events. Although patients in IRFs can be medically and functionally complex, providing more individualized, focused, and hands-on care often affords rehabilitation practitioners the opportunity to monitor more closely for incidents or actions that may lead to medical error. Nevertheless, complications do occur and, although there are no specific data identifying the rates of morbidity and mortality caused by medical error in the IRF, vigilance to decrease the opportunity for error can be fostered by the existing team approach to care. This approach includes universal precautions such as patient identification, checking for drug allergies, medication doses and forms, proper documentation and diligent surveillance of support lines, as well as rehabilitation-specific precautions such as proper use and maintenance of therapy equipment, mobility and orthotic devices (including restraints), dietary restrictions for dysphagic patients, and bowel and bladder management.

Medical errors can occur as isolated events or as the result of a chain of events, the latter becoming more common as more individuals are involved in the delivery of care, as is the case during rehabilitation. Minimizing error, in that human error is impossible to completely eliminate, involves ongoing, evolving, and tiered education so that all members of the rehabilitation team do not only act as an authority in their area of expertise but also as facilitators of information sharing to best meet each individual patient's needs. As such, it is imperative to have systems in place that not only prevent primary errors (education, proper documentation, organization) but also to prevent secondary errors (coordination or redundancy) by personnel as well as proper use of supplies, electronic and written records, and equipment.

In the IRF, medical errors that adversely affect patient outcomes could occur before admission, especially in the context of polytrauma and/or prolonged hospitalization with complex medical issues or severe debility. As stated earlier in this article, a thorough initial medical assessment and physical documentation is integral to initiating a successful recovery. This assessment includes a comprehensive review of previous diagnoses and interventions as well as review of medications, laboratory values, and radiographs. This task can be daunting, especially if the patient is coming from a noncontiguous facility. Although there are scant published data on delay of diagnoses, the incidence of such could have a great impact on patient safety. For example, fractures, pain, infections, metabolic derangements, nutritional deficiencies, end-organ damage, hydrocephalus, subclinical seizures, blood dyscrasias, and pressure sores are just a few of the things that may go unrecognized or undertreated before rehabilitation. If not recognized and addressed, all of these could affect the patient's potential for therapeutic participation and progression and, at worst, result in further injury or decline in function. In the setting of TBI, any missed or delayed diagnosis can be exacerbated by the inability of the patient to effectively communicate needs. Also, diseases that are not overtly visible may first present as change in sensorium, including agitation, which can place the patient at greater risk for injury or failure to progress.

Medication management is also integral to therapeutic participation and recovery and includes proper use, delivery, and monitoring. It is estimated that adverse drug events injure or kill more than 770,000 hospitalized patients annually.[28] Although no stratification is made regarding specific incidents during inpatient rehabilitation, the potential for medication mismanagement, especially if the patient is being transferred from an outside facility, is theoretically high. Documentation of drug and other allergies may also be difficult in this context, and the consequences of not knowing that information before initiating certain treatments could be dire. It is common for patients to come to the rehabilitation unit on multiple medications that have been changed in dosage or frequency from their home use or for which they previously had no need. These medications may include sedating medications or as-needed medications that may or may not be indicated once the patient has progressed to a less acute recovery phase. Medication reconciliation using a list of the patient's prehospital medications, current medications, patient (or family) interview, and, if possible, discussion with the referring medical or surgical service is the best way to prevent medication errors on admission. More than 40% of medication errors are thought to result from inadequate reconciliation in hand-offs during admission, transfer, and discharge of patients.[29] Of these errors, about 20% are thought to result in harm.[29,30] Many of these errors could be averted if formal medication reconciliation processes were in place. Polypharmacy in individuals with TBI can have dire consequences. For example, patients can suffer from worsening sleep-wake cycle disruption if they are placed on stimulants without understanding why the patient is having difficulty with arousal during the day. Likewise, medication for agitation can mask underlying injury, somatic or visceral pain, or chaining intracranial process. Before adding medications, it is best to evaluate the environment, accurately document the patient's daily behavior and response to current treatment. It is our recommendation that each brain injury rehabilitation facility formalize a medication reconciliation process to improve patient safety.

Posttraumatic epilepsy (PTE) is a well-recognized complication that generally occurs within 5 years after TBI. The incidence of PTE typically correlates with the severity of injury. Because poorly controlled epilepsy produces medical and social complications and uncontrolled seizures can be fatal, it is integral to patient safety that members of the rehabilitation team are not only familiar with the incidence and associated risk factors for PTE but also have some understanding of the acute and chronic management of seizure disorder. Medical complications caused by PTE are numerous and include alterations in neuronal connections that can lead to further/more severe seizures; aspiration, which can lead to pneumonia; heart rate and blood pressure changes; and disruption of respiratory and body temperature control. Likewise, seizure activity can cause injury through trauma, hyperthermia, hypoxemia, and further neuronal loss, all of which can have a dramatic impact on functional outcome.[31]

Patients also often present to the rehabilitation unit with tracheostomies, gastrointestinal or urologic ostomies and support lines such as peripherally inserted central catheters (PICC), peripheral intravenous catheters, feeding tubes, ports, shunts, fistulas, and urinary catheters. It is important to not only know when these devices were placed, but for what purpose, and to determine whether they need to be monitored, replaced, or discontinued. Medical staff knowledge of specialized medical equipment may also come into play on some specialized units, such as with the delivery of chemotherapeutic agents. Likewise, timely communication with the referring service that may have placed and/or managed the device or line previously is integral to patient safety.

Infection control is a ubiquitous challenge to patient health and safety in the general hospital setting but can be even more so in the IRF. Hospital acquired infections (HAI) have been estimated at approximately 1.7 million per year, resulting in approximately 98,000 deaths, more than 13,000 of these from urinary tract infection alone.[32] HAIs are among the most common adverse events in health care.[33] Methicillin-resistant *Staphylococcus aureus* (MRSA) and *Clostridium difficile* are two of the most prominent health care–associated infections and represent a major source of avoidable morbidity and mortality. Rates of MRSA isolates as high as 40% have been reported in US hospitals.[34] Patients generally participate in multiple therapies outside their hospital rooms, often in group settings, and using multiuse equipment. Infection control in this environment takes education of staff, patients, and family caregivers of the hospital and unit policy for specific pathogens. Extra care also must be taken to disinfect equipment such as therapy mats, multiuse orthotic devices, and assistive railings that can act as fomites. The community environment of the inpatient unit mandates even closer monitoring of high-risk patients such as those with compromised immune systems, open surgical wounds, or external fixation devices. Coordination of therapy interventions for these patients to avoid infectious transmission relies on effective communication from the medical team and implementation of simple but effective barriers to disease transmission, such as hand washing, proper use of disinfectant foams and gels, and selecting and disposing of appropriate barrier garments. In 2001, Mylotte and colleagues[35] evaluated the frequency of nosocomial infections in 493 consecutive admissions to a university-associated acute rehabilitation unit. They found that the most common infections were urinary tract infection, which accounted for 29.8% of the 94 nosocomial infections, followed by surgical site infection (17%), C difficile diarrhea (15%), and bloodstream infection (12.8%). Overall, 31 (26.5%) of 117 bacterial isolates from nosocomial infections showed antibiotic resistance. Nosocomial bacterial colonization and infection poses a significant health and safety risk to patients in the IRF and prevention requires a multifaceted approach involving everyone from the medical and therapy staff to pharmacy, laboratory, and environmental staff.

Interventional procedures performed on some rehabilitation units also present opportunity for medical error and the compromise of patient safety. Trigger point injections are minimally invasive and can provide focal muscular pain relief that allows improved range of motion and less stressful therapeutic interventions. Although generally safe, complications do occur and proper patient selection should include review of current medications, use of anticoagulants, patient tolerance of needles, and previous procedures. Vasovagal syncope, skin infection, pneumothorax, needle breakage, and hematoma formation are some of the documented adverse events.[36] Spasticity is also commonly seen on the rehabilitation unit after brain injury. Botulinum toxin and, less commonly, phenol injection can be used to lessen the pain and functional burden caused by spasticity. Although generally well tolerated and beneficial, a broad range of adverse outcomes has been reported and should be considered.[37] The safety implications of other invasive procedures that carry their own individual risks must also be considered, such as implanted intrathecal drug delivery system management and refills, PEG, tracheostomy and PICC line removal, pressure ulcer debridement, and suture/staple removal.

The emphasis on increasing patient mobility and independence also presents patient safety risks, especially when the patient has weight-bearing restrictions, delicate wounds, balance deficits, impulsivity, or decreased safety awareness. A patient's specific mobility challenges must be thoroughly understood by all members of the rehabilitation team to allow consistent and safe delivery of care. Again, communication and documentation are imperative. The most effective strategy for conveying this information is to have a centralized area for documenting functional and mobility limitations. This area can be maintained in the patient's room or in a staff report area and information should be updated regularly to reflect the patient's status. Mobility aids must also be regularly evaluated and maintained to ensure patient safety, including patient lifts, transfer aids, wheelchairs, and other power equipment that, if not functioning properly or in disrepair, pose a significant safety risk to patients and staff.

Individuals with TBI often require orthotic devices. These devices, including functional braces and adaptive equipment, can have a significant impact on patient safety if not managed appropriately. Although used for the ultimate goal of improving function and increasing independence, the variety of products available can create a challenge for proper and safe use, especially when the products or equipment can be donned/doffed by medical, nursing, therapy staff, or caregivers not entirely familiar with their use. These products must continually be reassessed for fit, proper use, and need to prevent injury, skin breakdown, or even interference with functional progression.[37]

Preventing falls is a ubiquitous goal across the spectrum of health settings because falls are a leading cause of morbidity and mortality, especially in elderly patients. The range of fall rates in the inpatient rehabilitation patient population has been reported as averaging 8.0 to 19.8 per 1000 bed days, with injury rates in excess of 48%.[38,39] Risk factors for falls are diverse and include many modifiable entities such as impaired balance, muscle weakness, missing or non–weight-bearing limbs, impulsivity, overuse or underuse of medications, and environmental hazards. The routine use of evidence-based interventions such as the Morse Fall Scale risk assessment, universal and individual fall risk precautions, environment and equipment audits, medication audits, staff training, and patient and family education can result in quantifiable decreases in patient fall risk and, therefore, an increase in overall patient safety.[40]

Unique challenges to medical and functional management are present when working with patients who are minimally or noninteractive; have communication deficits (aphasias or dysarthrias); have cognitive/awareness deficits; or have somnolence, restlessness, combativeness, emotional lability, or attention deficits, to name a few. These patients require an extra level of checks and balances to prevent medication and treatment errors because they are unable to advocate for themselves or reliably direct their own care. In this situation, extra attention must be paid to skin, ostomy, and bowel and bladder issues. This information must be well documented and communicated appropriately to avoid confusion about or failure to deliver an adequate level of care.

Management of patients with brain injury in the IRF can often entail judicious use of physical restraints to prevent patient harm to self, lines, or equipment. These patients often present to the inpatient unit with highly variable fluctuations in agitation, restlessness, and/or poor sleep-wake cycles that can most often be managed with appropriate medications, environmental controls, and timely redirection. These methods are occasionally inadequate to ensure patient safety and some form of physical restraint or monitoring device is required. It is imperative that medical, nursing, and therapy staff be trained in the appropriate use of available restraint and monitoring devices to ensure patient safety and also to facilitate progression through the rehabilitation process. Devices such as bed rail pads, low beds, floor mats, and enclosure beds along with medications are the preferred first-line approach to agitated or restless patients who do not respond to environmental adjustments or redirection. One-to-one or video surveillance supervision is also a viable option if staffing or technology allows. Bed or chair alarms, abdominal binders (to prevent feeding tube manipulation), soft mitts, and soft boots can provide less restrictive protection before consideration of the most restrictive devices such as torso straps or soft wrist restraints. Escalation of restraint type requires constant reassessment of patient needs and daily documentation, and justification for the use of restraints is the best way to ensure appropriate use and patient safety. It is advisable that facility policies incorporate an interdisciplinary approach to the management of agitated patients with brain injury.

Protecting privacy is also a vital component of patient safety. The community environment of the IRF, often with less strict visitation policies and increased patient mobility, creates the opportunity for unintentional lapses in patient privacy. The policy on sharing of patient information must be well known and practiced by all those involved in patient care. Likewise, the patient's wishes regarding who has access to their medical information must be well documented. Medical and therapy staff must be careful in discussing medical issues in therapy areas or hallways, and patients should be encouraged to request privacy when they have questions about their care, even if that involves waiting until the patient is in a more protected setting.

Appropriate recognition and evaluation of the deterioration of medical or mental status and the timely escalation of care are essential safety standards on the IRF, especially in free-standing rehabilitation units because the proper care may involve physical transfer to an acute medical center. Barriers to escalating care include failure to recognize deterioration, failure to properly investigate medical or mental status changes, and possible difficulty in obtaining specialist involvement or delay in medical testing (STAT laboratories, radiology examinations, and so forth.) Barriers to escalation may also include interpersonal and communication issues in which nurses or therapists are not comfortable presenting their concerns to the medical staff. In academic environments, this could also include the reluctance by house staff to escalate care because of not wanting to seem incompetent or not having the knowledge to know when escalation is needed. All of these situations present a significant safety risk to patients.

Medical, therapy, and ancillary staff education about the unique needs of patients with brain injury is imperative to maintaining an environment of safety. Nursing staff certification training in rehabilitation and brain injury should be encouraged and should include ongoing in-service updates involving the medical, nursing, and therapy staff to ensure not only patient safety but also staff safety. High rates of work injury and illness that create absences from work and discontinuity in patient care are well documented in the health care environment overall.[41,42] In a 2001 US survey, more than three-quarters of nursing staff reported that unsafe conditions interfered with their ability to deliver high-quality care.[43] Because of the hands-on approach to care required in the IRF, the variety of provider skill sets (nurses, aids, therapists), and the growing use of mobility aids and equipment, the chance for staff injury is increased. Moving and positioning patients creates the potential for staff musculoskeletal injuries[44] that can be reduced by the proper use of lifts and transfer devices. The reduction of this potential also translates directly into the safety of the patient and has been shown to increase the overall satisfaction and sense of security experienced by the patient being moved.[45] Attention to staff safety and its translation to patient safety is an integral part of overall safety culture on a rehabilitation unit. The successful implementation of lifts, adaptive equipment and clothing, and attention to the impact that provider mental and physical health can have on patient care can have far-reaching effects.

In addition, conveying medical and therapeutic information to patients and family is a more complex process than is typically appreciated, and deficiency in addressing this can have a significant impact on patient safety during, and often long after, the inpatient stay. Health literacy and the patient's and caregiver's ability to understand and comply with medical and therapeutic recommendations are multifactorial and highly variable but must be considered as an integral part of the rehabilitation process. Factors that can have significant bearing on effective communication in this setting include level of education, language, culture, previous health care experiences, socio-economics, family/caregiver dynamics, and psychosocial issues. More than 43% of American adults are unable to read, understand, and act on basic health information.[46] This deficiency can be amplified in the patient with brain injury and the family/caregiver's ability to cope with an injured loved one, especially in the rehabilitation environment when the goal is to transition the patient home, therefore transferring the burden of care from clinical and therapy staff to the caregiver. It is an essential task of the rehabilitation team to actively seek out the medical literacy of the patient and family to ensure effective communication regarding disease states, medications, treatments, and therapies.

Creating and maintaining a culture of safety in the IRF is a formidable undertaking that requires a malleable but solid framework of medical and therapy staff attention and commitment. It is only on a solid foundation that the intricate balance of medical management, therapeutic progress, and care coordination can be successful. Communication, education, shared goals, and effective leadership are the building blocks of that framework.

[Tags: patient safety, inpatient rehabilitation facility (IRF), communication, medical error, medication reconciliation, posttraumatic epilepsy (PTE), infection control, prevention, privacy, education].

PATIENT SAFETY AFTER BRAIN INJURY: TRANSITIONAL REHABILITATION FACILITIES

The purpose of transitional rehabilitation units in brain injury is to provide specialized rehabilitation treatment programs for individuals with TBI who have progressed to the point at which they no longer require intensive inpatient rehabilitation services but continue to have residual cognitive, behavioral, and physical impairments that significantly limit their ability to function independently in their community.[47] These programs are designed to provide care to individuals who are on their way to independence at the highest level allowable by their injury while maintaining physician and nursing supervision in a controlled setting. Although no specific literature exists in regard to patient safety in transitional brain injury units, some general safety concerns can be addressed by applying literature regarding SNFs, as well as long-term care facilities. There are several themes that permeate such literature and address medical, communication, education, and transition of care issues as factors affecting patient safety.

In the initial phase of admitting a patient into such a facility, the transition of care is of utmost importance. One of the first aspects is building a team of physicians, therapists, clinical case managers, and neuropsychologists to establish criteria for admission to a particular unit. Without clear understanding of the capabilities and limitations of each unit, prospective patients may be placed in jeopardy if their needs do not match those capabilities. Other facets of the transition of care is developing close relationships with both referral sources for the program to establish a clear understanding of what each program is able to offer the patient, as well as relationships with nearby, and best of all affiliated, acute medical institutions for emergent patient management should a medical complication outside the scope of the transitional unit arise. In general, the ability to share patient information accurately and quickly between different institutions results in increased patient safety.[48]

As mentioned earlier, medication reconciliation is vital during transitions of care. It is estimated that at least 1 medication discrepancy is found in more than 70% of patients in SNFs on transfer, and about half of admitted patients have a discrepancy between discharge summaries and medication reconciliation forms.[49] Another aspect of improving patient safety in terms of medications is the role of a clinical pharmacist on a transitional rehabilitation team to assist in the initial coordination and management of these records for proper transfer of care. Clinical pharmacy services have been shown to reduce mortality in hospitals.[50] Our experience with this matter has been that having a clinical pharmacist available to provide consultation is helpful in maintaining patient safety. Another tool we have found to be invaluable in the brain injury population has been close relationships with referral sources because we are able to quickly communicate with the referring physicians to elucidate the need and current clinical use for particular medications, if it is not clear from available documentation. This tool is especially important in brain injury medicine because medications are often used off label, based on clinical experience and ongoing research.

Other safety concerns stem from the nature of the transitional programs. The environment is a low-supervision setting, especially after therapy hours, which increases the risk of falls, inappropriate use of appliances, wandering, and so forth; thus, staff members need to be vigilant given the patient's level of independence. Because physicians do not see patients daily, close communication between all staff is important in maintaining patient safety. It is therefore advisable to build a patient-centered team with a unified mission and goals for each patient.

In the transitional setting, the main safety concerns are similar to those of the IRF, but are modified by both decreased perceived medical needs and increased patient independence. The most effective measures to mitigate adverse events and provide a safe patient environment are those of close communication in the interfacility and intrafacility settings, with the goal of ongoing patient and staff education and involving family members in the care process for ongoing safety once patients are discharged back into the community.

[Tags: patient safety, transitional rehabilitation, community reintegration, pharmacy, independence].

PATIENT SAFETY AFTER BRAIN INJURY: SNF

Individuals with TBI frequently transition to an SNF if it is determined that they are unable to tolerate intensive inpatient rehabilitation. However, there are approximately 8 million adverse events in US nursing homes each year.[51] These incidents include falls, pressure wounds, and medical errors. Because individuals with TBI are a vulnerable population, they are at high risk of harm from these types of adverse events. Wagner and colleagues (2011) recently found that adverse event reporting in nursing homes varies widely, except in cases of abuse in which there is more than a 95% rate of reporting.[52] This group also found that more than 70% of falls and medication errors are reported to states, but that 30% are unreported.

Because major medical illnesses are rarely diagnosed in SNFs, most individuals with medical decline are transported to emergency departments or their primary care physician's office for work-up. This process lends itself to lack of timely diagnosis of medical problems. Also, many providers practicing in an SNF do not see patients more than once per week. The infrequency of visits can lead to misdiagnosis of medical problems or exacerbation of conditions. As in other settings, on admission to an SNF an appropriate and thorough patient assessment should be undertaken, which allows comparison if a new sign or symptom is revealed. Because individuals with brain injury are a heterogeneous population with regards to functional and cognitive status, it is important to understand the nuances of the individual from the onset of care.

Just as communication is important in every other rehabilitation setting, on discharge to SNF from acute care hospitals, individuals should be sent with a discharge narrative. This narrative alerts the staff at the SNF to critical issues involved with the care of the patient. For the patient with TBI, the discharge narrative should include patient demographics; names of rehabilitation physicians; date in injury, admission, and discharge; principal and secondary diagnoses; history of present illness; past medical history; past surgical history; detailed social history; admission and discharge physical examination with detailed neurologic examination; admission and discharge functional examination detailing cognitive status; pertinent laboratories; hospital course with detailed environmental or behavioral treatment plan; diet; precautions; condition on discharge; disposition; follow-up appointments and therapies; and list of provided durable medical equipment. Appropriate communication between providers at each facility leads to improved patient care. However, this rarely occurs because discharge narratives are often completed after the time of discharge and there is difficulty obtaining contact information for other providers. In the TBI population, this relative lack of communication can lead to unnecessary transfers from the SNF back to acute care hospitals. For instance, if a particular stimulus induces agitation in a person with TBI and this information is not communicated to the staff at the SNF, then SNF staff may think that the agitation after the stimulus is a new finding and send the patient to the emergency department.

Sanders (1997) reported that improper communication between SNF and emergency departments led to unnecessary procedures and improper patient care.[53] In

2009, consensus standards to address gaps in care during these transitions were created.[54] Because of this, there have been many studies reviewing the need for data transfer systems between SNFs and hospitals.[55–60] To date, there is no standardized system that addresses this need, although there is much progress in the area. The Veterans Health Administration, Department of Defense, and private partners are currently piloting a virtual lifetime electronic record (VLER) that will create a centralized repository of administrative and medical information. The goal is for more efficient processing of benefits, better-informed clinicians, service, and care providers; improved continuity and timeliness of care; enhanced awareness among all involved parties; and elimination of gaps in records.[61] In addition, appropriate education and communication to SNF staff from acute care providers will allow prevention of injury or disease. For instance, an understanding of sleep-wake cycles in the TBI population allows nursing staff at the SNF to alert physicians when a patient off their schedule requires additional intervention to prevent cognitive decline. In addition, knowledge of agitation management in the brain-injured patient allows SNF providers to reduce the use of restraints and medications that can cause adverse events.

As in other settings, medication-related risks are a danger in the TBI population. It becomes a greater risk in those individuals in an SNF because there is often a lack of expertise of TBI care in these facilities. These patients are often seen by multiple providers and can be prescribed various medications; thus, medications must be reconciled on each visit with a physician and drug-drug interactions evaluated. If there is cause for concern, the staff at the SNF should be notified of signs and symptoms that may present. Family members of the patient are often available to act as liaisons between the provider and the SNF, but they should not be relied on to provide adequate detail to SNF staff, because they are not medical providers. If procedures are performed during physician visits, SNF personnel must be notified of the procedure, the outcome, complications, and any signs or symptoms to monitor for complications. SNF staff are often unfamiliar with procedures such as botulinum toxin injection, intrathecal drug delivery system implantation, and electrical stimulation, so ample education should be undertaken before and after the intervention. Any medically implanted device should be accompanied by written identification of the device for emergency purposes. In the case of intrathecal baclofen, oral baclofen should be prescribed to prevent withdrawal, in the event of device malfunction.

As mentioned earlier, because there is an infrequency of visits by physician providers in the SNF setting, family members are often unable to discuss their questions in a timely fashion. It may be beneficial to allow extra time during visits to entertain questions or to provide family members with appropriate staff contact information for questions that may arise between visits.

In the past decade, there has been an emphasis on reduction of infections in SNFs.[62] As noted in earlier, individuals with TBI are at risk for aspiration pneumonia. This risk may be more evident in SNFs because staff may not consistently work with a particular patient or be adept at safe swallowing techniques. There is also a high risk of incontinence in the nursing home population.[63] However, catheters and adult diapers are easier to use than timed voiding and bowel programs, but that ease of use comes at a price. This population is at risk for urinary tract infections if an indwelling or external catheter is used to manage continence. They are also at risk for skin breakdown because diapers allow containment of moisture that can macerate skin and lead to wounds.[64] Because of the population density in SNFs, patients are at risk for transmittable disease; therefore, it is important for neurologically impaired patients to be provided appropriate vaccinations.

Tinetti and colleagues (1991) reported on characteristics of SNF residents in whom restraints were initiated.[65] Those characteristics include older age, cognitive impairment, dependence in dressing, greater participation in social activities, nonuse of antidepressants, unsteadiness, agitation, and wandering were the most frequently cited reasons for initiation of restraints. Many of those same variables are seen in individuals with TBI (ie, cognitive impairment, dependence in dressing, unsteadiness, agitation, and wandering). As described earlier, the use of restraints in individuals with TBI increases the risk of agitation, and thus it can have a paradoxic effect.

Patient safety after TBI in the SNF setting is similar to each of the other settings described earlier, although there may be a need for increased education for SNF staff by the TBI specialist, because these staff members are not experts in brain injury medicine. As in the IRF setting, it may be beneficial for staff at the SNF to become certified in brain injury. The Academy of Certified Brain Injury Specialists provides a national certification program that reviews various aspects of brain injury including demographics, continuum of care, anatomy, physiology, functional impairment, treatment, psychosocial, and systems issues.[66]

[Tags: skilled nursing facility (SNF), medical error, communication, medication error, medication reconciliation, education, restraints].

PATIENT SAFETY AFTER BRAIN INJURY: COMMUNITY

As in each of the other settings, once people with TBI are at home, they continue to be at risk. A 2007 study, showed that individuals with TBI are at increased risk of mortality up to 8 years after injury.[67] Depending on the functional level of the patient, the onus is now on the patient or family to provide an adequately safe environment. It is at this time that the education and communication described in earlier comes into play. Patients and family draw on this knowledge to live their lives to the fullest, but in the safest possible manner.

Despite preparation for community integration, individuals with TBI may experience progressive isolation caused by cognitive and functional deficits.[68,69] This isolation may produce further psychological sequelae that can affect a person's safety in the community. A recent study found that major and minor depression occurred in approximately 50% of individuals with brain injury, 1 year after injury.[70] Teasdale and Endberg[71] found that individuals with TBI have higher rates of suicide up to 14 years after injury. For this reason, the outpatient brain injury specialist must inquire about the patient's life outside their perceived deficits and engage the patient and family in a manner that encourages them to discuss these problems with the provider. These psychological sequelae can point to further disorders in this population. As many as 50% to 60% of persons with TBI experience problems with alcohol and/or other drugs.[72–74] However, many of these persons had difficulties with substances before their traumatic injury.[72,75–79] Only a few studies have evaluated efficacy of screening instruments in this population. Those tested are the Brief Michigan Alcoholism Screening Test (BMAST), the Substance Abuse Subtle Screening Inventory (SASSI) and the CAGE questionnaire. Ashman and colleagues[80] found both the BMAST and SASSI to have high sensitivity and specificity in 1 study. This group also found the CAGE to have high specificity, but low sensitivity in the same study. These tools should only be used as a screening method to determine a negative impact of substance use; they should not be used as a substitute for the clinical interview.

As in other settings, persons with TBI living in the community are at risk for falls. A recent study from the Veterans Health Administration evaluated caregiver reports of subsequent injuries after discharge from inpatient TBI/polytrauma rehabilitation programs.[81] In this study, Carlson and colleagues[81] found that 32% of patients reported postdischarge, medically treated injuries. Of those with injuries, falls accounted for the most (49%), followed by motor vehicle accidents (37%), assaults (16%), and burns (12%). In addition, persons with TBI continue to be at risk for adverse effects of polypharmacy. These persons continue taking many of the medications from their acute hospital or rehabilitation stay. Without appropriate patient/caregiver education, patients or caregivers may improperly discontinue or combine various medications in a nonrecommended manner. Also, if the person with TBI has limited family resources, they may have a lower level of supervision than is necessary; this places them at risk for injuries, medication error, and high-risk/unsupervised behavior. In addition, if their caregiver is not available during medical provider appointments, there may be a disconnect between physician-recommended care and the care provided. Therefore, it is essential that the TBI specialist engages with the patient's family or caregiver to determine the risk for adverse event inside the home or in the community.

The person with TBI may consider returning to driving. In this population, there is considerable concern if the person experiences posttraumatic seizure disorder. If a person with TBI experiences seizures, physicians should check with the state department of motor vehicles to determine reporting requirements. Patients should also be disallowed from driving until they are seizure free, usually for 6 months, but each state may have different recommendations. If the person with TBI is seizure free and there are no gross cognitive, functional, medical, or psychological concerns, then the physician should consider recommending a driving evaluation. Although costly, a driving evaluation provides objective and subjective data as to the readiness of the patient.

[Tags: community, mortality, long-term outcome, community reintegration, depression, isolation, suicide].

PATIENT SAFETY AFTER BRAIN INJURY: THE MILITARY AND VETERAN SPECIAL POPULATION

On October 7, 2001, in swift response to the September 11 terrorist attacks, the United States began combat operations in Afghanistan, referred to as Operation Enduring Freedom (OEF). In addition, in March 2003, the United States engaged in military operations in Iraq, referred to as Operation Iraqi Freedom (OIF). These wars now account for the longest military campaign in US history, with close to 1.8 million troop deployments. Compared with other military engagements, there has been an increase in the level of morbidity compared with mortality. More powerful improvised explosive devices (IEDs) produce multiple organ system injuries, with the signature injury being TBI.[82]

During the last decade, brain injury has been one of the most prevalent injuries sustained by US military personnel while on deployment overseas during the current conflicts. As of December 27, 2011, there have been 47,383 casualties, including more than 2500 moderate-severe TBIs.[83–85] Estimates show that up to 15% to 20% of deployed services members sustain mTBI caused by blast exposure.[86,87] Between April 2007 and October 2009, more than 66,000 veterans were identified as possibly having TBI following deployment in OEF/OIF; more than 24,000 were confirmed to have sustained a TBI.[88] These numbers indicate that TBI is a major injury in the military population returning from combat. From January 2000 to November 2011, more than 225,000 active duty service members sustained a TBI.[89] Of these, 77% are mild, 17% are moderate, and 1% are severe.[89] The preponderance of nonpenetrating injury stems from the high incidence of IEDs, mortar attack, and other blast-producing weapons systems used by combatants.

After returning from a tour of duty, active duty service members are routinely screened for TBI and posttraumatic stress disorder (PTSD) with the Postdeployment Health Assessment (PDHA). This questionnaire is used to identify individuals with exposure to injury that resulted in a loss or alteration of consciousness. It helps to identify those service members who are at risk of developing symptoms from undiagnosed TBI. Hoge and colleagues[87] found that mTBI was associated with PTSD. Vanderploeg and colleagues[90] corroborated this finding in 2009 when they found that more than one-third of soldiers with mTBI were diagnosed with PTSD.

From 2008 to 2010, the suicide rate in army personnel exceeded that of the general population.[91,92] The 2010 army report also states that more than 45% of unsuccessful suicide attempts involved the use of illicit substances or alcohol.[92] It is because of these findings and the connection between PTSD and mTBI that this population is at high risk. Thus, medical providers need to be cognizant of the risk (**Box 4**).

[Tags: military, veteran, war, combat, improvised explosive device (IED), mild TBI (mTBI), posttraumatic stress disorder (PTSD), substance abuse, suicide].

OTHER CONSIDERATIONS

To date, there is no specific research agenda for patient and community safety in the TBI population, but there are many safety concerns. Research into return to work, school, and sports continues to be an area of interest. In the military population, returning to use firearms is an issue without good answers, but would benefit from

---

Box 4
Clinical pearls

- Prehospital and acute care
  - Field and trauma documentation of loss of consciousness and Glasgow Coma Scale
  - Vigilant neurochecks and acute reimaging
  - Management of ICP and hyperglycemia
- IRF
  - Medication reconciliation
  - Seizure and deep venous thrombosis prophylaxis
  - Functional communication, equipment needs
  - Patient and caregiver education
- Transitional unit
  - Proper patient selection for level of care
  - Establish good specialist relationships
- SNF
  - Detailed summary of deficits and needs on admission
  - Education of SNF care providers
  - Appropriate vaccinations because of patient density
- Community
  - Focus on ongoing caregiver education
  - Close surveillance for depression

specific research. One area for discussion includes the ethical issue of how to manage risks of noncompliance in the incapable patient. In addition, more research needs to be completed in the area of caregiver abuse of the incapable patient, specifically the study of physical, emotional, and financial abuse.

SUMMARY

Patient safety in rehabilitation after TBI is important. Thorough assessment on initial evaluation, vigilance for medical and procedural errors, appropriate communication between medical professionals, and evaluation of systems-based practices increases patient safety. It is the responsibility of the rehabilitation treatment team to ensure that appropriate measures are taken to reduce the risk of adverse events. This article is intended to promote discussion of patient safety after TBI within rehabilitation teams and to help improve outcomes throughout the recovery spectrum.

REFERENCES

1. Faul M, Xu L, Wald M, et al. Traumatic brain injury in the United States: emergency department visits, hospitalizations, and deaths. Atlanta (GA): Centers for Disease Control and Prevention, National Center for Injury Prevention and Control; 2010.
2. Finkelstein E, Corso P, Miller T, et al. The incidence and economic burden of injuries in the United States. New York: Oxford University Press; 2006.
3. Hyder AA, Wunderlich CA, Puvanachandra P, et al. The impact of traumatic brain injuries: a global perspective. NeuroRehabilitation 2007;22:341.
4. Injury prevention and control: traumatic brain injury. Centers for Disease Control and Prevention.
5. Rockhill CM, Jaffe K, Zhou C, et al. Health care costs associated with traumatic brain injury and psychiatric illness in adults. J Neurotrauma 2012. [Epub ahead of print].
6. Bombardier CH, Fann JR, Temkin NR, et al. Rates of major depressive disorder and clinical outcomes following traumatic brain injury. JAMA 2010;303:1938.
7. Fann JR, Hart T, Schomer KG. Treatment for depression after traumatic brain injury: a systematic review. J Neurotrauma 2009;26:2383.
8. van Velzen JM, van Bennekom CA, Edelaar MJ, et al. Prognostic factors of return to work after acquired brain injury: a systematic review. Brain Inj 2009;23:385.
9. Harrison JF, Cooke MW. Study of early warning of accident and emergency departments by ambulance services. J Accid Emerg Med 1999;16:339.
10. The Joint Commission. Root causes of sentinel events, 1995-2004. Oakbrook Terrace (IL): Joint Commission on Accreditation of Health Care Organizations; 2004.
11. Aiken LH. Evidence-based management: key to hospital workforce stability. J Health Adm Educ 2001;(Spec No):117.
12. D'Amour D, Ferrada-Videla M, San Martin Rodriguez L, et al. The conceptual basis for interprofessional collaboration: core concepts and theoretical frameworks. J Interprof Care 2005;19(Suppl 1):116.
13. Borrill C, West W, Shapiro D, et al. Team working and effectiveness in health care. Br J Healthc Manag 2000;6:364.
14. Gioia GA, Collins M, Isquith PK. Improving identification and diagnosis of mild traumatic brain injury with evidence: psychometric support for the acute concussion evaluation. J Head Trauma Rehabil 2008;23:230.

15. Espinosa-Aguilar A, Reyes-Morales H, Huerta-Posada CE, et al. Design and validation of a critical pathway for hospital management of patients with severe traumatic brain injury. J Trauma 2008;64:1327.

16. Jagoda AS, Bazarian JJ, Bruns JJ Jr, et al. Clinical policy: neuroimaging and decisionmaking in adult mild traumatic brain injury in the acute setting. Ann Emerg Med 2008;52:714.

17. Chun KA, Manley GT, Stiver SI, et al. Interobserver variability in the assessment of CT imaging features of traumatic brain injury. J Neurotrauma 2010;27:325.

18. Chang EF, Meeker M, Holland MC. Acute traumatic intraparenchymal hemorrhage: risk factors for progression in the early post-injury period. Neurosurgery 2007;61:222.

19. Douketis JD, Berger PB, Dunn AS, et al. The perioperative management of antithrombotic therapy: American College of Chest Physicians evidence-based clinical practice guidelines (8th edition). Chest 2008;133:299S.

20. Rangel-Castillo L, Robertson CS. Management of intracranial hypertension. Crit Care Clin 2006;22:713.

21. Bullock R, Chesnut RM, Clifton G, et al. Guidelines for the management of severe head injury. Brain Trauma Foundation. Eur J Emerg Med 1996;3:109.

22. Lv LQ, Hou LJ, Yu MK, et al. Risk factors related to dysautonomia after severe traumatic brain injury. J Trauma 2011;71:538.

23. Lombard LA, Zafonte RD. Agitation after traumatic brain injury: considerations and treatment options. Am J Phys Med Rehabil 2005;84:797.

24. Kahn DM, Cook TE, Carlisle CC, et al. Identification and modification of environmental noise in an ICU setting. Chest 1998;114:535.

25. Granberg Axell AI, Malmros CW, Bergbom IL, et al. Intensive care unit syndrome/delirium is associated with anemia, drug therapy and duration of ventilation treatment. Acta Anaesthesiol Scand 2002;46:726.

26. Langley G, Schmollgruber S, Egan A. Restraints in intensive care units–a mixed method study. Intensive Crit Care Nurs 2011;27:67.

27. Velji K, Baker GR, Fancott C, et al. Effectiveness of an adapted SBAR communication tool for a rehabilitation setting. Healthc Q 2008;11:72.

28. Lesar TS, Lomaestro BM, Pohl H. Medication-prescribing errors in a teaching hospital. A 9-year experience. Arch Intern Med 1997;157:1569.

29. Rozich JD, Howard RJ, Justeson JM, et al. Standardization as a mechanism to improve safety in health care. Jt Comm J Qual Saf 2004;30:5.

30. Gleason KM, Groszek JM, Sullivan C, et al. Reconciliation of discrepancies in medication histories and admission orders of newly hospitalized patients. Am J Health Syst Pharm 2004;61:1689.

31. Chen JW, Ruff RL, Eavey R, et al. Posttraumatic epilepsy and treatment. J Rehabil Res Dev 2009;46:685.

32. Klevens RM, Edwards JR, Richards CL Jr, et al. Estimating health care-associated infections and deaths in U.S. hospitals, 2002. Public Health Rep 2007;122:160.

33. Leape LL, Brennan TA, Laird N, et al. The nature of adverse events in hospitalized patients. Results of the Harvard Medical Practice Study II. N Engl J Med 1991; 324:377.

34. Verhoef J. Stopping short the spread of methicillin-resistant *Staphylococcus aureus*. CMAJ 2001;165:31.

35. Mylotte JM, Graham R, Kahler L, et al. Epidemiology of nosocomial infection and resistant organisms in patients admitted for the first time to an acute rehabilitation unit. Clin Infect Dis 2000;30:425.

36. Alvarez DJ, Rockwell PG. Trigger points: diagnosis and management. Am Fam Physician 2002;65:653.
37. Naumann M, Jankovic J. Safety of botulinum toxin type A: a systematic review and meta-analysis. Curr Med Res Opin 2004;20:981.
38. Morse JM. Enhancing the safety of hospitalization by reducing patient falls. Am J Infect Control 2002;30:376.
39. Halfon P, Eggli Y, Van Melle G, et al. Risk of falls for hospitalized patients: a predictive model based on routinely available data. J Clin Epidemiol 2001;54:1258.
40. O'Connor P, Creager J, Mooney S, et al. Taking aim at fall injury adverse events: best practices and organizational change. Healthc Q 2006;9(Spec No):43.
41. Yassi A, Ostry AS, Spiegel J, et al. A collaborative evidence-based approach to making healthcare a healthier place to work. Hosp Q 2002;5:70.
42. Koehoorn M, Lowe G, Kent V, et al. Creating high quality healthcare workplaces. Ottawa (ON): Canadian Policy Research Networks; 2002.
43. American Nurses Association. Health and safety survey, vol. 32. Silver Spring (MD): American Nurses Association; 2001.
44. Hoogendoorn WE, van Poppel MN, Bongers PM, et al. Physical load during work and leisure time as risk factors for back pain. Scand J Work Environ Health 1999; 25:387.
45. Ronald LA, Yassi A, Spiegel J, et al. Effectiveness of installing overhead ceiling lifts. Reducing musculoskeletal injuries in an extended care hospital unit. AAOHN J 2002;50:120.
46. Kindig D, Affonso D, Chudler E, et al. Health Literacy: a Prescription to End Confusion. Institute of Medicine Committee on Health Literacy. Washington, DC: National Academies Press; 2004.
47. Cifu D, Mcnamee S, Gater D, et al. The Polytrauma Rehabilitation System of Care Programs at the Richmond Veterans Administration Medical Center. Crit Rev Phys Rehabil Med 2009;21:197.
48. Carstens D, Patterson P, Laird R, et al. Task analysis of healthcare delivery: a case study. J Eng Tech Manag 2009;26:15.
49. Tjia J, Bonner A, Briesacher BA, et al. Medication discrepancies upon hospital to skilled nursing facility transitions. J Gen Intern Med 2009;24:630.
50. Bond CA, Raehl CL. Clinical pharmacy services, pharmacy staffing, and hospital mortality rates. Pharmacotherapy 2007;27:481.
51. Gurwitz JH, Sanchez-Cross MT, Eckler MA, et al. The epidemiology of adverse and unexpected events in the long-term care setting. J Am Geriatr Soc 1994;42:33.
52. Wagner LM, Castle NG, Reid KC, et al. U.S. Department of Health Adverse Event Reporting Policies for Nursing Homes. J Healthc Qual 2011. [Epub ahead of print].
53. Sanders AB. Emergency care for patients in long-term care facilities: a need for better communication. Acad Emerg Med 1977;4:854.
54. Snow V, Beck D, Budnitz T, et al. Transitions of care consensus policy statement American College of Physicians-Society of General Internal Medicine-Society of Hospital Medicine-American Geriatrics Society-American College of Emergency Physicians-Society of Academic Emergency Medicine. J Gen Intern Med 2009; 24:971.
55. Kelly NA, Mahoney DF, Bonner A, et al. Use of a transitional minimum data set (TMDS) to improve communication between nursing home and emergency department providers. J Am Med Dir Assoc 2012;13(1):85, e9–85, e15.
56. Terrell KM, Hustey FM, Hwang U, et al. Quality indicators for geriatric emergency care. Acad Emerg Med 2009;16:441.

57. Terrell KM, Brizendine EJ, Bean WF, et al. An extended care facility-to-emergency department transfer form improves communication. Acad Emerg Med 2005;12:114.
58. Terrell KM, Miller DK. Challenges in transitional care between nursing homes and emergency departments. J Am Med Dir Assoc 2006;7:499.
59. Madden C, Garrett J, Busby-Whitehead J. The interface between nursing homes and emergency departments: a community effort to improve transfer of information. Acad Emerg Med 1998;5:1123.
60. Cortes TA, Wexler S, Fitzpatrick JJ. The transition of elderly patients between hospitals and nursing homes. Improving nurse-to-nurse communication. J Gerontol Nurs 2004;30:10.
61. Virtual lifetime electronic record. 2011.
62. Flanagan E, Chopra T, Mody L. Infection prevention in alternative health care settings. Infect Dis Clin North Am 2011;25:271.
63. Sgadari A, Topinkova E, Bjornson J, et al. Urinary incontinence in nursing home residents: a cross-national comparison. Age Ageing 1997;26(Suppl 2):49.
64. Maklebust J, Magnan MA. Risk factors associated with having a pressure ulcer: a secondary data analysis. Adv Wound Care 1994;7:25.
65. Tinetti ME, Liu WL, Marottoli RA, et al. Mechanical restraint use among residents of skilled nursing facilities. Prevalence, patterns, and predictors. JAMA 1991;265:468.
66. Academy of Certified Brain Injury Specialists.
67. McMillan TM, Teasdale GM. Death rate is increased for at least 7 years after head injury: a prospective study. Brain 2007;130:2520.
68. Dikmen SS, Machamer JE, Powell JM, et al. Outcome 3 to 5 years after moderate to severe traumatic brain injury. Arch Phys Med Rehabil 2003;84:1449.
69. Lew HL, Poole JH, Guillory SB, et al. Persistent problems after traumatic brain injury: the need for long-term follow-up and coordinated care. J Rehabil Res Dev 2006;43:vii.
70. Hart T, Brenner L, Clark AN, et al. Major and minor depression after traumatic brain injury. Arch Phys Med Rehabil 2011;92:1211.
71. Teasdale TW, Engberg AW. Suicide after traumatic brain injury: a population study. J Neurol Neurosurg Psychiatry 2001;71:436.
72. West SL. Substance use among persons with traumatic brain injury: a review. NeuroRehabilitation 2011;29:1.
73. Kolakowsky-Hayner SA, Gourley EV 3rd, Kreutzer JS, et al. Post-injury substance abuse among persons with brain injury and persons with spinal cord injury. Brain Inj 2002;16:583.
74. Taylor LA, Kreutzer JS, Demm SR, et al. Traumatic brain injury and substance abuse: a review and analysis of the literature. Neuropsychol Rehabil 2003;13:165.
75. Bogner JA, Corrigan JD, Mysiw WJ, et al. A comparison of substance abuse and violence in the prediction of long-term rehabilitation outcomes after traumatic brain injury. Arch Phys Med Rehabil 2001;82:571.
76. Corrigan JD. Substance abuse as a mediating factor in outcome from traumatic brain injury. Arch Phys Med Rehabil 1995;76:302.
77. Corrigan JD, Bogner JA, Mysiw WJ, et al. Life satisfaction after traumatic brain injury. J Head Trauma Rehabil 2001;16:543.
78. Kreutzer JS, Witol AD, Marwitz JH. Alcohol and drug use among young persons with traumatic brain injury. J Learn Disabil 1996;29:643.
79. Ruff RM, Marshall LF, Crouch J, et al. Predictors of outcome following severe head trauma: follow-up data from the Traumatic Coma Data Bank. Brain Inj 1993;7:101.
80. Ashman TA, Schwartz ME, Cantor JB, et al. Screening for substance abuse in individuals with traumatic brain injury. Brain Inj 2004;18:191.

81. Carlson KF, Meis LA, Jensen AC, et al. Caregiver reports of subsequent injuries among veterans with traumatic brain injury after discharge from inpatient polytrauma rehabilitation programs. J Head Trauma Rehabil 2012;27:14.

82. Alvarez L. War veterans' concussions are often overlooked. New York: New York Times; 2008. p. A1.

83. Jones B, editor. Report to Congress on mild traumatic brain injury in the United States: steps to prevent a serious public health problem. Atlanta (GA): Centers for Disease Control and Prevention (CDC), National Center for Injury Prevention and Control; 2003.

84. Casualty status. Washington, DC: US Department of Defense; 2011.

85. Fischer H. U.S. military casualty statistics: Operation New Dawn, Operation Iraqi Freedom, and Operation Enduring Freedom. Washington, DC: Congressional Research Service; 2010.

86. Sayer NA, Cifu DX, McNamee S, et al. Rehabilitation needs of combat-injured service members admitted to the VA Polytrauma Rehabilitation Centers: the role of PM&R in the care of wounded warriors. PM R 2009;1:23.

87. Hoge CW, McGurk D, Thomas JL, et al. Mild traumatic brain injury in U.S. soldiers returning from Iraq. N Engl J Med 2008;358:453.

88. Vanderploeg R, Cornis-Pop M. Traumatic brain injury: independent study course. Washington, DC: Department of Veterans Affairs; 2008. p. 7.

89. DoD worldwide numbers for traumatic brain injury. Defense and Veterans Brain Injury Center; 2011.

90. Vanderploeg RD, Belanger HG, Curtiss G. Mild traumatic brain injury and post-traumatic stress disorder and their associations with health symptoms. Arch Phys Med Rehabil 2009;90:1084.

91. Kuehn BM. Military probes epidemic of suicide: mental health issues remain prevalent. JAMA 2010;304:1427.

92. Health promotion, risk reduction, suicide prevention. United States Army; 2010.

Patient Safety in the Rehabilitation of the Adult with a Spinal Cord Injury

Matthew Shatzer, DO

KEYWORDS

• Spinal cord injury • Patient safety • Complications

There are approximately 12,000 new cases of traumatic spinal cord injury annually. In 2010, there were approximately 265,000 individuals living with SCI. Over time, the average age of people with SCI has steadily risen, and it is now 40.7 years. Males (80.7%) are more likely to suffer from an SCI. The most common cause of SCI is motor vehicle crash (40.4%), followed by falls (27.9%), violence (15.0%), and sports injuries (8.0%). While the life expectancy of someone with an SCI has steadily increased over the years, there is still a decrease in overall life expectancy. This depends on the level of injury and completeness of injury.[1]

There are multiple medical complications that are commonly seen in individuals with SCI. These include, but are not exclusively limited to, pneumonia, decubiti ulcers, undiagnosed fractures, urinary tract infections (UTIs), autonomic dysreflexia, deep venous thrombosis, and pulmonary embolism.

SAFETY RISKS IN ADULTS WITH SPINAL CORD INJURY

Individuals with spinal cord injury have multiple impairments that may pose safety risks. The following sections describe impairments and safety risks that are involved as a result of such impairments and some general recommendations to minimize the safety risk.

Sensory Loss

Almost all people who have sustained an injury to the spinal cord will have resultant sensory dysfunction. This can result in significant safety risks. For one, lack of sensation in the extremities can result in falls, as proprioceptive feedback will be impaired. Additionally, a person with decreased sensation will be at higher risk for burn from

Disclosure: None.

Department of Physical Medicine and Rehabilitation, Hofstra- North Shore-LIJ School of Medicine, Great Neck, NY, USA

E-mail address: Mshatzer@NSHS.edu

Phys Med Rehabil Clin N Am 23 (2012) 371–375

doi:10.1016/j.pmr.2012.02.010

1047-9651/12/$ – see front matter © 2012 Published by Elsevier Inc.

modalities. Due to this, these patients should not use plug-in heating pads and should be supervised when using heat modalities to prevent burns. Anecdotally, individuals with SCI have also sustained burns secondary to laptop computers. Patients should be counseled not to place laptop computers or other devices on their laps.

Weakness

Individuals who sustain SCI have varying degrees of weakness, depending on their American Spinal Injury Association (ASIA) impairment scale and level of injury. Weakness of the extremities will increase risk of falls, musculoskeletal injury, and skin breakdown. The risk of occurrence of sequelae secondary to weakness that occurs from an SCI can be minimized several ways. Use of appropriate assistive devices and orthotics may be appropriate for an individual with an incomplete injury. For individuals with complete injuries or incomplete injuries who are unable to ambulate, evaluation of an appropriate wheelchair is necessary. Patients with complete injuries should also be turned every 2 hours to prevent development of skin breakdown.

Pulmonary

Individuals with SCI have baseline respiratory compromise. As a result of weakness, these individuals have difficulty with secretion management, atelectasis, and hypoventilation. This is a result of compromised innervation to the intercostal muscles. In individuals with a T5 to T12 neurologic level of injury, the abdominal muscles and intercostal muscles are weakened, and the patient is unable to forcefully cough. From the T1 to the T5 level, there is even worse weakness, and even silent respiration may be impacted. Due to this, an individual with an SCI will have restrictive pulmonary disease with a decrease in all lung volumes. As a result, spinal cord injured individuals will have a lower threshold of pulmonary wellness and may more easily develop pneumonia.

PATIENT ASSESSMENT WITH AN EMPHASIS ON SAFETY

By using the ASIA Classification for Spinal Cord Injury, one can stratify the risks involved in developing complications. The following information regarding level and classification of injury may be helpful in determining risks.

An individual with a complete injury (ASIA A) will have an increased risk of developing pressure ulcers as well as burns. This is due to the fact that these individuals are insensate below the level of the injury and therefore are unaware of a developing ulcer. As well, these individuals have no motor function below the level of injury and are unable to offload;therefore they cannot prevent breakdown as easily.

ASIA classification is also of use when stratifying risk for autonomic dysreflexia (AD). AD is present in individuals with ASIA A T6 and above injuries. This is due to the fact that this level is above the major splanchnic outflow; therefore parasympathetic flow is limited.[2]

Incomplete spinal cord injured individuals may actually have a higher risk for falls as a result of relative weakness of the lower extremity. Additionally, individuals with incomplete SCIs are at higher risk of suicide.[3]

Safety Risk to Adults With SCI Along the Health Care Continuum

Adults with SCI are cared for in a variety of health care settings including acute medical/surgical wards, inpatient rehabilitation facilities, subacute rehabilitation facilities, outpatient facilities, and even the home of the patient. As increasing numbers of adults with SCIs are living longer and more active lifestyles, they will periodically need health care. Risks for their safety can be encountered as the adult with SCI moves along the continuum of health care. The multiple transition points through different health care settings and multiple health care providers pose a challenge to the care of the SCI patient. Some of the issues include

Communication-related issues, especially at transition points such as admissions and discharges

Limited knowledge about the care of this population among health care providers

Limited education of patients and their families on being effective advocates for their needs

Fragmented social support systems and

Limited education and financial resources.

It is therefore very important that first and foremost, patients and their immediate family members are properly educated about SCI and its short-term and long-term consequences and recognition and management of commonly seen conditions in this population. It is also equally important that health care providers have a working knowledge about the care of the SCI patient. Health care providers should consider using a checklist format to ensure that all possible consequences of SCI are adequately addressed regardless of location of care along the health care continuum (Appendix A). Communication at time of transition points should follow a structured format with appropriately documented admission notes and discharge summaries with pertinent medical and surgical information relevant to the patient's care.

PREVENTION

Safety risks may be avoided with appropriate preventative measures.

Pressure Ulcers

Turning a spinal cord injured individual every 2 hours will help decrease the risk of decubiti ulcers. Side-lying the patient at a 30° angle is most efficacious in relieving pressure.[4] This is based on research, which has recognized that individuals with SCI can develop pressure ulcers within 2 hours of maintaining continued pressure.[5]

Urinary Tract Infections

Appropriate management of neurogenic bladder will also prevent development of UTI. Patients with SCI should have regular evaluation of bladder function with urodynamic testing to optimize management. Frequently, this is done annually for the first several years after the injury. If no problems are identified, bladder surveillance should be done every other year.

Deep Vein Thrombosis

Individuals with SCI are at high risk to develop deep venous thrombosis (DVT). Appropriate prophylaxis for DVT is necessary to prevent this complication. Typical DVT prophylaxis involves the use of low molecular weight heparin and compression devices. According to the Consortium for Spinal Cord Medicine, an individual with a motor incomplete injury should have prophylaxis for 8 weeks for ASIA C injury, and for the length of hospitalization for an ASIA D injury. Motor complete injured individuals should have prophylaxis for 8 weeks, unless there is another associated risk factor, in which case prophylaxis should be for 12 weeks. The patient must be monitored closely for lower extremity edema and erythema, which may be indicative of a DVT. Additionally, if there is no obvious source for a fever, a DVT should be part of the differential diagnosis.

Aspiration Pneumonia

It is important for the individual with an SCI to maintain the ability to clear secretions to prevent the onset of pneumonia. There are several interventions that can be used. In the acute phase, a rotating bed may be used. Aggressive suctioning is necessary to prevent build up of secretions. As well, the patient should receive chest physiotherapy. Other techniques used are assisted cough and mechanical insufflation–exsufflation.

TREATMENTS

Early intervention of the potential complications from SCI is very important to minimize the risk of further decline in the patient's well being.

A UTI should be suspected if the patient has a change in the frequency or color of his or her urine. Additionally, UTI should be part of the differential diagnosis if the patient has other signs such as fever, increase in spasticity, increase in frequency of required catheterization, or change in status of urinary continence. A urine analysis as well as culture should be done to identify the appropriate antibiotic to use.

Pressure ulcers must be treated immediately to prevent worsening of the patient's condition. Ulcers with necrotic slough must be debrided. This can be performed chemically with a topical enzymatic medication. Other options are mechanical debridement with a wet-to-dry dressing and sharp debridement with a scalpel.

Deep Vein Thrombosis

Individuals with a DVT should be treated with anticoagulation, typically with coumadin with a goal international normalized ratio of 2.0 to 3.0. An inferior vena cava filter should be considered if the patient was already on anticoagulation when they developed a DVT or there is a contraindication for treatment with medications.

SUMMARY

Adults with SCI often live with multiple impairments associated with their underlying injury. The combination of these impairments, coupled with the lifelong need to interface with the health care system, poses several risks to the safety of individuals living with SCI. Physiatrists are often called upon to participate and lead in the care of this population and thus should assume a leadership role in minimizing the safety risks to patients.

REFERENCES

1. Spinal cord injury facts and figures at a glance. University of Alabama Birmingham. Available at: http://www.nscisc.uab.edu. Accessed February 22, 2012.
2. Braddom R. Physical medicine and rehabilitation. 4th edition. Saunders; 2007.
3. Kirshblum S. Spinal cord injury medicine. 1st edition. Lipincott Williams WIlkins; 2002.
4. Defloor T, Schoonhoven L, Katrien V, et al. Reliability of the European pressure ulcer advisory panel classification system. J Adv Nurs 2006;54(2):189–98.
5. Dinsdale SM. Decubitus ulcers: role of pressure and friction in causation. Arch Phys Med Rehabil 1974;55(4):147–52.

APPENDIX A: SCI PATIENT SAFETY CHECKLIST

1. Physical health
   a. Cardiac disease
   b. Pulmonary disease
      i. Aspiration pneumonia

    c. Skin: pressure ulcers

    d. Urinary tract infections

    e. Osteoporosis and fracture risk

    f. Appropriate screening for age specific medical problems (ie, cancer screening, kidney and bladder evaluations, diabetes, hypertension)

    g. Weight change (weight loss or weight gain)

    h. Pain

    i. Spasticity management

    j. Range-of-motion restrictions and heterotopic ossification

    k. Autonomic dysreflexia

    l. Falls and near-falls in ambulators

    m. Polypharmacy

2. Mental health

    a. Depression and suicidal ideation

    b. Substance abuse

3. Socioeconomic:

    a. Changes in support system, living arrangements, and financial resources

4. Functional level

    a. Changes in ability to perform activities of daily living and transfers

5. Evaluation of adaptive equipment, orthotics and wheelchair

Patient Safety in the Rehabilitation of the Adult with an Amputation

Gail Latlief, DO[a,b,*], Christine Elnitsky, PhD, RN[a,c,d,e],
Stephanie Hart-Hughes, PT, MSMS, NCS[a,c],
Samuel L. Phillips, PhD, CP[a,c,f], Laurel Adams-Koss, OT[a],
Robert Kent, DO, MHA[b], M. Jason Highsmith, DPT, CP[g]

KEYWORDS

- Patient safety • Limb loss • Falls • Prosthetics • Wound care
- Physical therapy • Transfers • Patient handling

The number of individuals with amputation(s) in the United States has increased in recent decades. In the United States in 1996, the estimated prevalence of major limb amputation was 1.2 million persons.[1] In 2008, the estimated prevalence increased to 1.6 million persons.[2] The prevalence of amputation is predicted to continue to increase at least at this rate and possibly faster. In the United States, transtibial amputations represent approximately 26% of lower limb amputations performed every year, with cost estimates ranging from $27,000 to $50,000 per transtibial amputation.[3–6] As of December 2011, approximately 1,420 patients with amputations from the Operation

Disclosures: (1) Contents do not represent the views of the Department of Veterans Affairs nor the US Government. (2) This material is the result of work supported with resources and the use of facilities at the James A. Haley Veterans Affairs Hospital, Tampa, FL.

[a] HSR&D RR&D Center of Excellence, James A Haley Veterans Hospital, 8900 Grand Oak Circle, Tampa, FL 33637, USA
[b] Department of Neurology, College of Medicine, University of South Florida, Tampa, FL, USA
[c] VISN 8 Patient Safety Center of Inquiry, Tampa, FL 33620, USA
[d] Colleges of Nursing, University of South Florida, 12901 Bruce B. Downs Boulevard MDC Box 22, Tampa, FL 33612, USA
[e] College of Behavioral and Community Sciences, University of South Florida, 13301 Bruce B. Downs Boulevard MHC 1110, Tampa, FL 33612-3807, USA
[f] Department of Mechanical Engineering, College of Engineering, University of South Florida, Tampa, FL 33620, USA
[g] School of Physical Therapy & Rehabilitation Sciences, College of Medicine, University of South Florida, 12901 Bruce B. Downs Boulevard, MDC077, Tampa, FL 33620, USA
* Corresponding author. HSR&D RR&D Center of Excellence, James A Haley Veterans Hospital, 8900 Grand Oak Circle, Tampa, FL 33637.
E-mail address: Gail.Latlief@va.gov

Key Points

Safety considerations are numerous for persons with amputations. Key considerations include:

- Ensuring open communication between members of the rehabilitation team as well as with the patient and caregivers
- Considering the effect of prosthesis selection
- Therapy plan including a falls assessment
- Continuous monitoring of pain management and wound care
- Education and training of the patient and caregiver
- Appropriate management of the complex patient; including multilimb and multitrauma
- Identifying comorbidities, secondary complications, and long-term outcomes

---

Iraqi Freedom/Operation Enduring Freedom/Operation New Dawn campaigns have been treated in all military treatment facilities.

Rehabilitation of adults with limb amputations as a result of dysvascular conditions or traumatic events can be affected by comorbid medical conditions such as diabetes and cardiovascular or heart disease. It may be difficult to regain mobility and function, and patients may choose to use a wheelchair, when they have an above-the-knee or through-the-knee artificial limb (prosthesis) fitted. Discomfort, functionality, reliability, ease of use, previous mobility, and the amount of exertion needed to use a prosthesis are important factors that affect a patient's mobility or function. Fear of falling, number of falls, social circumstances, and help and support from other people are also important influences.[7] Amputation of a limb or limbs is known to be associated with a myriad of overuse syndromes, degenerative conditions, and injuries. In addition, because of the high number of persons with amputation who are infirm and mobility impaired, caregivers and health care providers who routinely care for these persons are likely at an increased risk of injury. Patients with amputations may experience complications with wound healing, pain, edema, contractures, and additional surgery, resulting in limited return to function and satisfaction and high rehabilitation costs.[4,8,9]

This article reviews the evidence in patient safety issues encountered in the course of rehabilitation of adults with amputation and identifies recommendations for clinical prevention and future research directions. Specifically, safety issues in the following areas are discussed: the prosthesis, falls, wound care, pain, and treatment of complex patients.

We conducted a search of several electronic databases. The sources that we searched to obtain data for this review were PubMed (from 1960 to December 2011), Index Medica using MEDLINE (from 1960 to December 2011), reference lists from the articles obtained, and personal communication with content experts. The terms used in the search were amputation rehabilitation and safety and cited author cross-references. Studies were included if the article was in English and used human subjects. Expert opinion from the staff and colleagues of the Tampa Regional Amputation Center was sought and included.

METHODOLOGIC ISSUES

Comparisons of published study results for safety in amputation rehabilitation from descriptive studies or controlled studies are limited by the number and type of studies available and lack of a standard definition for safety outcome points in time to measure success and failure of different interventions. Published studies included original research articles, case reports, and review articles. Published studies are limited by sample size and methodical design.

SAFETY AND THE PROSTHESIS

Receiving the prosthesis is often a focal point early in the rehabilitation of the person with amputation. Before receiving the device, there can be safety issues. Commonly, postoperative compressive and limb-shaping strategies are used. In some cases, incision lines can be stressed if attempting to don a shrinker when the scar is not closed. Poorly fit shrinkers can lead to improperly shaped limbs that are prone to skin breakdown. With regard to use of compression wrapping, potential concerns include a constrictive tourniquet effect with transverse, circularly applied wraps. Further, compressive wrap fasteners are sharp and there is an obvious concern for use with people whose sensation and circulation are compromised. A safer method of stump wrapping is the is the figure eight technique with use of tape for closing ends of elastic compression wrap.

In some cases, immediate postoperative prostheses or rigid dressings can be furnished. The purpose of these devices is to manage limb volume and provide closely supervised and early preprosthetic weight-bearing capabilities. They also have a secondary function of providing protection to the limb from external trauma and preventing knee contractures. There are numerous benefits such as limb conditioning and acclimation to donning a definitive device. However, these preprosthetic devices can be a source of safety concern. If supervision is inadequate, fitting is poor, structural strength is insufficient, and so forth, these devices can lead to skin and limb trauma, material failure, falls, and other problems. The literature is mixed on the use of these devices, with a generally positive view.[10] A large retrospective review of literature spanning 1960 to 2002 compared measures of safety, efficacy, and clinical outcomes of various strategies of postoperative dressing and management in transtibial amputation.[10] Analysis of 10 controlled studies supported only 4 of the 14 claims cited in the uncontrolled, descriptive studies reviewed. Postamputation dressing and management strategies aim to improve wound healing, control pain, allow early prosthetic fitting, and enable a quick return to function.

Once the time has come and prosthetic component selection proceeds, prescription is necessary. Risks are associated with underprescription and overprescription of components. In terms of underprescription, the active user who receives components below their functional capabilities is at risk of either experiencing poor performance from their prosthesis or potentially catastrophic component failure. The opposite phenomenon (overprescription of components) is equally problematic because higher-level components may require a more aggressive pattern of use to optimize function. This situation could introduce nonoptimal forces to the amputated residual limb. In addition, higher functioning components may introduce the possibility of participating in higher-level activities. For instance, some microprocessor knees may offer reciprocal stair descent (or ascent). Some users may feel obligated to attempt these activities to their detriment and without adequate training, strength, conditioning, and so forth.

With regard to the prosthesis itself, there are inherent safety issues with most elements of the prosthesis. For example, the socket has the complex task of supporting the residual anatomy and structurally interfacing with the components transferring forces between the body and environment. Socket fit can be poor because of anatomic challenges such as birth anatomy, and acquired and developed variations such as heterotopic ossification. Socket issues are one of the most common prosthetic problems.[11,12]

The skin of the residual limb in lower limb amputees is prone to problems. The skin of the residual limb was not designed for load bearing, but that is what is required when using a lower extremity prosthesis. The skin of the residual limb is exposed to shear and stress forces, increased moisture, and prolonged exposure to the prosthesis. Consequently, various skin problems may develop. Frequently, treatment of skin-related prosthetic issues involves a period of time of not using the prosthesis. This situation increases the falls risk. It has been suggested that once the issue has been resolved, continued prosthetic use does not affect healing.[13]

There is limited research on incidence of skin problems associated with amputation. One literature review in 2006 found only a single article describing the incidence and prevalence of skin problems in lower limb amputees.[14] Observational studies have begun to describe potential determinants of skin problems of the residual limb in these individuals.[11,14,15] Prevalence of skin problems ranges from 36% to 63%.[11,14,16] Some features identified in the literature as associated with increased incidence of skin problems are increased prosthetic use, poor residuum or prosthetic hygiene, use of antibacterial soap, smoking, and individuals with transtibial residual limbs. Conversely, some published factors associated with reduced incidence of skin problems were higher age, amputation caused by peripheral arterial disease or diabetes, and use of a single-point cane or no walking aid compared with another type of walking aid.[14] Reasons for these associations are clinically unclear; however, these seemingly contradictory findings may be caused by decreased use of the prosthesis or differences in reporting. Thus far, no relationship between the incidence of skin problems and socket design or prosthetic components has been identified. Further research is clearly needed to better understand the incidence of skin issues in the amputee population.

Suspension is an important component to evaluate. Beyond the obvious risk of suspension failure, pistoning or vertical prosthesis movement on the residual limb causes the prosthetic side to be effectively longer during swing. In addition to contributing to gait deviations, this situation can lead to the prosthesis catching on the floor or other objects and to trips and falls. Poor suspension also frequently leads to skin irritation this is due to friction or pistoning of the residual limb within the socket.

In addition to their contribution to gait deviations, poor fit, suspension, or alignment can make the prosthesis less stable, potentially reducing a user's balance. The factors may also affect the user's confidence in the prosthesis. If the user does not have confidence in the prosthesis, they may act tentatively, which can alter gait mechanics and hamper operation of safety features. For example, weight-activated safety features require a certain amount of body weight applied through the prosthesis. If the user fails to apply sufficient load through the prosthesis, the safety feature does not activate.

In regard to safety relative to prosthetic feet, some amputees adopt an ankle strategy to assist with postural control and balance. In order to effectively use an ankle strategy, ankle stiffness must be appropriately selected.[17] Both ankle stiffness and the number of degrees of freedom available at the prosthetic ankle are factors during gait on prevailing terrain. In addition, during gait, the keel lever can affect knee stability. For instance, a keel lever that is too soft can result in a premature loss of anterior stability and knee buckling in terminal stance.

There are some situations in which a specialized prosthesis is required. For example, most prostheses are not designed for use in a wet environment. Showers, pools, and water sports may require a customized water prosthesis.

As stated earlier, the prosthesis is often a focal point in the rehabilitation of the amputee. Therefore, it is important that the entire health care team is involved with determining patient goals and expectations. It is equally important that the prosthesis includes correctly prescribed components such that safety issues are appropriately balanced with ambulatory and mobility demands. Furthermore, to optimize prosthetic function, appropriate training and rehabilitation on the functional implementation are crucial. Because of the prevalent rate of dependency for transfer and mobility early in the course of rehabilitation, there is increased risk of injury to members of the health care team and the patient's caregivers. This subject is discussed next.

SAFETY OF THE HEALTH CARE TEAM AND CAREGIVERS

Rehabilitation after amputation is a process. Involved in this process are several people, including health care team members and relatives and friends of the amputee. Commonly, patients need greater assistance early in the rehabilitation process as they are learning mobility and transfer skills without an anatomic connection to the floor. This situation requires new strategies for transferring into/out of chairs, cars, bed, bathtubs, and other environments, depending on previous function and goals. At times, in the early phase, family and friends may be tempted to provide high levels of assistance, introducing risk of injury to all involved. Considerable rates of injury are known to exist among rehabilitation professionals in association with patient-handling activities.[18,19] It is plausible that the risk of injury in family caregivers of dependent loved ones such as amputees is greater, given that most of these individuals are untrained and the environment is likely ill equipped for safe handling and transfers.

Gait training the amputee has inherent safety considerations as well. Because amputees are known to have a pervasive rate of falls and balance compromise at high levels of function, those learning to ambulate may be at increased risk of falls. Thorough gait training should include a progression of not only skills (eg, weight shifting, stepping) but also a variety of environments. According to 1 study, most amputees (87%) experience at least 1 barrier in the environment.[20] Gait training environments should include necessary therapeutic situations (eg, harness systems, treadmills) but also flat ground, prevailing terrain, ramps/hills, and stairs.[21] Each new environment should ideally be practiced with progressively less support, introducing greater mobility; however, the potential for safety risk thereby increases. Stairs and ramps present unique challenges for amputees because of the altered forces on the prosthesis. It is important for the rehabilitation team to understand the functional capabilities of the particular prosthetic components as well as the individual to select the proper method of stair climbing or descending for that individual. Alternative methods such as seated stair handling may be considered for balance-impaired individuals or early in rehabilitation.[22] In addition, if these environments, and others the amputee faces in the community, are not addressed, then ambulatory safety is not optimized for that patient.

FALLS AND LOWER EXTREMITY AMPUTATION

Lower extremity amputation is known to compromise gait, balance, and overall capacity to react to slips and trips.[23–26] Thus, falls are pervasive and often seen as normal events in these individuals. In addition, when a limb is lost to vascular disease, several additional comorbidities and risk factors are in place that further increase the likelihood of falls.[27–29] These factors include probable advanced age, presence of neuropathy, partial foot ulcerations or amputation on the sound side, and likely visual impairment.[30]

The literature reports variation in fall incidence in individuals with lower extremity amputation based on clinical setting. Approximately 20% of lower extremity amputees fall while receiving inpatient rehabilitation acutely after limb amputation. Eighteen percent of those patients experience a fall-related injury.[28] Wheelchair use, specifically self-transfers and reaching activities, have been identified as playing a major role in these falls.[30] Risk factors associated with increased fall risk while undergoing inpatient rehabilitation have been identified[28] and include age of 71 years or greater, prolonged length of stay (between 22 and 35 days), presence of 4 or more comorbidities, cognitive impairment, and use of benzodiazepines or opiates.

The incidence and risk factors associated with falls in individuals with lower extremity amputation in other care settings are less defined in the literature. Miller and colleagues[25] reported that 52% of unilateral amputees living in the community fell within a 1-year period. Given that an estimated 1.8 million persons in the United States are living with limb loss, with that number expected to double by the year 2050,[31] there is a great need for further work in this area. Specifically, efforts need to be made to acquire a greater understanding of fall-specific mechanisms, refine fall risk assessment, and develop an evidenced-based repertoire of fall-specific interventions customized to this patient population.

Despite the need for further research, some evidence does exist to guide health care providers in the management and treatment of fall risk in individuals with lower extremity amputation. Interventions showing promise include specialized componentry (ie, microprocessor knees), wheelchair design and user training, physical therapy intervention for gait/balance training, and the use of injury-reducing devices.

In a recent review of the literature by Highsmith and colleagues[23], safety, energy efficiency, and cost efficacy of C-Leg use for transfemoral amputees was summarized and reported. These investigators identified 7 articles pertinent to the topic of safety that met their established assessment criteria for methodologic quality and bias risk. These studies provided a grade B recommendation that after an accommodation period with a C-Leg, previous nonmicroprocessor knee users experience a decrease in the number and frequency of recalled stumble and fall events in addition to improved balance.

High fall incidence after limb amputation in the acute inpatient rehabilitation setting, which has been in large part related to wheelchair use, renders wheelchair skills training attractive as a fall prevention intervention. Dyer and colleagues[30] reported preliminary data pertaining to a multidisciplinary fall prevention program implemented in this setting. This program included a multifaceted approach that spanned several risk domains to include overall risk assessment, environmental assessment, medication management, customized alteration of care plans in response to fall events, and continuous patient wheelchair skills training. Although the incidence of falls was reduced only marginally with this intervention in place, there was a marked reduction in the severity of falls and the incidence of repeat falls. This finding was encouraging given the scope of this problem in the inpatient rehabilitation setting after lower limb amputation.

Exercise intervention, specifically balance training, has been identified by many as a key element of any fall prevention program.[32] A 20-minute balance training program performed on 5 consecutive days using a novel balance-specific mechanical apparatus on individuals with transtibial amputations was reported by Matjacic.[33] Findings indicated improved performance on all functional outcome measures after intervention. Although falls was not an end point, the positive effect measured on balance and gait outcome is encouraging and investigation as to whether translation of these benefits to fall reduction warrants further study.

Many amputees require some type of assistive device when ambulating. Choices include single-point canes, quad-tip canes, forearm crutches, 2-wheeled walkers, and 4-footed walkers. In general, it is recommended to go from gait training in parallel bars to an appropriate assistive device to full weight bearing as quickly as possible. If walkers are to be used, a study by Tsai and colleagues[34] of 20 persons found that 2-wheeled walkers allow individuals with lower limb amputations to walk more quickly and with less interruption. In addition, their walking was deemed no less safe than walking with a 4-footed walker.

Given the prevalence of falls and additional comorbidities that further increase fall risk in individuals with lower limb amputation, emphasis on injury prevention is imperative. Devices such as rigid dressings, stump protectors, and hip protectors should be considered for all individuals with lower limb amputations especially in those individuals at high risk for falls whose risk factors are not modifiable.

There are many needs and safety issues that are unique to persons with upper extremity amputations. Some of these issues include body image concerns, social isolation, overuse syndrome, significant impact on functionality of tasks/difficulties with activities of daily living (ADL), and skin integrity issues frequently caused by traumatic loss of the limb.

After any amputation, a person must deal with many psychosocial and adjustment issues. For a person with an upper limb amputation, these issues are magnified because of the inability to completely conceal an upper extremity prosthesis or missing limb. Upper extremities are visible in social situations and day-to-day activities (ie, shaking hands, eating, talking with hand gestures). Even if wearing an upper extremity prosthesis, a person may feel uncomfortable in social situations, because the prosthesis looks and functions noticeably different from a sound arm. Further complicating body image and other psychological issues, a person with an upper limb amputation may also be dealing with posttraumatic stress disorder, because upper limb amputations are frequently the result of traumatic loss. These issues may lead to low participation and social reintegration for some persons with upper extremity amputations.

Social isolation is yet another concern that persons with upper limb amputation may face. Because the number of persons with upper extremity amputation is significantly lower than those with lower extremity amputations, the person may not encounter others with an upper extremity limb loss, or not someone with the same level of amputation. Educational materials and support groups may be unintentionally focused on persons with lower extremity amputations because the numbers are so much greater. There is a wide range of potential levels of upper extremity amputation, so it may be difficult to find a peer visitor with the same level of limb loss.

Another concern is overuse syndrome. Many people with unilateral upper extremity amputations are at risk of developing a repetitive stress injury or problems associated with overuse of the contralateral limb. This situation can be caused by not wearing a prosthesis and performing all tasks, including tasks meant to be bilateral, using only the sound limb. Even those regularly using a prosthesis can encounter overuse issues, because the prosthesis is usually used as a tool, and the sound limb continues to function as the prime mover for all tasks. Some injuries associated with repetitive use/overuse are rotator cuff injuries, tendonitis, lateral/medial epicondylitis, and carpal tunnel syndrome. The frequency of overuse injuries has been reported as high as 50%.[35] Another factor that affects overuse is the high rate of abandonment for persons with upper extremity amputations. The rejection or nonwear rate has been reported between 20% and 44%.[36–39]

Although most persons with an amputation experience some change to or difficulty in task/ADL performance, there seems to frequently be a great impact on persons with upper extremity amputation. When a person with an upper extremity amputation loses the dominant arm, they have to relearn how to perform their basic ADL tasks. Many functional and ADL/instrumental ADL tasks are bilateral tasks, or tasks that require great hand and finger dexterity. Many of the tasks need to be performed by a different method or by using adaptive equipment and techniques. Upper extremity amputation makes it more difficult to use an assistive device for mobility, so for those with multiple injuries, the upper extremity amputation can exacerbate lower extremity mobility issues.

Because upper limb loss is frequently traumatic, it is not uncommon for a person with upper extremity amputation to have significant skin integrity issues, including burns, nonhealing wounds, repeated surgical/residual limb revisions, and extensive scarring. This situation can create multiple concerns for the person, including pain management, body image, psychological problems, ability to cope with and accept the amputation, infection, and difficulties being fitted for and wearing a prosthesis.

These are all potential concerns for any person with any amputation, but those with an upper extremity amputation may be at increased risk. These issues should be addressed early in the rehabilitation phase and should continue to be addressed throughout the rehabilitation process by all team members.

WOUND CARE AND PAIN MANAGEMENT

Wound care and pain management are a challenge in the rehabilitation of patients with amputations. Wound care and pain management generally proceed in systematic phases. In the case of a traumatic amputation, the typical approach consists of the following phases: preclosure of the residual wound and then definitive closure of the residual limb.[40] The goal of wound management during the preclosure phase is to promote healing of the underlying soft tissue and to treat or reduce the risk of infections. Blast injuries that lead to amputation often result in skeletal injuries to remaining limbs. The goal of wound management during the definitive closure phase is to prepare the residual limb for prosthetic fitting. For the first 14 to 21 days, the patient has sutures in place, closing the surgical wound. After sutures are removed, adhesive strips are applied during final wound closure. Throughout the definitive stage of wound healing, compression dressings are applied to reduce swelling and shape the residual limb for prosthetic fitting. There are 2 types of compression dressings: rigid and soft. Rigid compression dressings, made of casting material, are changed as swelling of the residual limb decreases. Soft compression dressings are elastic bandages applied to reduce the swelling at the distal portion of the residual limb.

Stansby and colleagues[41] tested a new negative pressure wound therapy system in a pilot study of diabetic patients with postamputation wounds to assess reduction in wound depth and area. Patients with postamputation wounds in both acute and home settings had dressings changed 3 times per week for 4 weeks. Results showed general trends in reduction of wound area and depth as well as controlled pain and exudates, as well as ease of use reported by patients and providers. Five of the 14 patients had adverse events: further surgical revision of postamputation wound, ulceration on plantar aspect, methicillin-resistant Staphylococcus aureus, or wound deterioration. Although results were believed to be promising, the study had a small sample size and lacked a comparison, hence efficacy could not be addressed.

Managing pain related to amputation is one of the greatest challenges for the patient and the amputation rehabilitation care team. Pain is one of the most common complaints among persons with amputations; it is reported in as many as 80% of amputees. Although pain directly does not apply to amputee safety, indirectly pain is an important safety consideration. Pain can lead to poor biomechanics, increased osteoarthritis, and improper use of the prosthesis, resulting in skin breakdown, gait deviations, increased risk of falls, and prosthetic abandonment.

Pain generally falls into 2 categories: residual limb pain and phantom limb pain.[40] Moreover, pain in this population is commonly associated with slower walking, difficulty using a prosthesis, and a lower quality of life. Pain assessment and treatment using pharmacologic and nonpharmacologic means for pain control should start in the preoperative phase and continue throughout the process of rehabilitation and prosthetic training. Understanding how persons with amputation self-manage pain is important for providers who advise them about maximizing function and participation in family, societal, and community roles.

Additional sources of pain after amputation include the residual limb, prosthetic device, and altered body mechanics. Pain in the residual limb may be related to infection, hematoma, edema, bone spurs or abnormal bone growth, neuroma, or mechanical effects of wearing a compression device.[40] Pain may occur during prosthetic fitting and adjustments to fit a socket over a residual limb while it is healing. Pain may also occur during physical or occupational therapy. Normal body mechanics (eg, the way one lies, sits, or moves) are altered after amputation, resulting in pain in the back, neck, and other limbs.

A current Cochrane review sought to clarify the uncertainty in optimal pharmaceutical management of phantom limb pain by summarizing the evidence on effective interventions up to September 2011.[42] The outcomes considered were change in pain intensity, function, mood, sleep, quality of life, satisfaction, and adverse effects. Because of the wide variability in the studies, a qualitative description and narrative summary of results were prepared based on analysis of 13 studies involving 255 participants and 6 groups of medications (N-methyl-D-aspartate receptor antagonists, antidepressants, anticonvulsants, anesthetics, opioids, and calcitonin). Results suggest selected pharmaceuticals (morphine, gabapentin, and ketamine) showed trends of analgesic efficacy in short-term administration. The adverse effects of ketamine were more serious and included loss of consciousness, sedation, hallucinations, hearing and position impairment, and insobriety. Gabapentin side effects included somnolence and dizziness.[42] Ten studies were high quality and 3 were moderate quality. Results must be cautiously interpreted because the review was based on a small number of studies with limited sample sizes that varied considerably and lacked long-term efficacy and safety outcomes.

Investigators explored pain management strategies used by patients with physical disabilities who were all using adaptive means of mobility.[43] During 54 in-depth interviews, 28 adults with physical disabilities (amputation, cerebral palsy, spinal cord injury) distinguished between usual and unexpected pain. Usual pain was experienced on a consistent basis and was generally associated with need to get more rest, exercise, or freedom from stress and could be self-managed using preventive techniques or scheduling/pacing activities. Unexpected pain was periodic and self-managed using immediate response and changes in ADL.

RECOMMENDATIONS FOR CLINICAL PREVENTION

Given that the average number of lower limb amputations performed on persons in acute hospitals between 1989 and 1992 was 105,000 and that most are preceded by a minor traumatic event that is often related to footwear, footwear solutions have been offered by the Department of Veterans Affairs (VA).[44] A robust preventive program is an important component of any amputation care plan.

Advising and encouraging patients to make proactive plans for managing each kind of pain episode they experience helps them better manage pain so they can increase their overall participation levels. Multiple and flexible approaches may be needed. For example, simplifying the work to be done and strategies for conserving energy for high-priority activities can be used. Persons with disabilities may choose to find ways to use personal assistance. They may need guidance in how to schedule or pace tasks; assistive technologies and devices can be used. Studies indicate strategies for self-management of usual pain may include hopes for prevention, deliberate planning, and realistic decision making about activities and participation.[44] Strategies for managing unexpected pain may include attempts to dissociate the mind and body and put in place safety nets (support circle of friends, medications) for help or relief.[43]

TREATING COMPLEX PATIENTS

At the James A. Haley VA Hospital, the diversity in conditions that lead to amputations or exist as comorbidities can complicate the rehabilitation process. Multitrauma patients, such as patients who sustain blast injuries, motor vehicle accidents, or gunshot wounds with concomitant traumatic brain injuries, pose particular safety concerns. As for patients who suffer traumatic brain injuries along with amputation of 1 or multiple limbs, understanding and identifying key safety features in the rehabilitation process is integral to patient safety. These patients are prone to falls from having cognitive impairment that is compounded by an amputation, along with further issues such as spasticity, visual impairment, impulsivity, or vestibulocochlear deficits. Another important consideration is patients who undergo craniectomy after the initial event, which leads to increased possibility of severe injury if a fall were to occur. Although wearing a helmet is not usually a consideration for a noncomplicated amputee, it is our practice to always have a helmet in place during gait training in any patient with a craniectomy. Along with fall issues, understanding the cause and ramifications of the patient's other injuries is important in mapping out a safe rehabilitation process. Patients with multiple injuries may have an amputation along with weight-bearing restrictions on other joints that complicate safety issues. When progressing weight bearing, the use of a tilt table or overhead tracts and harness systems allows for offloading weight to continue to work on balance, mobility, and upright tolerance.

Polypharmacy is a major concern in patients with traumatic brain injuries and this is compounded when a patient has an amputation. The use of sedating medications such as many pain medications, neuromodulators, and antispasticity medications can affect cognitive therapies and ability to participate as well as decrease safety in cognitively impaired patients. Heterotopic ossification of joints and soft tissue can cause pain, skin integrity, and mobility issues. The treatment of heterotopic ossification can also be limited by the presence of other healing fractures. This is an important area for prosthetists to work closely with therapists and providers to make socket modifications, such as windows, to identify pain with increased weight bearing or any skin breakdown that may result from underlying heterotopic ossification. Working with in an interdisciplinary team approach to manage these patients is of utmost importance to identify safety concerns and catch issues as early as possible. Working within these teams, educating family members of patients with amputations with concomitant cognitive deficits needs to be a focus to ensure safety and help prevent complications. Patients' families need to be educated on issues such as skin monitoring, stump sock management, donning and doffing prosthesis, residual limb hygiene, and componentry inspection and maintenance.

Another complex subset of amputee patients are those with spinal cord injuries. These injuries can be cervical, thoracic, or lumbar, complete or incomplete, with varying degrees of ability to tolerate prosthetics, ambulation, skin complications, and level of independence or expected independence. Working closely with the patient's primary spinal cord injury team is integral to optimal safety for these patients. Identifying team and patient goals, often dictated by their level of injury, is important for choosing the most appropriate prosthesis. Whereas some patients may wish to have a prosthesis only for cosmesis, other patients may be able to progress to future ambulation and the most appropriate prosthetic limb for their individual situation helps them safely attain these goals. Working within an interdisciplinary team is in the patient's best interests. Identification of pain issues, early skin issues, progress of limb shaping, and changes in independence need to be monitored to assure the highest level of safety for these patients while they progress through rehabilitation.

Renal patients are of special concern to providers who deal with amputations as well and they offer their own specific complexities. Although the list of comorbidities can be extensive, patients with amputations secondary to dysvascular issues are more likely to have renal impairment as well. With changes in limb size because of fluctuating edema, prosthetic fit needs to be monitored closely to identify early skin breakdown or further complications such as pistoning, which could also lead to falls. Medication dosing has to be monitored as well. Close attention should be paid to medications that are cleared by the kidneys, and creatinine clearance should be monitored; it is also important to work closely with the patient's nephrologist, including keeping updated scheduling of dialysis if the patient's renal issues have progressed to that point. One important medication that is often used in phantom limb pain, gabapentin, needs especially close attention because it can cause further renal damage and the dosing changes depending on clearance issues. Comorbidities such as visual impairment, diabetes mellitus, cardiovascular issues, and metabolic demand should all be closely monitored in patients with severe renal disease as well to optimize safety. Patients who are brittle diabetics should also have glucose regularly checked to identify extreme changes in blood sugar that could compromise safety.

Coronary artery disease is prevalent in patients with lower extremity peripheral vascular disease, especially among those who go on to amputation. The use of dipyridamole-thallium imaging in these patients may improve the ability to diagnose asymptomatic coronary artery disease before initiating an exercise program, thereby allowing adequate treatment and preventing complications during rehabilitation.

Exercise testing using lower extremity exercise has been the gold standard for screening for coronary artery disease, but many patients with peripheral vascular disease and those with amputations have difficulty performing this type of exercise. Arm ergometry is a safe and effective exercise alternative for detecting asymptomatic coronary disease in those unable to exercise their lower extremities and can be used to determine safe upper extremity exercise levels in poorly conditioned patients and those with known coronary disease. Arm ergometry testing is also useful for providing prognostic information concerning functional outcome after a rehabilitation program. Exercise testing is therefore indicated in all vascular amputee patients before beginning an exercise training and prosthetic rehabilitation program. Exercise training can safely and inexpensively enhance the functional capacity of amputee patients with peripheral vascular disease.

SUMMARY

Interdisciplinary team assessment and management throughout all phases of care leads to the best and safest outcomes. Communication is integral to the interdisciplinary team approach. A comprehensive patient-centered treatment plan should be developed early in the course of rehabilitation process. Safety considerations should be considered with the treatment plan, with open lines of communication of team members and ongoing education of patients and caregivers. Environmental barriers and access to care considerations should be addressed early in rehabilitation.

Future Research Directions

It is evident from the studies reviewed in this article that there is a lack of formal controlled evaluations or scientific evidence for the effectiveness of preventive measures for reducing the occurrence of injuries and reinjury in amputation rehabilitation. Further studies are needed to understand the causes of amputation injuries so that randomized controlled or prospective cohort studies can be designed to evaluate the effectiveness of potential countermeasures. In the light of the gaps in current knowledge, specific recommendations for future countermeasure research and development include:

- Definitive evidence to support the benefit of any single postoperative care technique is lacking.[41] There have been numerous descriptive case series reports on the different types of management strategies but relatively few randomized comparative studies.[10] The current literature primarily is descriptive and does not provide sufficient evidence to support clinical decisions of (1) when to fit a cast with a prostheses and (2) when to begin weight bearing, especially in patients with peripheral vascular disease.
- Studies need to control for other variables besides dressing techniques that might have a greater impact on outcome.
- Further controlled, randomized studies are needed to directly compare different management strategies.
- Future studies need to consistently define their outcome measures, detail rates, and the impact of complications; use a more sensitive measure of postoperative pain, and quantify any savings of health care use and rehabilitation costs.
- Future studies need to more accurately document and control for variables such as amputation-level selection, surgical skill and technique, healing potential, comorbidity, nutrition, immune status, and functional ability.
- Prospective investigation of the temporal incidence of skin problems among lower limb prosthesis users and what factors are associated with skin problems among patients using a prosthesis are needed.[11]
- The impact of patient factors, prosthetic socket design, and prosthetic component selection on residual limb skin issues needs further elucidation.
- Questionnaires such as the one developed by Meulenbelt and colleagues[14] and continuing research on outcome measures for prevention and treatment of residual stump skin problems among users of a prosthesis play an important role. Biomechanical research into the mechanism(s) of injury is also crucial to the understanding of this critical issue.
- Pharmaceutical interventions for phantom limb pain: the direction of efficacy of calcitonin, anesthetics, and dextromethorphan needs further clarification. Larger and more rigorous randomized controlled trials are needed to make stronger recommendations about which medications are useful for clinical practice.[42]
- Investigation into the role of education for both providers and patients as well as caregivers to improve their knowledge and management about risk prevention strategies is needed.
- Investigation into providers' skills, attitudes, knowledge, and behavior in relation to safety risk is needed.
- Formal evaluation of preparticipation screening programs and an investigation into the role of health care personnel and rehabilitation programs on the incidence of injury and reinjury are needed.

Areas to Assess to Assure Optimal Safety	Extra Considerations
Vision	Changes, deterioration
Skin 　Residual limb 　Contralateral limb 　Pressure wounds in other areas for 　　patients with limited mobility	Limb preservation
Balance	Change, risk of falls
Range of motion (ROM) and restrictions 　Hip flexion 　Knee flexion 　Lumbar spine flexion and extension 　Cervical spine ROM 　Shoulder ROM	Observe for contractures, strength 　Consider Thomas test 　Flexion contractures 　Effects on gait, osteoarthritis development 　Able to see ground, survey surroundings 　Catch deficits early, rotator cuff monitoring 　　especially in those patients who continue 　　to use a wheelchair part time
Safe transfers	Identify gaps in knowledge or training as well 　as physical ability, review patient's current 　mobility, aids
Prosthesis 　Fit 　Function	Identify areas of irritation to skin, assess pain, 　discuss changes in limb shape, pistoning, 　time on prosthesis Working properly, aligned with patient's 　physical abilities and activities Ensure appropriate donning and doffing
Comorbidity review 　Diabetic 　Peripheral vascular disease 　Cardiac issues 　Pulmonary 　Osteoarthritis 　Osteoporosis 　Renal disease 　Cognitive issues such as dementia	Hypoglycemic events, adequate glucose 　control, lack of sensation, skin Contralateral limb issues, pain Progression, increased metabolic demand, 　appropriate medications, orthostasis, 　review cardiac testing, cardiac 　precautions Safe to ambulate, alternate mobility Change in gait, antalgic gait, include back 　pain assessment Increased risk for significant injury with falls, 　hip pads, level of ambulation Assess fluid fluctuations, review dialysis 　schedule if pertinent, identify medica 　tions such as neuromodulators that can 　affect renal function or medication 　dosing Assess for any decline from baseline
Precautions	Identify necessary related or unrelated 　precautions such as fall, seizure, weight 　bearing, or swallow precautions
Gait assessment	Check gait, including axial movements, shoe 　wear, prosthesis height, stability, antalgic, 　Trendelenburg Two-minute, 'get up and go', and L tests
Early limb shaping and safety	Residual limb protector, figure of 8 elastic 　compression wrap, limb shaping, 　edema fluctuations, wound healing, 　early fall education

(continued on next page)

Areas to Assess to Assure Optimal Safety	Extra Considerations
Medication review	Identify any unnecessary medications Review pain, hypertensive and diabetic medications
Pain assessment	Phantom limb pain and need for neuromodulators Back pain Residual limb pain Joint pain from abnormal stresses

Complex patients
  Traumatic brain injury
  Spinal cord injury
	Weight bearing, healing fractures, hetero topic ossification, other wounds, spasticity emotional/psychosocial status
	Review cognitive status, inhibition and compulsivity, need for helmet if status after craniectomy, vision, balance, and vestibulocochlear issues
	Ambulation status, need for thoracolumbo sacral or cervicothoracolumbosacral orthosis and affect on safety and mobility, transfers, any symptoms of urinary tract infection

- Further research into cause, treatment, acute management, and long-term impact on the patients with heterotopic ossification is needed.
- Further research into causes, treatment, and measure of volume changes within the residual limb is needed.
- For upper extremity and multilimb amputee populations the sample sizes are small, making research challenging. Multisite or nonexperimental approaches may be beneficial in these populations.
- The interdisciplinary expertise required and geographically diverse population suggest research into care through telemedicine or other remote means is required.
- More studies are needed to understand the full effects of exercise testing and training on specific cardiac variables, cardiovascular risk factors, and functional capacity for patients with peripheral vascular disease after amputation.

REFERENCES

1. Adams PF, Hendershot GE, Marano MA. Current estimates from the National Health Interview Survey, 1996. Vital Health Stat 10 1999;200:1–203.
2. Zeigler-Graham K, Mackenzie EJ, Ephraim PL, et al. Estimating the prevalence of limb loss in the United States: 2005 to 2050. Arch Phys Med Rehabil 2008;89(3): 422–9.
3. Eneroth M, Apelqvist J, Troeng T, et al. Operations, total hospital stay and costs of critical leg ischemia. Acta Orthop Scand 1996;67:459–65.
4. Green GV, Short K, Easley M. Transtibial amputation, Prosthetic use and functional outcome. Foot Ankle Clin 2001;6:315–27.
5. Larsson J, Apelqvist J. Towards less amputations in diabetic patients. Incidence, causes, cost, treatment, and prevention–a review. Acta Orthop Scand 1995; 66(2):181–92.

6. Reiber GE. Epidemiology and health care costs of diabetic foot problems. In: Veves A, Giurini J, LoGerfo FW, editors. The diabetic foot. Totowa (NJ): Humana Press; 2002.

7. Cumming J, Barr S, Howe TE. Prosthetic rehabilitation for older dysvascular people following a unilateral transfemoral amputation. Cochrane Database Syst Rev 2006;4:CD005260.

8. Cutson TM, Bongiorni DR. Rehabilitation of the older lower limb amputees: a brief review. J Am Geriatr Soc 1996;44:1388–93.

9. Ehde DM, Czerniecki JM, Smith DG, et al. Chronic phantom sensations, phantom pain, residual limb pain, and other regional pain after lower limb amputation. Arch Phys Med Rehabil 2000;81:1039–44.

10. Smith DG, McFarland LV, Sangeorzan BJ, et al. Postoperative dressing and management strategies for transtibial amputations: a critical review. J Rehabil Res Dev 2003;40(3):213–24.

11. Dudek NL, Marks MB, Marshall SC, et al. Dermatologic conditions associated with use of a lower-extremity prosthesis. Arch Phys Med Rehabil 2005;86:659–63.

12. Pezzin LE, Dillingham TR, Mackenzie EJ, et al. Use and satisfaction with prosthetic limb devices and related services. Arch Phys Med Rehabil 2004;85(5):723–9.

13. Salawu A, Middleton C, Gilbertson A, et al. Stump ulcers and continued prosthetic limb use. Prosthet Orthot Int 2006;30(3):279–85.

14. Meulenbelt HE, Geertzen JH, Jonkman MF, et al. Determinants of skin problems of the stump in lower-limb amputees. Arch Phys Med Rehabil 2009;90(1):74–81.

15. Dudek NL, Marks MB, Marshall SC. Skin problems in an amputee clinic. Am J Phys Med Rehabil 2006;85(5):424–9.

16. Meulenbelt HE, Geertzen JH, Jonkman MF, et al. Skin problems of the stump in lower limb amputees: 1. A clinical study. Acta Derm Venereol 2011;91(2):173–7.

17. Nederhand MJ, Van Asseldonk EH, van der Kooij H, et al. Dynamic Balance Control (DBC) in lower leg amputee subjects; contribution of the regulatory activity of the prosthesis side. Clin Biomech (Bristol, Avon) 2012;27(1):40–5.

18. Waters TR, Rockefeller K. Safe patient handling for rehabilitation professionals. Rehabil Nurs 2010;35(5):216–22.

19. Campo M, Weiser S, Koenig KL, et al. Work-related musculoskeletal disorders in physical therapists: a prospective cohort study with 1-year follow-up. Phys Ther 2008;88(5):608–19.

20. Ephraim PL, MacKenzie EJ, Wegener ST, et al. Environmental barriers experienced by amputees: the Craig Hospital Inventory of Environmental Factors–Short Form. Arch Phys Med Rehabil 2006;87(3):328–33.

21. Kahle JT, Highsmith MJ, Hubbard SL. Comparison of nonmicroprocessor knee mechanism versus C-Leg on Prosthesis Evaluation Questionnaire, stumbles, falls, walking tests, stair descent, and knee preference. J Rehabil Res Dev 2008;45(1):1–14.

22. Highsmith MJ, Schulz BW, Hart-Hughes S, et al. Differences in the spatiotemporal parameters of transtibial and transfemoral amputee gait. J Prosthet Orthot 2010; 22(1):26–30.

23. Highsmith MJ, Kahle JT, Bongiorni DR, et al. Safety, energy efficiency, and cost efficacy of the C-Leg for transfemoral amputees: a review of the literature. Prosthet Orthot Int 2010;34(4):362–77.

24. Miller WC, Deathe AB, Speechley M, et al. The influence of falling, fear of falling, and balance confidence on prosthetic mobility and social activity among individuals with a lower extremity amputation. Arch Phys Med Rehabil 2001;82(9):1238–44.

25. Miller WC, Speechley M, Death B. The prevalence and risk factors of falling and fear of falling among lower extremity amputees. Arch Phys Med Rehabil 2001; 82(8):1031–7.

26. Yang J, Jin D, Ji L, et al. The reaction strategy of lower extremity muscles when slips occur to individuals with trans-femoral amputation. J Electromyogr Kinesiol 2007;17(2):228–40.

27. Gooday HM, Hunter J. Preventing falls and stump injuries in lower limb amputees during inpatient rehabilitation: completion of the audit cycle. Clin Rehabil 2004; 18(4):379–90.

28. Pauley T, Devlin M, Heslin K. Falls sustained during inpatient rehabilitation after lower limb amputation: prevalence and predictors. Am J Phys Med Rehabil 2006;85(6):521–32.

29. Roberts TL, Pasquina PF, Nelson VS, et al. Limb deficiency and prosthetic management. 4. Comorbidities associated with limb loss. Arch Phys Med Rehabil 2006;87(3 Suppl 1):S21–7.

30. Dyer D, Bouman B, Davey M, et al. An intervention program to reduce falls for adult in-patients following major lower limb amputation. Healthc Q 2008;11(3 Spec No):117–21.

31. Ziegler-Graham K, MacKenzie EJ, Ephraim PL, et al. Estimating the prevalence of limb loss in the United States: 2005 to 2050. Arch Phys Med Rehabil 2008;89(3): 422–9.

32. Shubert T. Evidence-based exercise prescription for balance and falls prevention: a current review of the literature. J Geriatr Phys Ther 2011;34(3):100–7.

33. Matjacic Z, Burger H. Dynamic balance training during standing in people with trans-tibial amputation: a pilot study. Prosthet Orthot Int 2003;27(3):214–20.

34. Tsai HA, Kirby RL, MacLeod DA, et al. Aided gait of people with lower-limb amputations: comparison of 4-footed and 2-wheeled walkers. Arch Phys Med Rehabil 2003;84(4):584–91.

35. Jones LE, Davidson JH. Save that arm: a study of problems in the remaining arm of unilateral upper limb amputees. Prosthet Orthot Int 1999;23(1):55–8.

36. Biddiss EA, Chau TT. Upper limb prosthesis use and abandonment: a survey of the last 25 years. Posthet Orthot Int 2009;31(3):236–57.

37. Datta D, Selvarajah K, Davey N. Functional outcome of patients with proximal upper limb deficiency–acquired and congenital. Clin Rehabil 2004;18(2):172–7.

38. McFarland LV, Winkler SLH, Heinemann AW, et al. Unilateral upper-limb loss: satisfaction and prosthetic-device use in veterans and servicemembers from Vietnam and OIF/OEF conflicts. J Rehabil Res Dev 2010;47(4):299–316.

39. Raichle KA, Hanley MA, Molton I, et al. Prosthesis use in persons with lower-and upper-limb amputation. J Rehabil Res Dev 2008;45(7):961–72.

40. Rossbach P. Military In-Step: wound and skin care. US Army Amputee Patient Program and Amputation Coalition of America. 2005. Available at: http://www. amputee-coalition.org/military-instep/wound-skin-care.html. Accessed December 20, 2011.

41. Stansby G, Wealleans V, Wilson L, et al. Clinical experience of a new NPWT system in diabetic foot ulcers and post amputation wounds. J Wound Care 2010;19(11):496–502.

42. Alviar MJ, Hale T, Dungca M. Pharmacologic interventions for treating phantom limb pain. Cochrane Database Syst Rev 2011;12:CD006380.

43. Dudgeon BJ, Tyler EJ, Rhodes LA, et al. Managing usual and unexpected pain with physical disability: a qualitative analysis. Am J Occup Ther 2006;60:92–103.

44. Reiber GE, Smith DG, Boone DA, et al. Design and pilot testing of the DVA/Seattle Footwear System for diabetic patients with foot insensitivity. J Rehabil Res Dev 1997;34(1):1–8.

Patient Safety in the Rehabilitation of Children with Traumatic Brain Injury and Cerebral Palsy

Rajashree Srinivasan, MD

KEYWORDS

- Traumatic brain injury • Cerebral palsy • Patient safety
- Rehabilitation

NM is a 10-year-old boy who sustained traumatic brain injury (TBI) after a motor vehicle accident. He was an unrestrained front seat passenger while returning from school when the car was T-boned on the passenger side by a pickup truck. He sustained a right temporoparietal fracture, subdural hematoma, right humeral fracture, and right femur fracture. His Glasgow Coma Score at the scene was three. He was taken emergently to the operating room, where he underwent a craniectomy, placement of skull in abdomen, open reduction and internal fixation of the femur fracture, and cast placement for the fractured humerus. He was found on secondary survey to have cervical ligamentous laxity, and was placed in a cervical collar for 12 weeks. His father was deceased and his mother, who was also in the accident, experienced a TBI. His maternal grandmother was involved in his care. The patient was admitted to the rehabilitation unit after being medically stabilized.

At admission, the patient was reported to be in a coma (Ranchos Los Amigos scale level II), was non–weight-bearing on the right side, and was wearing a cervical collar. He was also noted to be hemiparetic on the left side and dependant for all his care. During inpatient rehabilitation, NM was treated for agitation, spasticity, aggressive behavior, and autonomic instability. He was noted to have an electrolyte imbalance and was taking phosphenytoin for prophylactic management of seizure risk.

TBI is termed the *silent epidemic*, with an estimated 10 million people being affected annually worldwide.[1] The prevalence of TBI in children that is severe enough to require hospitalization is estimated to be 70 per 100,000. Head trauma constitutes approximately 80% of traumatic pediatric injuries, with 5% dying at the scene of accident and 5% to 10% discharged to long-term care facilities. Nonaccidental trauma is most common in infants, whereas falls and sports-related injuries are seen in toddlers

Department of Rehabilitation Medicine, Baylor University Medical Center, 3301 Swiss Avenue, Dallas, TX 75204, USA
E-mail address: RajashrS@BaylorHealth.edu

Phys Med Rehabil Clin N Am 23 (2012) 393–400
doi:10.1016/j.pmr.2012.02.012
1047-9651/12/$ – see front matter © 2012 Elsevier Inc. All rights reserved.

and school-aged children, respectively. Motor vehicle accidents are seen in young adults, with an increasing incidence of concussion in amateur and professional athletes.[1] Demographics, development, epidemiology, and dependency for care make safe and efficient care challenging to provide. Concussion is a separate topic and is not addressed in this article.

Most patients have been already been medically stabilized by the time they reach the rehabilitation setting. Hence, this article discusses the rehabilitation aspects, with an emphasis on patient safety. The goal of rehabilitation is to maximize current function, enable patients to be self-sufficient, and teach compensatory strategies to achieve the new potential and educate families about these functions.

A detailed history must be obtained from the caregivers when the patient is admitted to the rehabilitation unit. Practitioners must recognize that families are under a lot of stress and hence may not be able to provide an accurate history, and therefore a secondary history must be obtained a day or two later when they are more ensconced in the setting. A history of attention deficit hyperactivity disorder (ADHD) is important in children with a TBI, because a 10% to 20% prevalence of preinjury ADHD exists.[2] The family must also be included in the goal-setting and be provided with a detailed explanation of the rehabilitation process. Information about the patient should be obtained before admission to accommodate any medical needs. **Box 1** outlines key points in the safe inpatient rehabilitation of children with a TBI.

The weight-bearing status must be noted to ensure proper transfer techniques and ambulatory processes. Identification and documentation of the stages of coma is important to assess the efficacy and safety of medications being used. Use of neurostimulants has been studied, although some studies were retrospective as opposed

---

Box 1
Key points important in the safe inpatient rehabilitation of children with a TBI

History and physical examination on admission to unit: includes detailed description of patient's injury; medical and surgical treatments rendered; past medical, developmental, and birth history; pertinent allergies; medications; family history; previous level of function and performance in school (if applicable)

Medication reconciliation: review medications for potential drug–drug interactions and polypharmacy

Transition in care: review discharge summary from previous hospital and double-check treatment plan to ensure safe transition from one facility to another

Rehabilitation prescription with safety precautions (ie, seizure risk, fall risk, weight bearing status, range of motion restrictions)

Education: patient and family/caregiver on TBI and its treatment

Communication: between rehabilitation team members and between medical and surgical specialists involved in the patient's care, especially at transition points in care, including hand-offs

Monitoring: laboratory value abnormalities, infections (urinary tract, pneumonia), missed fractures, agitation (Rancho Los Amigos scale, Rappaport scale, impulsivity, bowel/bladder function, swallowing function, skin breakdown, sleep-wake cycle)

Spasticity management (range of motion, splinting, casting, medications, chemodenervation, operative procedures [intrathecal baclofen, dorsal root rhizotomy], contracture release)

Deep vein thrombosis prophylaxis

Transition discharge with appropriate discharge summary

to prospective. Hence, the use of neurostimulants should be judicious, with close attention being paid to variations in autonomic instability.

Cognitive status is delicately balanced after any injury to the brain. As sleep-wake cycles are altered, mental status is precipitously balanced, and use of medicines in arousal and sleep should be vigilant. Use of medications such as N-methyl D-aspartate antagonists (amantadine) should be used carefully because they promote apoptosis through blocking excitatory effects of glutamate in young rats.[3] Use of other medications, such as bromocriptine, methylphenidate, and donepezil, requires close monitoring because their efficacy is still unclear.[4]

Altered mental status, either agitation or somnolence, should prompt a search for cause. **Box 2** lists some common causes to consider. Laboratory tests should be obtained, such as complete blood cell count, chemistry and blood culture, chest radiographs, urine analysis, and culture studies. Use of imaging studies such as non-contrast CT or MRI may be ordered; however, radiation exposure from CT and radiographs should be considered before these tests are ordered.

Physical aggression, verbal aggression, and explosive anger are associated with agitation. Agitation has been defined as the "subjective evidence of one or more of the following behaviors: restlessness, derogatory or threatening demands, verbal abusiveness, sexually inappropriate comments or actions, or attempts at physical violence of sufficient severity to disrupt nursing care or therapy."[5] Because no one medication has been shown to manage agitation better, the risks and benefits of each medication should be considered before use. **Box 3** lists medications used to treat agitation.

Risk of fall should be considered as consciousness improves. Impulsivity, lack of attention, lack of executive functioning, lack of insight into deficits, lack of safety awareness, urinary urgency, lack of balance, and lack of assistance at moment of wanting to go to the bathroom are a few factors that can add to the risk of falls. Once patients are able to verbalize their needs, a voiding schedule must be established. Families should be educated about weight-bearing status and taught to perform safe transfers, using gait belts as needed. Ambulation should be assessed before patients begin walking based on their weight-bearing status. Either a "one-to-one sitter" or family members must be with the patient to provide reminders of safety awareness. Depending on a hospital's resources or policies, a safety enclosure bed can sometimes be used.

Spasticity is defined as a velocity-dependant resistance of a muscle to stretch[6] and is a sign of upper motor neuron injury. Scales commonly used to grade spasticity include the Ashworth, modified Ashworth, and Tardieu scales. Treatment of spasticity

---

Box 2
Causes of altered mental status and agitation

Hydrocephalus

Infection: urinary tract infection, tracheitis, meningitis, pneumonia

Electrolyte imbalance

Venous thrombosis

Occult fracture

Environmental factors: overstimulation, altered sleep-wake cycle

Neurogenic bowel and bladder

Perforated bowel

Box 3
Medications used to treat agitation

Benzodiazepines: lorazepam, diazepam, and clonazepam

ß-blockers: propranolol (not approved by the U.S. Food And Drug Administration [FDA] in children)

Anticonvulsants: valproic acid, carbamazepine, and lamotrigine

Antidepressants/selective serotonin reuptake inhibitors: sertraline, paroxetine, citalopram, fluoxetine, and amitriptyline

Antipsychotics: propranolol, clozapine (not FDA-approved in children), ziprasidone, quetiapine, and olanzapine

---

in the acute setting is to prevent development of contracture. Range of motion exercises, stretching, use of positioning devices, and use of modalities are helpful in treating spasticity. Use of splinting or casting must be monitored carefully because skin breakdown can occur when the splint/cast remains on for a long time and when the cast is removed. Close attention must be paid to positioning. The patient should be positioned on the side with hips flexed past 90° and with neck flexion.[7] Medications used to treat spasticity should be based on the goals: pain relief, proper positioning, caregiver ease, and hygiene issues. Many patients use their spasticity to help with positioning, transfers, maintenance of muscle tone, and prevention of deep vein thrombosis.

Pharmacologic agents used to treat spasticity include baclofen, benzodiazepines, dantrolene sodium, clonidine, and tizanidine.[8] Chemodenervation with botulinum toxin and phenol can also complement the use of stretching, splinting, and casting. Phenol and botulinum toxin injections can be used together to target a larger number of muscles if severe spasticity is present. However, the FDA has not approved the use of botulinum toxin in children younger than 12 years in the United States, although it has been approved for use in Canada, Australia, and other countries.[9] The potential risk of distant spread of toxin should be discussed with the patient and families before use. Furthermore, a conversion factor for different toxins does not exist, because the units of biologic activity among the products are not equivalent. The medication guide for using the toxin should be provided to caregivers. For safety reasons, the lowest possible dose should be used, based on weight.[10] Botulinum toxin injections are easy to perform and commonly injected once every 3 months. Phenol injections can also be used to treat spasticity. However, these can be painful and are associated with a risk for deep vein thrombosis, and the effects are permanent. Factors to consider when deciding whether to use chemodenervating agents should include cost and risks and benefits; patients must be at the center of the care process and not the diagnosis.

The intrathecal baclofen (ITB) pump is an effective method of treating spasticity of cerebral origin, especially cerebral palsy.[11] It has also been used to treat spasticity from acquired brain injury.[12] The pump is usually implanted after the patient has had an ITB trial, helping families see the decrease in spasticity. The decision to implant an ITB pump should not be made lightly, because the consequences of improper maintenance can result in death. Importance of refilling the ITB pump should be stressed to the family, because if in the absence of commitment to regular follow-up, this procedure can be dangerous. Families should be trained to recognize signs and symptoms of baclofen overdose and withdrawal, which are outlined in **Box 4**. Clinicians should be skilled in recognizing and troubleshooting malfunctioning pumps, including mechanical failure from rotor stall, computer error, no/low drug in reservoir,

---

Box 4
Signs and symptoms of baclofen overdose and withdrawal

Baclofen overdose: gross reduction in tone, loss of skills after change in dose, somnolence, altered mental status

Baclofen withdrawal: fever, irritability, itching, increased spasticity; extreme cases involve rhabdomyolysis and onset of seizures resulting in death

---

battery failure, catheter malfunction from migration, fracture, kink/occlusion, disconnection from pump, human error from programming error, and refill error.[13]

Sensory deficits associated with TBI can also cause safety concerns. Anosmia is seen in 5% to 65% of patients, depending on the severity of injury.[14] Parents and caregivers must be trained to look for other signs of danger (eg, gas burner left on, which is a fire hazard).

Conductive hearing loss recovers spontaneously in 3 weeks. If a delay occurs, a repeat audiogram and evaluation for middle-ear pathology is recommended. Vision impairment can present as hemianopsia, cortical visual impairment, cranial nerve palsies, and diplopia. Vision screening with the appropriate care provider is important to identify the deficit so an effective strategy can be implemented. Both vision and hearing impairments can pose safety risks to the patient (falls), and these should be taken into account when writing the rehabilitation prescription and educating the family or caregiver.

When more than one health care provider is involved in patient care, the potential exists for a lack of effective communication, especially at transition points in the patient's care (ie, changes in duty shifts among nurses and physicians). Appropriate handoffs between staff are important for effective and safe patient care. Use of checklists can be helpful in decreasing the risks of errors. Also, holding staff accountable for safety is important in reducing errors.

Occasionally, misunderstanding between caregivers and insurance companies occur with respect to the patient's medical benefits (coverage for durable medical equipment; number of days allowed in an acute rehabilitation setting). Having a well-functioning team is critical, with members effectively communicating and keeping the entire team informed of the patient's benefits.

In teaching institutions, residents must be well supervised and trained properly to ensure safety in care.

Discharge planning is a key factor in rehabilitation, which should begin when the patient is admitted to the hospital. Care must be coordinated with the family and school to ensure ongoing success of the rehabilitative process. Families must be trained in the medical and nursing care of the child, which often adds an extra layer of strain for the family. Discharge disposition must be determined as early as possible. A home evaluation may be necessary to ensure that the patient equipment will fit through the doors and to provide recommendations regarding home modifications. Caregivers must be identified and training begun as soon as possible. In this era of managed care and accountable health care organizations, resources are limited and therefore must be used wisely. Long-term care facilities for pediatric patients are limited and must be well explored before placement.

Schools must be part of the care plan to integrate an individual educational plan, including any modifications regarding any school work (eg, note-taking with a computer or recorder; use of an extra set of books; exemption from taking written tests). This plan can be achieved with the assistance of a trained licensed pediatric neuropsychologist or the school counselor. The school also must be aware of any medications being taken and any restrictions regarding participation in physical education. If the child has an ITB, the school must be aware of it and the school nurse must be able to recognize signs and symptoms of malfunction. Families and schools must be aware of the diagnosis of TBI and be watchful for any behavioral problems.

The mode of transportation that will be used at discharge must be discussed with the family. The patient must be safely positioned in either a wheelchair with tie downs or placed in the seat of the vehicle with appropriate restraints. If there is insufficient head control, a soft cervical collar may be needed to help support the neck while upright. The family must practice car transfers before discharge. If spasticity is an issue and the patient cannot be positioned appropriately, transport in a van/stretcher may be necessary. The child may need frequent rest if there is increased sensory stimulation, or if they have greater medical needs, like frequent suctioning or uncontrolled seizures.

Medication reconciliation at admission and discharge is crucial because a lot of changes occur during hospitalization. A list of the medications at discharge, follow-up appointments, and in-hospital procedures is helpful in keeping track of patient's hospital stay. Ongoing follow-up with various specialists can place a great deal of stress on the families. Hence, support should be offered in the form of counseling, social work support, or respite care. Outpatient therapies will also need to be set up in a way that is feasible for family members to take the patients and also care for other family members. Involving the primary care physician at discharge is important because this cements the medical home model, providing continuity of care.

A frequent question asked is: "When can I start driving?" Return to driving should be addressed by a driving rehabilitation specialist to ensure assessment of vision and cognitive and motor skills, and should include an on-road evaluation.[15]

CEREBRAL PALSY

Cerebral palsy is defined as a group of disorders affecting the development of movement and posture, causing activity limitation, which are attributed to nonprogressive disturbances that occurred in the developing fetal or infant brain. The motor disorders of cerebral palsy are often accompanied by disturbances of sensation, cognition, communication, perception, and/or behavior, and/or by a seizure disorder.[16] Cerebral palsy is the leading cause of childhood disability,[17] and has a prevalence of 2 to 3 per 1000 live births.[18]

The medical history should include a record of prenatal and pregnancy complications; maternal illnesses; exposure to toxins, drugs, or alcohol; prenatal care; fetal movements; and history of trauma. It should also include information about the perinatal period, including gestational age at delivery, delivery type and presentation, birth weight, and Apgar score, and a full developmental history.

A motor delay prompts the family to seek medical care, which leads to the diagnosis. Although static, patient presentation changes with growth and development of the child, and can present as spasticity; seizures; cognitive delay; speech and language problems; sensory changes; gait abnormalities; and musculoskeletal problems, such as contractures and hip subluxation/dislocations; nutritional deficiencies from improper intake; and oromotor problems.

Management of spasticity includes proper positioning, range of motion exercises, and medications, and treatment is important for preventing contractures. A neurosurgical procedure used in treatment of spasticity is the selective dorsal root rhizotomy, which can improve gait and range of motion but has residual motor control problems.[19] Good outcomes are dependent on proper patient selection, with criteria including age of 3 to 6 years, good trunk control, and good underlying strength.[20]

Growth and nutrition are affected in cerebral palsy. Dysphagia, spasticity (causing a high energy-requiring state), poor oromotor control, and oral aversion cause maladaptive eating patterns, affecting nutritional status and growth. Drooling from poor oromotor control and poor head control with decreased sensation can cause skin irritation and breakdown, social embarrassment, and decreased social integration. Medications used to treat drooling include glycopyrrolate, cetirizine, and scopolamine.[20]

Growth is also affected in children who are nonambulatory, have spastic quadriplegia, or experience seizures, causing them to be shorter, which is thought to be from the causes of cerebral palsy.[20]

Musculoskeletal problems seen include scoliosis, hip dislocations, and contractures. Their presence may pose safety risks to the child through increasing the risk of falls and pressure ulcers, and may restrict their mobility. Primitive reflexes may persist and protective reflexes are absent.[21]

All children are entitled to a free and appropriate education, including special education at public expense. Education should be in the least-restrictive environment as possible.[20] Baseline neuropsychological evaluation is helpful in making school recommendations and any modifications at school.

Transition to adult care is important. Patients with cerebral palsy have lived with their parents all their lives, and therefore must be trained to be independent. This ability is dependent on the degree of disability, with less-disabled individuals being able to obtain advanced education and jobs. Vocational rehabilitation is a concept that should be introduced early to patients and caregivers. They also need to be taught about the medical condition and impairments, effective strategies to address these, and preventive measures to minimize safety risks. They should also be educated on how to navigate the health care system and advocate for any needs. Health care providers who are trained and comfortable taking care of patients with cerebral palsy must be identified to ensure a proper transition from a pediatric care provider. Importance of health maintenance should be stressed to patients and caregivers.[20]

Families often attempt complementary and alternative medicine to address patient issues. Health care providers must be able to set aside their personal opinions and work in a nonjudgmental manner toward providing the patient with sound information so that an informed decision can be made.

Abuse in individuals with special needs such as cerebral palsy or TBI are recognized and can pose a significant safety risk. Inability to leave an abusive situation because of mobility impairments or dependency on caregivers can place individuals with disabilities with women in particular being at risk for abuse, because they have a fear of retaliation if they report it.[22] Children with physical limitations, cognitive deficits, and visual/hearing impairments are also at risk for injury secondary to fire, poison, and water-related accidents. Information on fire safety, poison prevention, and water safety is available for children with visual or hearing impairment, physical limitation, and cognitive deficits.[23]

REFERENCES

1. Gean AD, Fischbein NJ. Head trauma. Neuroimaging Clin N Am 2010;20:527–56.
2. Levin HS, Hanten G. Executive functions after TBI in children. Pediatr Neurol 2005;33:79–93.
3. Pohl D, Bittigau P, Ishimaru MJ, et al. NMDA antagonists and apoptotic cell death triggered by head trauma in developing rat brain. Proc Natl Acad Sci U S A 1999; 96:2508–13.

4. Pangilinan PH, Giacoletti- Argento A, Shellhaus R, et al. Neuropharmacology in pediatric brain injury: a review. PM R 2010;2:1127–40.

5. Mysiw WJ, Jackson RD, Corrigan JD. Amitriptyline for post traumatic agitation. Am J Phys Med Rehabil 1988;67:29–33.

6. Sanger TD, Delgado MR, Gaebler-Spira D, et al. Classification and Definition of disorders causing hypertonia in childhood. Pediatrics 2003;111(1):e89–97.

7. Alexander M, Mathews D. Pediatric Rehabilitation: Principles and Practices. 4th edition. New York: Demos Publishing; 2009.

8. Crooks CY, Zumsteg JM, Bell KR. TBI: a review of practice management and recent advances. Phys Med Rehabil Clin N Am 2007;18(4):681–710.

9. Quality Standards Subcommittee of the American Academy of Neurology and the Practice Committee of the Child Neurology Society, Delgado MR, Hirtz D, et al. Practice parameter: pharmacologic treatment of spasticity in children and adolescents with cerebral palsy. Report of the Quality Standards Subcommittee of the American Academy of Neurology and the Practice Committee of the Child Neurology Society. Neurology 2010;74:336–43.

10. Apkon SD, Cassidy D. Safety considerations in the use of botulinum toxins in children with cerebral palsy. PM R 2010;2:282–4.

11. Albright A, Cervi C, Singletary G. Intrathecal Baclofen for spasticity in cerebral palsy. JAMA 1991;265:1418–22.

12. Francisco GE, Latorre JM, Ivanhoe CB. Intrathecal baclofen for spastic hypertonia in chronic traumatic brain injury. Brain Inj 2007;21:335–8.

13. Francisco GE, Saulino MF, Yablon SA, et al. Intrathecal baclofen therapy: an update. PM R 2009;1:862–8.

14. Doty RL, Yousem DM, Pham LT, et al. Olfactory dysfunction in patients with head trauma. Arch Neurol 1997;54(9):1131–40.

15. Lane AK, Benoit D. Driving, brain injury and assistive technology. NeuroRehabilitation 2011;28(3):221–9.

16. Bax M, Goldstein M, Rosenbaum P, et al. Proposed definition and classification of cerebral palsy. Dev Med Child Neurol 2005;47:571–6.

17. Stanley FJ. Cerebral palsy trends: implications for perinatal care. Acta Obstet Gynecol Scand 1994;73:5.

18. Nelson KB, Ellenberg JH. Epidemiology of cerebral palsy. In: Schoenberg BS, editor. Advances in Neurology, vol. 19. New York: Raven Press; 1978. p. 421–35.

19. Wright FV, Sheil EM, Drake JM, et al. Evaluation of selective dorsal root rhizotomy for the reduction of spasticity in cerebral palsy: a randomized controlled trial. Dev Med Child Neurol 1998;40:239–47.

20. Green LB, Hurvitz EA. Cerebral palsy. Phys Med Rehabil Clin N Am 2007;18:859–82.

21. Paine RS, Oppe TE. Neurologic examination of children. Clinics in Developmental Medicine (UK): William Heinemann Medical Books; 1966. p. 279.

22. Young ME, Nosek MA, Howland C, et al. Prevalence of abuse in women with physical disabilities. Arch Phys Med Rehabil 1997;78:S34–8.

23. Available at: http://www.safekidsusa.org. Accessed December, 2011.

Patient Safety in the Rehabilitation of Children with Spinal Cord Injuries, Spina Bifida, Neuromuscular Disorders, and Amputations

David Cancel, MD, JD[a], Jaishree Capoor, MD[b],*

KEYWORDS

- Pediatric rehabilitation • Pediatric spinal cord injury
- Spina bifida • Pediatric amputee • Patient safety

Pediatric patient safety continues to challenge both pediatricians and pediatric physiatrists. While there is a trend toward developing general patient safety initiatives, there is little research on pediatric patient safety. This article identifies major areas of general safety risk, with a focus on timely diagnosis and care coordination to prevent secondary complications that compromise health, function, and quality of life in pediatric neuromuscular disease, spinal cord disorders, and amputation.

ASSESSMENT OF THE PEDIATRIC PATIENT IN THE REHABILITATION SETTING, WITH AN EMPHASIS ON SAFETY

Assessment of the pediatric patient should contain information about the child in the variety of environments in which he or she lives and receives care. The most commonly encountered settings are home, school, therapy gym, and medical facilities.

Medical History

This section should describe the child's principal diagnosis and include pertinent information about the events that led to the present condition in chronologic order

[a] Department of Rehabilitation Medicine, Kingsbrook Rehabilitation Institute, 585 Schenectady Avenue, Brooklyn, NY 11203, USA
[b] Children's Rehabilitation Center, 317 North Street, White Plains, NY, USA
* Corresponding author.
E-mail address: jc1058@columbia.edu

Phys Med Rehabil Clin N Am 23 (2012) 401–422
doi:10.1016/j.pmr.2012.03.001
1047-9651/12/$ – see front matter © 2012 Elsevier Inc. All rights reserved.

(ie, trauma that led to spinal cord injury or brain injury; cancer that necessitated lower limb amputation). The historian should be a reliable source. Key points of the medical history, with an emphasis on safety, are briefly discussed here.

Birth and developmental history
Birth and developmental history include prenatal care, perinatal and neonatal events, prematurity, and age onset of major developmental milestones. It is important to distinguish between steady delay and skills regression for accuracy of diagnosis.

Medical and surgical history
It is important to determine the child's general health status, and review hospitalizations, providers, allergies, and immunizations. A systemic approach to disease-specific complications is helpful. Seizures, visual and hearing impairments, and behavioral issues are more common in static and progressive diseases of the central nervous system. History of past or present respiratory complications should be explored in disabilities such as spina bifida, muscular dystrophy, cerebral palsy (CP), spinal cord injury (SCI), and spinal muscular atrophy. Frequent infections or failure to thrive may indicate chronic aspiration. Other examples of disease-specific complications and interventions include: recurrent aspiration, malnutrition, antispasticity, and orthopedic management in CP; central ventilatory dysfunction, syringobulbia, tethered cord, autonomic dysreflexia, pressure ulcers, urinary tract infections, and latex allergy in spinal cord disorders; nightmares, sweating, insomnia and fatigue consistent with hypercapnia, or exercise dyspnea from cardiomyopathy in advanced muscular dystrophy. Pressure ulcers may be related to weight changes, contractures, malnutrition, and incontinence, in addition to ill-fitting braces and poor positioning. Caregivers should have a high index of suspicion and be educated about signs of occult fracture in children with mobility issues.

Medication safety risks
Children with disabilities often require several different classes of medications including antiepileptics, antispasticity agents, antidepressants, and opiates. These medications may be prescribed by several different providers in several different environments (ie, acute rehabilitation units, long-term care facility, school, patient's home), and also have significant side effects and drug-drug interactions. There is a high risk for medication-related errors in dosing and administration. A common risk factor is weight-based dosing and off-label use. Prescribers often deviate from standardized medication dosing.[1] Medication side effects should be monitored and dosages adjusted as weight changes. The most common adverse drug reactions are associated with skin-related complications.[2]

Neuromusculoskeletal Problems

Contractures and deformities of the extremities and spine secondary to weakness, spasticity, and pain can all contribute to loss of functions such as ambulation and self-care, and this in turn can lead to additional problems such as skin breakdown. Growth and decreased motor function may be associated with increased energy costs, contractures, and muscle stiffness.[3] Spinal deformity secondary to scoliosis and the rate of increasing curvature must be well documented to help plan surgical intervention. Manual dexterity is also of significant importance because limited use of the hands can adversely affect the ability to propel a wheelchair, don/doff a prosthesis or orthosis, perform activities of daily living, and self-catheterize the bladder. Children with hemiplegia should also be assessed for functional deficits in the nonhemiplegic hand.[4]

Current and Prior Level of Function

Current and prior level of function includes 5 major domains, including physical development (such as transfers and ambulation), and cognitive, communication, social, and adaptive/self-care skills. The amount of personal assistance and equipment needed for maximal independence should be documented. Screening tools commonly used to identify developmental delays include Denver II, CAT/CLAMS,[5] or Developmental Assessment of Young Children (DAYC).[6] A functional decline associated with new neurologic impairments may be a sign of myopathy, or cord tethering in spina bifida, or myelopathy in Down syndrome.[7]

Poorly fitting orthotics, prostheses, and equipment

It is important for the clinician to inquire about orthotics, prostheses, and equipment. Questions regarding poor fit, pain with use, skin irritation, recent weight changes, and integrity and function of the devices are important in determining safety with application. Orthotic or prosthetic devices used by children with neurologic or sensory deficits can increase the risk of injury or skin breakdown. The child should be evaluated at home and school for assistive devices and adaptive equipment that can maximize safety and access to the environment (ie, wheelchairs/mobility/gait aids, standers, adaptive/feeding chairs, hospital bed, augmentative communication devices, grab bars, tub benches, bedside commodes, hand-held showers, raised toilet seats).

Impaired cognition

The cause of impaired memory, attention span, and judgment can be multifactorial in origin. Factors that can contribute include: underlying neurologic disorders; effects of medications such as antiepileptics, spasticity agents, and pain medications; infections and metabolic disorders; and attention-deficit disorder. Impaired cognition can delay acquisition of motor skills and affect performance in school and activities of daily living, as well as safety with outdoor play.

Impaired swallowing, feeding, and communication

Inability to swallow effectively can increase the risk of aspiration pneumonia and malnutrition. It is important to review dietary history as well as history of swallowing abnormalities and diagnostic testing results; one should monitor for aspiration signs, such as coughing with feeds or when asleep. Children may need positioning strategies for feeding.[8] Caloric requirements in children need to be adjusted based on growth curves adjusted for height and weight, and activity patterns consistent with specific disability. It is important to monitor growth velocity as well as actual growth itself. It is especially important to elicit dietary history as active children transition to wheelchairs.

Impaired adaptive skills: dressing, toileting, and hygiene

The ability of the child to perform self-care should be recorded. The child may need undergarments to protect skin maceration secondary to soiling. The use of indwelling catheters should also be recorded because they can predispose a child to urinary tract infections.

Education and Socioeconomic Issues

It is important for rehabilitation clinicians to have a good understanding about the child's level of family, financial, and community support, including educational services, environmental accommodations, service coordination, and adequacy of home health aide and nursing services. It is also important to evaluate the level of understanding of the child and caregiver about the child's medical diagnosis and impairments. Language barriers should also be identified.

Physical Examination

It is important to perform a comprehensive physical examination of the child living with a physical disability, and attention should be given to neuromuscular and functional impairments that can exacerbate or create safety risks in the rehabilitation setting. The same diagnosis may require different examination techniques as the child with disability grows and develops. For example, in neonatal brachial plexus injury (BPI), the examination focus is on spontaneous movements, primitive reflexes, and tone, whereas in older children with persistent weakness attributable to BPI, the examination focus is on contractures, shoulder instability, and compensatory movements and function. Examiners must be familiar with age-appropriate milestones and developmental trajectories in various disabilities. A child-friendly environment is required for cooperation with examination. The most informative and accurate part of the examination often occurs while the child plays in the waiting room or proceeds into the examination room. Hands-on examination should occur last. The following are some key areas to be examined that are relevant to the patient's safety.

Neurologic system

1. Cognitive and behavioral evaluation: the level of the child's alertness, awareness, attention, behavior, and cooperation should be recorded.
2. Cranial nerve examination should focus on vision, hearing, smell, facial symmetry, and tongue movements. Bedside swallowing evaluation can be beneficial.
3. Motor strength can be tested in key muscles of the upper and lower limbs in school-aged children. Spontaneous active movements should be observed at rest initially, and may be elicited in infants using primitive reflexes and position changes. Quality of movement, asymmetries, postures, weakness, incoordination, and reflex abnormalities may reflect motor deficits and should be recorded.
4. Sensory evaluation may include assessment of light touch, pain/temperature, proprioception, and vibration if indicated and when possible. When accurate sensory examination in young children is limited, behavior changes and motor response to sensory stimulation should be recorded.
5. Presence of tone, spasticity, posturing, persistent primitive reflexes, and absent protective reactions should be noted, as they can potentially lead to contractures and increased risk for falls. Monitoring for changes in tone and spasticity should be carried out, using a standardized instrument such as the modified Ashworth Scale or Tardieu scale, respectively.
6. Evaluate balance in both sitting and standing positions if possible.

Musculoskeletal system: limb and spinal deformities

Bone configuration and joint mobility can change over time. Posture, alignment, passive and active ranges of motion should be recorded for the upper and lower extremities and spine. Contractures should be recorded for each of the involved joints. Limb length discrepancies and painful/tender areas should also be identified. If the child has a lower limb amputation, then the residual limb shape, length, circumferential measurements, integrity of suture line and painful/tender areas should be recorded as well as any hip or knee contractures. Redness and swelling of an extremity after exertion may be the sign of a fracture.[7]

Skin

The skin should be thoroughly checked for any evidence of skin breakdown or irritation in the affected limb or trunk of a child wearing an arm, leg, or thoracic orthosis. The skin of the residual limb should also be checked in the child using a prosthesis, especially over pressure-sensitive areas such as the tibial tuberosity. Nonambulatory children who are bed-bound, or spend a significant amount of time in a wheelchair and have significant spasticity, should have their skin checked at the following bony prominences: sacrum, greater trochanters, ischial tuberosities, heels, medial knees, thoracic spine, and occiput (especially in infants and young children with disproportionately large heads).

GENERAL PEDIATRIC REHABILITATION PRESCRIPTION CONSIDERATIONS TO MAXIMIZE PATIENT SAFETY
Precautions

Universal precautions are generally practiced during therapy. However, there are certain precautions that pediatric physiatrists may need to consider when writing a prescription for rehabilitation. Some examples include: (1) seizure precautions; (2) fracture/fall risk (ie, amputee, osteopenia, balance, cognitive disorder); (3) cardiac and fatigue precautions (ie, neuromuscular disease); (4) surgery-related precautions (ie, weight bearing and range-of-motion restrictions); (5) risk for autonomic dysreflexia, orthostasis, pressure sores, temperature regulation, and sensory precautions in children with spinal cord injuries; (6) impaired communication and cognition (can pose a risk if modalities such as heat, cold, and electrical stimulation are being considered); (7) risk for atlantoaxial instability (ie, Down syndrome, juvenile idiopathic arthritis, skeletal dysplasia); (8) visual-spatial deficits (ie, spina bifida); (9) behavioral issues (ie, aggressive behavior); (10) pulmonary precautions (ie, aspiration risk, need for positioning and supplemental oxygen or monitoring for oxygenation levels); (11) thermoregulation precautions with exercise; (12) shunt precautions and need for protective headgear (used to maximize safety in the child with cranial defects, unsafe gait, or previous brain injury).

Exercise Regimen

An important principle in the planning of rehabilitation therapies includes the timing of therapy sessions to minimize patient fatigue secondary to other treatments or comorbidities (ie, chemotherapy, radiation, and dialysis). There are several different types of exercises including aerobic, resistance, and flexibility. Aerobic exercises are the mainstay of rehabilitation and the least controversial. Resistive exercises are controversial because of the risk of muscle injury during this type of exercise, and are discussed further in the section on muscular dystrophy. Resistance training machines are safer than free weights because they allow a fixed pattern of movement and are easier to learn. Equipment must also have proper sizing to avoid joint and muscle malalignment.[9]

IMPACT OF CARE COORDINATION AND TRANSITIONAL PLANNING ON PATIENT SAFETY
Transitions in Care

Rehabilitation clinicians involved in the care of children with disabilities should also consider factors such as transition points in the care of the child as potential safety risks. Examples of transitions in care include: medical care on medical/surgical wards of hospitals; transfer from hospital to rehabilitation ward or facility; transfer from rehabilitation facility to home or long-term care facility; and transitioning from pediatric to adult care.[10] Health care providers must identify necessary transition services, coordinate care, and ensure timely referral before transition, as well as enhance patient knowledge, autonomy, and involvement in clinical decision making.[11]

Coordination of care among multiple different clinicians and settings can be challenging given the multitude of clinical and nonclinical providers, including family, physicians, teachers, therapists, nurses, coaches, paraprofessionals, service coordinators, and home attendants. Among the most common reasons for failure to receive continued medical care is lack of recommendation by acute care doctors or schools.[12] Effective transmission of information remains challenging, especially when surgical interventions are planned and informed consent is needed.[13] Communication among providers at various points in the continuum of health care is important to ensure that information exchange occurs and care is not compromised as the child moves back and forth along this continuum. Communication extends to all caregivers of the child, and should take into account that caregivers rely on multiple sources of information in deciding on a plan of care.[14] Portable care notebooks facilitate effective communication.[15,16] Collaboration between acute care and community social workers and case managers can result in better patient-centered care.[17] Children with special health care needs provided with care coordination in medical homes benefit from increased access to specialty care, higher rates of school attendance, decreased hospital use, fewer unmet needs, and decreased financial burden on the family.[18,19]

PATIENT SAFETY IN CHILDREN WITH NEUROMUSCULAR DISORDERS

This section addresses patient safety issues common to children with neuromuscular disorders. While these conditions have varied physiologic causes, they all share characteristic patterns of functional disability and common safety risks. This section focuses on dystrophinopathies and spinal muscular atrophy (SMA).

Dystrophinopathies represent a heterogeneous group of neuromuscular disorders occurring within the sarcolemma. The muscle cells undergo repeated cycles of necrosis and regeneration, with fibrous tissue infiltration of the affected tissue. Eventually the muscle cells are no longer able to regenerate, resulting in a clinical and functional decline. Death usually results from respiratory failure. The most common dystrophinopathy is Duchenne muscular dystrophy, affecting 1 in 3500 males. In Duchenne, the abnormality occurs via an out-of-frame mutation at the Xp21 gene loci, producing a nonfunctional protein. In its milder form, Becker muscular dystrophy, the defect is in an in-frame mutation of the X chromosome that produces some functioning dystrophin, with varying degrees of clinical and functional decline. Full review of dystrophinopathies is beyond the scope of this article; however, the topic has been discussed elsewhere in the literature.[20] **Table 1** outlines common impairments and secondary complications associated with Duchenne muscular dystrophy.

SMA represents an autosomal recessive motor neuron disorder of variable expressivity characterized by a deficiency in the Survival Motor Neuron Gene 1 (SMN1) of Chromosome 5q11. SMA has an incidence of about 1 in 10,000 live births and a carrier frequency of 1 in 50. There are currently 3 clinical subtypes of SMA, with the recent addition of a fourth subtype with onset in the fourth decade. SMA type I (Werdnig-Hoffman or infantile-onset SMA) is characterized by severe neuromuscular deficits, inability to attain independent sitting, and life expectancy of approximately 2 years. SMA type II (intermediate-onset SMA) is characterized by onset of symptoms at 6 to 18 months of age. Children fail to achieve ambulation without assistance, but have a life expectancy into young adulthood. SMA type III (Kugelberg-Welander or juvenile-type) is characterized by onset after 2 years of age with impaired ambulation and full life expectancy, with limitations dependent on the onset and severity of symptoms. SMA type IV (adult-onset SMA) is a fairly recent category of SMA with autosomal dominant or recessive inheritance. There is a progressive decline beginning in the fourth decade and presenting with milder symptoms. A full review of the genetic causes of SMA, its subtypes, and pathology is given by Alexander and Matthews.[20]

COMMON SAFETY CONCERNS IN CHILDREN WITH NEUROMUSCULAR DISORDERS
Anesthesia and Cardiac Risks

General safety guidelines for anesthesia in Duchenne calls for preoperative cardiac workup with electrocardiography and echocardiography to evaluate for cardiomyopathy, pulmonary function testing, and creatine kinase levels. General sedation is often recommended, and intravenous or local anesthesia can be used. If inhaled anesthesia is to be given, practitioners must be prepared for possible rhabdomyolysis.[21]

Fracture Risk

Children with neuromuscular disorders generally share common risk factors secondary to osteoporosis and decreased mobility. In dystrophinopathies, there is an increased risk for fractures as disease progression makes ambulation more difficult. Although falls are a common mechanism for fracture, many develop fractures from even minor trauma or aggressive stretching. It is important to recognize the risks at specific developmental milestones, considering age-appropriate guidelines for care and fall avoidance. This guidance should include transfer, stair, curb, and playground training.

Obesity

Children with neuromuscular conditions become more reliant on wheelchair mobility after a decline in ambulation or because of a fear of falling. Children are either gradually unable to ambulate, or limit their ambulation because they are afraid of falling. There is a decline in lean body mass and an increased risk of osteoporosis and fractures. Medical comorbidities can also worsen. In particular, increased abdominal girth can worsen respiratory limitations by reducing diaphragmatic excursion.

Scoliosis

Increased spinal deformity is associated with puberty and cessation of ambulation. Worsening of scoliosis contributes to decreased pulmonary function in curves over 100°.[22] With spinal orthoses, there is also an increased risk of pressure sores and respiratory compromise from the constrictive nature of the brace. Bracing does not affect scoliosis progression in Duchenne muscular dystrophy.[20] In SMA, spinal orthoses are often used to slow progression of scoliosis until corrective surgery. When surgical correction is desired, there is also the additional consideration of adverse limitations in function. A child with contractures of the upper extremities may have been able to use the abnormal curvature for positioning during self-care.[22]

Pulmonary

Respiratory complications are the leading cause of mortality in this group. Such complications can develop slowly or acutely. Children with neuromuscular dystrophy should have regular pulmonary function testing to follow disease progression.[20] Children with neuromuscular disorders will generally have a decrease in pulmonary function over time. Nocturnal hypoventilation may initially present with daytime somnolence and fatigue. Sleep studies and noninvasive ventilation may be helpful. Pulse oximetry during therapy may be used to monitor oxygenation. Pulmonary toilet and secretion clearance are also important.[20,23] Ventilatory muscle training can reduce respiratory muscle fatigue in chest wall disorders. Neck or glossopharyngeal (frog) breathing can be taught as both an alternative to ventilation or as a rescue method for ventilator failure.[23]

Table 1
Duchenne muscular dystrophy

History, Signs, Symptoms	Safety Risk	Consultation/Diagnostic Tests/Intervention
Proximal muscle weakness, calf pseudohypertrophy, Gower sign, waddling gait	Falls due to progressive neuromuscular weakness	Physiatry: for multidisciplinary care coordination of neuromuscular rehabilitation services across the home, school, hospital, and community settings
Shortness of breath/chest pain/palpitations/arrhythmias, orthopnea, pedal edema	Dilated cardiomyopathy, conduction abnormalities	Cardiology: echo or cardiac MRI by age 10 years and repeated annually or biannually, ECG for conduction abnormalities, initial studies suggest ACE inhibitors and β-blockers show benefit in treating heart failure and cardiomyopathy
Shortness of breath, snoring, insomnia, daytime sleepiness	Atelectasis, restrictive lung disease, respiratory failure	Pulmonary: baseline PFTs prior to wheelchair confinement, then twice-yearly pulmonary evaluations after FVC <80%; PFTs dictate management of scoliosis more so than the magnitude of the curve Incentive spirometry to prevent atelectasis
Lateral curvature of the spine, asymmetric shoulders, pelvic obliquity	Scoliosis	Spine surgery: close monitoring with serial radiographs around adolescent growth spurt. Indication for surgery: before the primary curve >25°–40° and FVC >50% of predicted Radiology: communicate proper positioning technique to place children as upright as possible to prevent erroneous scoliosis curve measurements
Loss of muscle/joint range of motion, decreased strength and endurance, impaired mobility, impaired activities of daily living, poor trunk control, falls, history of steroid use	Progressive, painful contractures of iliotibial band, hip, and knee flexors; overuse weakness; osteopenia; fractures; falls; pressure ulcers	Physical and occupational therapy: for passive stretching exercises to prevent contractures; for sitting balance, trunk strength, and standing/weight-bearing exercises, gait training, wheelchair mobility, energy-conservation techniques, and parental home exercise program instruction. Therapy programs should be yearlong because contractures rapidly progress after wheelchair dependence develops Board of Education/Individualized Education Program (IEP): an IEP evaluation should be expedited to assure timely delivery of PT, OT, paraprofessional services, adaptive physical education, transportation, and neuropsychological evaluation Durable medical equipment clinic: supine or prone stander, standing frame (EZ Stander) bathroom chair, semielectric hospital bed, manual and motorized wheelchairs, Hoyer lift Orthotics: posterior leaf spring, AFO while ambulatory, solid AFO when nonambulatory; orthotic sneakers, balanced forearm orthosis, night splints. It is important to understand the types of orthotics applied with DMD progression. Orthopedic surgery: for contracture release surgeries and fracture evaluations

Fever, cough	Infections: primarily pneumonia and influenza	Primary care: for basic medical care follow-up. The American Thoracic Society recommends that patients with DMD receive the pneumococcal and annual influenza vaccination
Weight loss, dysphagia, constipation, abdominal pain, heartburn, obesity	Decreased gastric motility causing dysphagia and GERD	Nutrition and GI: for balanced diet rich in nutrition supplementation, particularly vitamin D and calcium
Hearing loss, visual/spatial difficulties, delayed developmental milestones	Sensorineural hearing loss, impaired retinal neurotransmission, speech and language delay	Audiology: for hearing test to evaluate for sensorineural hearing loss Ophthalmology: to evaluate for vision loss. Obtain vision test prior to motorized wheelchair prescription Neuropsychology: for cognitive rehabilitation focusing on compensatory strategies
Stress/anxiety due to cultural, psychosocial, and financial reasons for the patient and family	Psychosocial stress, insurance obstacles, cultural/language barriers	Social work and service coordination: for insurance obstacles, home therapy, and HHA services. Service coordinators provide home visits to alleviate caregiver stress and meet care coordination needs that hospital social workers are unable to provide Child Life: for recommendation to Make-a-Wish Foundation Translation services: to help bridge cultural and language barriers Muscular Dystrophy Association Clinic: grant information and care coordination Palliative care team

Abbreviations: ACE, angiotensin-converting enzyme; AFO, knee ankle foot orthosis; DMD, Duchenne muscular dystrophy; ECG, electrocardiography; FVC, forced vital capacity; GERD, gastroesophageal reflux disease; HHA, Hospital Housekeepers of America; MRI, magnetic resonance imaging; OT, occupational therapy; PFT, pulmonary function test; PT, physical therapy.

Swallowing

Neuromuscular disorders can present with bulbar dysfunction and fatigue, particularly in SMA. Deficits can present as difficulty feeding or failure to thrive. Adjustments can be made to feedings with techniques such as double swallow, chin tuck, head turning, or supraglottic swallow. Dietary modifications can be made to consistency and portion size of food. Placement of a percutaneous endoscopic gastrostomy tube may also be a consideration.

Exercise Regimen

Current guidelines recommend aerobic, low-resistance, submaximal, concentric exercises. Eccentric exercises are generally avoided in children with myopathies or dystrophinopathies. In Duchenne, muscle groups that perform eccentric activity have been noted to exhibit weakness early in the course of the disease process. These muscles are usually hip extensors, knee extensors, and ankle dorsiflexors.[20] Increased weakness or pain during exercise is often a sign of muscle overuse.[20] Although there are data on improvement in lower extremity function after moderate-resistance aerobic exercise, at this time there are insufficient data to recommend high-resistance exercise. There are concerns that high-resistance exercise may lead to muscle damage, through overuse in tissue that is already susceptible to mechanical injury, with a reversal of functional gains.[20] Submaximal aerobic activity is recommended at a level that improves cardiovascular capacity and oxygen use. Aquatic therapy in heated pools is recommended for nonambulatory children.[23] These concerns derive from the increased mechanical stress placed on inherently unstable muscle fibers during lengthening exercises.[20]

Equipment

Decreased ambulation may increase the risk for obesity, contractures, pressure sores, osteoporosis, and worsening of scoliosis. Improper or poorly functioning orthotics and adaptive equipment may further increase these risks. When acquiring a wheelchair, considerations of functional mobility include manual versus power wheelchairs. Communication between providers in the medical and educational settings facilitates timely management. Anticipation of progressive decline in function may warrant a power wheelchair before cessation of ambulation. To safely use a power chair, the child must have adequate cognitive ability (children as young as 2 years of age can learn to use a power chair) and coordination. With a progressive decline in mobility and self-care, the child may need to have a wheelchair with positioning elements such as tilt-in-space.[23] The child may also require a hospital bed for pressure relief, fitted with side rails or an overhead trapeze. Furniture should also be assessed in the home, with loose rugs or obstructions being cleared out.[23]

PATIENT SAFETY IN THE CHILD WITH AN AMPUTATION

The approach to the pediatric amputee is different from that of the adult in several aspects. The main clinical distinction is that pediatric amputees are still experiencing skeletal growth. As children grow, they will require multiple prostheses before reaching physical maturation. There is also concern over appositional bone growth that may require surgical revision, or may guide the initial level of amputation. In a very young amputee, the choice of prosthetic design will depend on the level of cognition and motor milestones. Children are also more active than their adult counterparts, placing a greater demand on the residual limb, supporting limbs, and the prosthesis. The child may also develop issues of body image that must be addressed, and the prosthesis should be designed to minimize the psychological impact on the wearer.

THE INITIAL EVALUATION OF A CHILD WITH A PROSTHESIS

For preamputation status, cognitive ability for prosthetic training, current level of function, and self-care to guide choice of prosthesis are assessed. Nutritional status is monitored to promote wound healing. family and financial support systems available are assessed.

Etiology of amputation can affect prognosis and follow-up. The most common causes of pediatric amputations are: (1) congenital limb deficiencies[23] (the clinician should be aware that the amputation may be part of a syndrome affecting multiple organs and that screening for cardiac, renal, or other systemic abnormalities may be warranted)[20,24]; (2) traumatic amputation (most commonly of the fingers); (3) tumors (osteosarcoma, sarcoma, neurofibromatosis); and (4) meningococcemia (septic shock with limb ischemia or infectious emboli can result in autoamputation of digits or extremities). Meningococcemia associated with epiphyseal growth plate necrosis can also occur.[25]

Common Safety Concerns in Children with Amputations

There are several areas that could pose a safety risk in children with amputations: (1) surgical site infections, wound dehiscence, and residual limb edema, all of which can lead to a delay in healing of the incision line and subsequent fitting of a prosthesis; (2) contractures; (3) trauma to the residual limb; (4) concurrent medical issues (limb salvage, radiation therapy, chemotherapy, metastatic disease, trauma- related brain injury, and fractures); (5) risk of falling; and (6) prosthesis-related complications (ie, poor socket fit, terminal appositional overgrowth, patellar tendon and growth plate traction injury).

To promote healing of the residual limb, debridement (if necessary) and wrapping with bandages can both be of benefit. Parents and child (if possible) should be able to demonstrate that they can wrap the residual limb in a figure-of-8 formation. To minimize the risk of contractures and trauma to the residual limb, a protective orthotic that encases the residual limb and maintains it in an extended position can be of benefit. Child and family should also be educated to avoid placing pillows behind the knee.

SPINAL CORD INJURIES

Because spinal disorders in the pediatric population are relatively rare, there is inadequate knowledge, experience, and expertise among pediatric physiatrists, orthopedists, neurosurgeons, and primary care pediatricians in the diagnosis and systematic management of spinal cord disorders. Secondary complications affected by early onset, growth, and development may include paralysis, sensory loss, neurogenic bowel and bladder, spasticity, pain, cardiovascular, endocrine and sexual dysfunction, as well as orthopedic deformities, such as contractures, scoliosis, and hip dysplasia. Because the spine attains near adult size by age 10 years, the assessment and care of children must be tailored to the patient's age, in addition to neurologic status, and type and level of injury. One of the major challenges in caring for children and adolescents with spinal cord injuries is to address the changing objectives of each developmental stage. In addition, spina bifida onset is in utero, with associated congenital malformations, as well as brain abnormalities, resulting in cognitive and behavioral impairments.

Table 2
Medical errors and patient safety risks in rehabilitation of children with spinal cord disorders (Vogel)

	Safety Risk	Evaluation	Preventive Interventions and Recommendations
1.	Urinary tract deterioration from neurogenic bladder	Urodynamics testing showing high leak point bladder pressures >40 cm or detrusor-sphincter dyssynergia (DSD)	Timely urology follow-up. Clean intermittent catheterization (CIC) should begin approximately at age 3 y or earlier if the child is experiencing recurrent urinary tract infections (UTIs) or exhibits renal impairment
			Children with adequate hand function should begin self-catheterizations when they are developmentally 5–7 y old
			Anticholinergic medications indicated if DSD or high leak point pressures
			Bladder augmentation if inadequate bladder capacity despite anticholinergic therapy in high-pressure, low-volume bladder
			Continent catheterizable conduit, Mitrofanoff procedure (umbilical appendicovesicostomy), or Vocare functional electrical stimulation (FES), if upper extremity/visuomotor deficits or developmental delay limit self-catheterizations
	Urinary tract infection, antibiotic resistance and risks	Limit antibiotic treatment to those with symptomatic UTIs with systemic toxicity, including fever, chills, dysreflexia, or exacerbation of spasticity; incontinence; or cloudy and foul-smelling urine	Limit prophylactic antibiotic use to recurrent and severe UTIs, obstructive uropathy or compromised renal function, including vesicoureteral reflux and hydronephrosis
			Fluoroquinolones contraindicated in children younger than 18 y because of theoretic adverse cartilage events
2.	Neurogenic bowel complications: diarrhea, constipation, impaction	Abdominal radiograph to rule out impaction	Initiation of bowel program at age 2–4 y
			Nutrition counseling
			Anterograde continence enema should be done prior to urologic procedures
	Laxative complications	—	Avoid prolonged, early use of anthraquinones (ie, Senna)

#	Risk	Details / Signs	Management
3.	Deep venous thrombosis (DVT), pulmonary embolus, and postphlebitic syndrome	—	DVT prophylaxis should include graduated elastic stockings for older children and adolescents as well as anticoagulation
	Uneven elastic wrapping may result in constrictions with venous obstruction	—	Smaller children may need custom-made lower extremity garments, such as Jobst stockings
	Allergy risk from latex-containing elastic wraps	—	See section on latex allergy
	Bleeding risk with anticoagulation therapy		Drug monitoring
4.	Hypercalcemia with complications of nephrocalcinosis, urolithiasis, and renal failure (higher risk in adolescent boys during first 3 months of injury)	Insidious onset of abdominal pain, nausea, vomiting, lethargy, malaise, polydipsia, polyuria, dehydration, behavioral changes or acute psychosis, elevated serum calcium	Monitor calcium; Management includes IV hydration, furosemide, and pamidronate
5.	Cardiovascular risks		
	Blood pressure measurement error	Consider developmental variations of blood pressure cuff sizes, varying cognitive and verbal communication ability, and dependency on parents and guardians	Determine BP regularly, use appropriately sized blood pressure cuffs
	Sympathetic overactivity due to autonomic dysreflexia (AD) in response to noxious stimulation below the zone of the SCI in patients with SCI at or above T6 level	Noxious stimuli to bladder-UTI, urolithiasis; ingrown toenail, pressure sore, syrinx, tethering; Preschool-aged children may present with vague symptoms; Adolescents in athletic competition may not report symptoms if they deliberately induce AD by clamping urinary catheters to improve performance	The mainstay of treatment is removal of noxious stimuli; Management should be conducted in a calm and reassuring atmosphere; Medical alert identification and education about diagnosis and management should be provided for caregivers and supervising adults in the home, school, and community, including teachers, school nurses, therapists, coaches, and health care providers
6.	Cardiopulmonary risks		
	Risk for respiratory failure related to sleep apnea in children with cervical SCI	Signs: headache, restless sleep, snoring, daytime sleepiness and mental dullness. Higher risk in obese, younger children, especially using baclofen or diazepam	Supplemental noninvasive ventilatory support systems, such as biphasic positive airway pressure and airway secretion management

(continued on next page)

Table 2
(continued)

	Safety Risk	Evaluation	Preventive Interventions and Recommendations
	Failure to thrive and upper airway obstruction risk in young children during phrenic nerve pacing	—	Tracheostomies
	Decreased cardiovascular adaptations to exercise in SCI at T6 or higher	Signs: decreased cardiac output, exertional hypotension, and hyperthermia	Orthostasis precautions with exercise, including tilt tables, gradient stockings, abdominal binder, salt tablets
7.	Hyperhidrosis (excessive sweating) below the zone of the SCI in patients with SCI at or above T6 level. May increase the risk for pressure ulcers through maceration of skin	—	See pressure sores section
8.	Poikilothermia with hypothermia or hyperthermia in SCI at T6 or above due to sympathetic dysregulation of lower body muscles. Increased vulnerability of infants and children with SCI to temperature extremes because of their relatively large surface area and their variable communication and cognitive and problem-solving skills	—	Air conditioning and heating are considered medically necessary for vulnerable children; functional cooling suits are recommended for children who are unable to participate in summer outdoor activities
9.	Fever risk higher in children with acute SCI	Thorough history and physical examination as well as diagnostic studies guided by clinical evaluation. Rule out common pediatric problems such as otitis media Keep high index of suspicion for SCI-specific problems, such as fracture or heterotopic ossification manifested by limited range of motion or swollen extremity or scrotal swelling consistent with epididymitis Abdominal disorders require high index of suspicion in the presence of fever, anorexia, abdominal distension, and nausea and vomiting.	Monitoring and education about accurate diagnosis and management

10a.	Pain can be very disabling and can negatively affect school, work, and social interactions. Self-mutilation may be a manifestation of dysesthesia that usually resolves after a few months post-SCI onset; risk for headaches and postconcussion symptoms after combined SCI/TBI	Evaluation complicated by variable cognitive and communication abilities, compounded by lack of sensation or tenderness	Education that altered/absent sensation from SCI does not preclude pain. Diagnosis using pediatric-specific pain scales such as FACES and FLACC. Treat pain syndromes as dictated by underlying etiology. Monitor for postconcussion headache that may become more perceptible after neuropathic pain from SCI subsides
	Risk of overuse syndromes with inefficient compensatory patterns and malalignment affected by growth	Careful evaluation of posture, alignment, positioning, seating, equipment, bracing, changes in spasticity patterns, overuse patterns are required to identify pain	Prevention of overuse pain with early diagnosis and timely referral prior to irreversible loss of function. Proper positioning, seating, equipment, bracing, pain and spasticity management as dictated by underlying cause
10b.	Spasticity risks	A high index of suspicion and thorough evaluation are necessary to identify clinically obscure noxious stimuli that perpetuate spasticity, particularly in view of variable age-dependent communication skills	Prevention encompasses avoidance of inciting factors with establishment of good bladder, bowel, skin, stretching, range of motion, splinting, and positioning programs Spasticity management options include medications, intrathecal baclofen pump, selective dorsal rhizotomy, epidural spinal cord stimulation, and localized injection of botulinum toxin. (Pediatric spasticity management risks are discussed in article by Rajashree Srinivasan elsewhere in this issue)
	Side effects of treatments for pain and spasticity: burn risk with modalities; premature closing of growth plates with ultrasound; risk of off-label use of medications in children	—	Monitor dosages with off-label use of pain medications for children, monitor for cognitive side effects in children taking sedating medications, communicate precautions on use of modalities in children with SCI with physical and occupational therapists. Medication reconciliation

(continued on next page)

Table 2
(continued)

	Safety Risk	Evaluation	Preventive Interventions and Recommendations
11.	Latex allergy in 6%–18% pediatric SCI elicited by direct contact with latex through cutaneous, mucosal, intravenous or serosal routes or by airborne dissemination of latex antigens	Signs: localized or generalized urticaria, wheezing, angioedema or anaphylaxis.	Family and caregiver education about need for latex-free environment to minimize the risk for sensitization and to prevent allergic reactions
		Subtle clinical manifestations include rash with blowing up balloons or allergies to foods such as kiwi, banana, avocado, and chestnuts	—
		Risk of precipitating a severe allergic reaction with skin tests	Individuals allergic to latex should wear a medical alert identification and carry auto-injectable epinephrine
12.	Pressure ulcers are one of the most common complications for children and adolescents with SCI	Young children may be at risk for skin breakdown due to trauma with activities and play; compliance issues with pressure relief and precautions	Prevention education may include inspection, positioning and transfer techniques to avoid friction and shear, hygiene, dietary modification, periodic orthotic and equipment evaluation with pressure mapping to optimize pressure relief and accommodate growth, improved environmental accommodation
			Monitoring for changes in spasticity, continence, and deformities resulting in uneven seating. Automatic timers to remind children to perform pressure relief maneuvers. Pressure ulcer prevention must be developmentally based and responsibility must be progressively shifted from the parents to the children as they grow
			School staff must be aware of strict compliance with positioning recommendations to prevent new and recurrent sores, as well as proactive in communication with caregivers

13.	Orthopedic issues	—	Prevention and management of orthopedic complications is generally complicated and should be directed by clinicians experienced in caring for children and adolescents with spinal cord disorders. Communication between medical and education settings ensures compliance with precautions and protocols for optimal outcomes
	Heterotopic ossification (HO) and complications of treatments	Average onset of HO is reported as 14 months after pediatric SCI, which is later than in adults	Prophylaxis for HO using etidronate disodium is not routinely used in pediatric SCI population because of relatively low risk for HO. In addition, etidronate disodium may be contraindicated in prepubertal children because of the potential development of rachitic-like changes. Postoperative use of radiation therapy may be contraindicated in younger children because of long-term consequences of radiation
	Osteoporosis and fractures: osteopenia begins immediately after sustaining a SCI and plateaus 6 to 12 months later. Pathological fractures occur in about 14% of children and adolescents with SCI	Causes of fractures include gait training, range of motion, and minor trauma. Pathological fractures signs may include a warm, swollen extremity; fever; and subtle radiography findings, especially in the supracondylar femur and proximal tibia	Adherence to handling, positioning, range of motion, and weight-bearing precautions, especially with transfers and ambulation. Padded bivalve casts enable inspection to prevent pressure ulcers. Encouraging weight bearing with orthotics or FES, good nutrition, transfer training and adequate sunlight and equipment

(continued on next page)

Table 2
(continued)

Safety Risk	Evaluation	Preventive Interventions and Recommendations
Scoliosis: very high risk in childhood-onset SCI (98% with 67% requiring surgery)	Complications of scoliosis include pelvic obliquity, impaired use of the upper extremities, pressure ulcers, pain, poor fitting of orthotics, gastrointestinal and cardiopulmonary abnormalities, and TLSO interference with mobility, function and self-catheterization. Imaging studies to exclude hydrocephalus, hydrosyringomyelia, and tethered cord should be performed in children with spina bifida with progressive scoliosis or neurological changes such as progressive weakness or spasticity	Timely orthopedic and/or neurosurgical referral for bracing/surgery as indicated. Monitor scoliosis with periodic radiographs. TLSO prophylaxis in preadolescent children may delay curve progression. Timing of the surgical repair and the extent and type of spine fusion depend on the child's age, location, degree and flexibility of the curve, neurological level and ambulation status. The lumbosacral joint should not be fused in children who are ambulatory. Hip contractures should be corrected before spine surgery to avoid excessive torque to the spine fusion after surgery
Hip dislocation, subluxation, and contractures are especially common among young children with SCI	Monitor for early signs of hip instability with periodic radiographs, and examination for asymmetrical hip abduction, leg length discrepancy, spasticity, and gait and seating problems	Management must be individualized and based on the neurological level, presence of hip dysplasia, pain, and ambulation status. Foot deformities predispose to pressure ulcers must be carefully inspected. Discuss risks and benefits of surgery and coordinate decision making with patients, caregivers, and health care providers in various settings

#			
14.	Neurological complications in spina bifida: meningitis, ventriculitis, shunt malfunction, associated with cognitive abnormalities	Shunt malfunction symptoms in younger children: increased intracranial pressure, nausea, vomiting, and severe headache. Adolescents may present with irritability, decreased perceptual motor function, attention issues, headaches, poor school performance, weakness, or worsening scoliosis Chiari II malformation symptoms in infants and younger children may include feeding and swallowing abnormalities, stridor, vocal cord paralysis, weak cry, apnea, sleep-disordered breathing, nystagmus, opisthotonos, upper extremity weakness and spasticity. Adolescents may present with progressive scoliosis, decreased upper extremity function, neck pain, and depressed respiratory function	Monitoring and timely referral for neurosurgical evaluation
		Tethered cord syndrome	
		Worsening of weakness, sensory loss, spasticity, progressive scoliosis, bowel/bladder changes, pain, or orthopedic deformities in the lower extremities	Monitoring and timely referral for neurosurgical evaluation
15.	Lack of anticipatory guidance and transition planning	Frequent medical evaluation and diagnostic testing is needed to monitor progress throughout the lifespan	Must be provided in a developmentally sensitive manner to prepare children, adolescents, and their families for secondary complications and transitions. Transition planning should be initiated during childhood and increase in intensity as child approaches adulthood. Transition planning includes independent living, employment, finances, socialization, and health care
a.	Provision of comprehensive primary care, including preventative health care maintenance and management of intercurrent illnesses	Frequent medical evaluation and diagnostic testing is needed to monitor progress throughout the lifespan	Care notebooks facilitate coordination and communication: http://www. medicalhomeinfo.org/for_families/care_ notebook/

(continued on next page)

Table 2
(continued)

	Safety Risk	Evaluation	Preventive Interventions and Recommendations
b.	High risk for obesity in adolescents with decreased mobility, especially spina bifida	Cardiovascular risk assessment includes factors for obesity, sedentary lifestyle, smoking, hyperlipidemia, hypertension, and family history. Screening for hyperlipidemia after 2 years of age in those with a high-risk family history	—
		Monitor body mass index with skinfold thickness	Need developmentally based program to improve aerobic fitness, strength, endurance, and precautions to prevent injuries during exercise
c.	Disaster preparation	—	Emergency kit that contains urologic supplies, catheters, medicines, suppositories, cell phone, flashlight, back-up manual wheelchair if no power wheelchair
d.	Adolescents with SCI may be at a greater risk for substance abuse, psychological problems, suicide	—	Address psychological issues and sexuality and reproductive health issues in a developmentally appropriate manner with children, adolescents, and their parents
e.	Sexuality is often overlooked in children and adolescents with spinal cord disorders. About 10%–20% of individuals with spina bifida experience precocious puberty		Educate patients about sexuality and sexual development

SAFETY RISKS IN CHILDREN WITH SPINAL CORD INJURIES

To minimize safety risks to children with spinal cord injuries, continuity of care is very important. Children should be followed in clinics by providers familiar with the child or adolescent's baseline status and condition. This aspect is particularly important for early identification of secondary complications that are related to growth and development, such as scoliosis, hip dysplasia, tethered cord, and syrinx.

It is important to regularly document: (1) motor levels, sensory levels and reflexes; (2) presence and degree of pain, spasticity, and tone; (3) orthopedic malalignments (contractures and scoliosis); and (4) level of function, including onset of developmental milestones and acquisition of physical, cognitive, communication and adaptive skills.

There are several safety risks in children with spinal cord injuries, such as: (1) proper spinal stabilization in the acute care setting (ie, spine clearance and halo fixation); (2) use of interventions such as functional electrical stimulation for upright mobility in specific scenarios (ie, hip dislocation, lower extremity contractures, severe scoliosis, and following myocutaneous flaps surgery); (3) following surgery (ie, weight bearing and therapy clearance, tendon transfers, myocutaneous flaps for pressure ulcers); (4) risk for infections (ie, aspiration pneumonia, urinary tract infections); (5) risk of pathologic fractures (ie, secondary to osteoporosis); (6) risk of pressure ulcers; (7) risk of falls, compounded by age-related communication and cognitive skills; (8) risk of autonomic dysreflexia. Specific safety risks, their evaluation, and preventive/treatments are outlined in **Table 2**.[26–28] It is essential that all providers involved in the care of children with spinal cord injuries have a working knowledge of the various impairments, potential complications, effective treatments, and precautions.

Helpful websites:

www.unitedspinal.org
www.spinalcord.org
www.independenceexpo.org
www.thinkfirst.org
http://www.mdausa.org/clinics/

REFERENCES

1. Scheufele EL, Dubey A. Can de facto dosing practices bridge the knowledge gap in pediatric medication recommendations? AMIA Annu Symp Proc 2009; 2009:573–7.
2. Aagaard L, Christensen A, Hansen EH. Information about adverse drug reactions reported in children: a qualitative review of empirical studies. Br J Clin Pharmacol 2010;70(4):481–91.
3. Hanna SE, Rosenbaum PL, Bartlett DJ, et al. Stability and decline in gross motor function among children and youth with cerebral palsy aged 2 to 21 years. Dev Med Child Neurol 2009;51(4):295–301.
4. Mercuri E, Jongmans M, Bouza H, et al. Congenital hemiplegia in children at school age: assessment of hand function in the non-hemiplegic hand and correlation with MRI. Neuropediatrics 1999;30(1):8–13.
5. CATCLAMS. Available at: http://cpj.sagepub.com/content/33/7/404.abstract. Accessed February 24, 2012.
6. DAYC. Available at: http://portal.wpspublish.com/portal/page?_pageid=53,69524. Accessed February 24, 2012.
7. Wind WM, Schwend RM, Larson J. Sports for the physically challenged child. J Am Acad Orthop Surg 2004;12(2):126–37.

8. Bauer ML, Figueröa-Colon R, Georgeson K, et al. Chronic pulmonary aspiration in children. South Med J 1993;86(7):789–95.
9. Somarriba G, Extein J, Miller TL. Exercise rehabilitation in pediatric cardiomyopathy. Prog Pediatr Cardiol 2008;25(1):91–102.
10. Murphy NA, Carbone PS. Parent-provider-community partnerships: optimizing outcomes for children with disabilities. Pediatrics 2011;128(4):795–802.
11. Wang G, McGrath BB, Watts C. Health care transitions among youth with disabilities or special health care needs: an ecological approach. J Pediatr Nurs 2010; 25(6):505–50.
12. Slomine BS, McCarthy ML, Ding R, et al. Health care utilization and needs after pediatric traumatic brain injury. Pediatrics 2006;117(4):663–74.
13. Bernat JL, Peterson LM. Patient-centered informed consent in surgical practice. Arch Surg 2006;141(1):86–92.
14. Lashley M, Talley W, Lands LC, et al. Informed proxy consent: communication between pediatric surgeons and surrogates about surgery. Pediatrics 2000; 105(3 Pt 1):591–7.
15. Available at: http://www.denveriionline.com/denver. Accessed February 24, 2012.
16. Available at: http://www.medicalhomeinfo.org/for_families/care_notebook/. Accessed February 24, 2012.
17. Zimmerman J, Dabelko HI. Collaborative models of patient care: new opportunities for hospital social workers. Soc Work Health Care 2007;44(4):33–47.
18. Needs of children with disabilities addressed best through partnerships. 2010; 31(9). Available at: https://aapnews.aapublications.org. Accessed February 24, 2012.
19. Srinivasan R. Patient safety in rehabilitation of children with traumatic brain injury. Phys Med Rehabil Clin N Am 2012;23(2):393–400.
20. Alexander MA, Matthews DJ. Pediatric rehabilitation: principles and practice. 4th edition. New York: Demos Publishing; 2010. p. 277–360.
21. Birnkrant DJ, Panitch HB, Benditt JO, et al. American College of Chest Physicians consensus statement on the respiratory and related management of patients with Duchenne muscular dystrophy undergoing anesthesia or sedation. Chest 2007; 132(6):1977–86.
22. Driscoll SW, Skinner J. Musculoskeletal complications of neuromuscular disease in children. Phys Med Rehabil Clin N Am 2008;19(1):163–94, viii.
23. Braddom RL. Physical medicine and rehabilitation. 4th edition. Philadelphia: Elsevier Saunders; 2011. p. 741–54, 1041–63, 1097–132.
24. Edelstein JE, Moroz A. Lower limb orthotics and prosthetics: clinical concept. Thorofare (NJ): SLACK Incorporated; 2011. p. 184–96.
25. Buysse CM, Oranje AP, Zuidema E, et al. Long-term skin scarring and orthopaedic sequelae in survivors of meningococcal septic shock. Arch Dis Child 2009;94(5):381–6.
26. Pediatric Spinal Cord Disorders. In: Vogel L, Betz R, Mulcahey MJ, et al, editors. Spinal cord medicine. Philadelphia: Lippincott, Williams and Wilkins; 2000. p. 136–55.
27. The Faces Pain Scale—Revised. Pediatric pain sourcebook of protocols, policies and pamphlets. 2007. Available at: http://painsourcebook.ca/docs/pps92.html. Accessed February 24, 2012.
28. Merkel SI, Voepel-Lewis T, Shayevitz JR, et al. The FLACC: a behavioral scale for scoring postoperative pain in young children. Pediatr Nurs 1997;23(3):293–7.

Patient Safety in Interventional Pain Procedures

Samuel P. Thampi, MD[a],*, Vishal Rekhala, MD[a],
Travis Vontobel, MD[a], Vamsi Nukula[b]

KEYWORDS

- Pain management • Patient safety
- Interventional pain procedures • Human error

SCOPE OF ERRORS IN INTERVENTIONAL PAIN MANAGEMENT
Human Error

To err is human and as long as humans interact in providing care, there is the potential for human error. Human error can be classified into knowledge-based error, rule-based error, and skill-based error. Skill-based errors are a result of lack of judgment (eg, a physician who unintentionally orders 10 mg of dilaudid, instead of 1.0 mg of dilaudid), rule-based errors are a result of ignorance of rules related to a situation (eg, a physician who performs a cervical epidural injection instead of a lumbar epidural injection failing to do a time out to verify the type of procedure before starting the procedure), and knowledge-based errors are a result of incomplete or incorrect knowledge in a particular problem or situation (eg, a novice interventionalist who unknowingly heats up the annuloplasty canula in the spinal canal instead of the disc, while performing an intradiscal annuloplasty).[1]

Regardless of the type of error, medical errors in pain management can be catastrophic (ie, spinal cord injury after spinal injections or respiratory arrest after opiate overdose). Regrettably, in the practice of interventional pain management, a significant number of patients are victims of avoidable human error. In a closed claims study, Fitzgibbon and colleagues[2] found 97% of the closed claims in pain management malpractice suits in pain management were related to invasive procedures. Of the invasive

Financial Disclosure statement: The primary author or coauthors have no financial incentives with any device maker or drug manufacturing company. The primary author or coauthors have no financial incentives with any device maker or drug manufacturing company.

[a] Department of Physical Medicine and Rehabilitation, Kingsbrook Jewish Medical Center, 585 Schenectady Avenue, Suite 224, Brooklyn, NY 11203, USA
[b] St. George's University, University Centre, Grenada, West Indies
* Corresponding author.
E-mail address: mdspine@gmail.com

procedures, most of the complications were related to epidural steroid injections. Unfortunately, the patient who was a victim of error before the injury can also be prone again to medical errors in the hands of the pain management physician.

Technical Problems

Advances in the field of pain management have introduced several types of devices into clinical practice. These include (1) the fluoroscope and the fluoroscope table, (2) radiofrequency generator, (3) dorsal column stimulator, and (4) intrathecal drug delivery systems. The machines are not perfect; they break down, at times even during the procedure. For example, a recently inspected fluoroscope might fail during a procedure, requiring replacement in the middle of the procedure. This can create a safety hazard for the patient. The interventional pain management physician should be able to recognize when equipment is malfunctioning and implement procedures to remedy the situation in the event of a breakdown, without compromising patient safety.

Communication Problems

Interventional pain management requires teamwork, even for the solo practitioner. Pain management physicians work within a team that can also include pain management nurses, anesthesiologists, nurse anesthetists, radiology technicians, operating room technicians, physical therapists, occupational therapists, secretaries, pharmacists, and, most importantly, the patient. Effective communication is a key element in the successful completion of interventional pain procedures. Lack of communication or miscommunication among team members can contribute to patient safety errors.[3] Within the team, errors can occur when one team member is not able to perform his or her role adequately, thereby jeopardizing the patient's safety. For instance, a novice radiology technician who is not experienced with the use of the fluoroscope can produce poor radiological images that result in poor visualization of critical areas of the spine. There should be a good understanding of the terminology used in the procedure by all the team members (ie, "10° cephalad tilt" or "30° right oblique tilt"). Poor communication among the team members during the procedure can result in poor visualization of critical spinal anatomy during a spinal procedure. In another instance, lack of communication between the physician and the radiology technician can lead to a potentially catastrophic injury when the technician elevates the table on which the patient is lying to very close to the image intensifier, resulting in an instant spinal cord injury if the needle is still in the neck of the patient.

Regardless of years of clinical expertise, an interventional pain management physician can potentially make a "wrong patient/wrong side/wrong procedure" error while performing an interventional pain procedure secondary to improper communication at the team level. It is important to understand that errors happen at the most prestigious hospitals in the most experienced hands.

Characteristics of Patients With Pain Syndromes That Place Them at Increased Safety Risk During Interventional Pain Management Procedures

Elderly patients with pain syndromes can have comorbid diseases that require the use of anticoagulants. The use of anticoagulants just before the interventional pain management procedure can increase the risk for epidural hematomas with spinal injections.

TYPES OF MEDICAL ERRORS COMMONLY SEEN IN PAIN MANAGEMENT
Diagnosis-Related Errors

Diagnosis-related errors are typically the result of a medical condition that was mis-diagnosed or not diagnosed in a timely manner. Some examples are described in the following sections.

Neurogenic claudication versus vascular claudication
Performing an epidural steroid injection on a patient with misdiagnosed vascular clau-dication can occur as a result of not performing an adequate vascular assessment as part of the history and physical examination. Vascular claudication and neurogenic claudication have similarities and differences and clearly excluding a vascular claudi-cation is necessary before performing an epidural steroid injection for neurogenic claudication.

Cervical radiculopathy versus primary shoulder pathology
Regional joint pathology can manifest as neck pain with radiation to the ipsilateral shoulder and misdiagnosis can result in unnecessary injection to the cervical spine.[4–7]

Gluteal pain syndromes
Regional hip pathology can manifest as low back pain with radiation to the ipsilateral hip and misdiagnosis can result in unnecessary injection to the lumbar spine.[8] Misdi-agnosis of Piriformis syndrome and assuming a diagnosis of lumbar radiculopathy can result in an unnecessary injection.[9]

Headaches
Misdiagnosis of migraine versus intracranial lesions can result in an unnecessary injec-tion. Although the vast majority of patients with headaches do not have tumor, head-aches can occur in 50% of patients with intracranial tumors. Awareness of potential tumors as a cause of headaches is necessary to prevent a misdiagnosis. Neurologic evaluation can provide clues to mass lesion, such as seizures, focal findings, mass effect, and personality changes.[10]

Low back pain: malignancy versus lumbar spine degenerative joint disease
Elderly patients often present with low back pain secondary to osteoarthritis, from which they can benefit from epidural steroid injections. However, osteoporotic compression fractures or underlying metastatic disease are also part of the differential diagnosis and if present would require different treatments and prompt attention.

Treatment-Related Errors

There are several different types of treatment-related errors and some examples are described in the following sections.

Direct spinal cord injury
Patient sedation during an interventional procedure is helpful, as this can minimize patient anxiety and patient movement during the procedure, and allow efficient needle placement. Patient sedation, although useful, needs careful attention during cervical and thoracic epidural steroid injections. When relying solely on loss of resistance tech-nique, one can run the risk of the Touhy needle advancing farther anteriorly, as the lig-amentum flavum can be incomplete in some patients. Deep sedation during epidural steroid injection is risky if the needle inadvertently enters the spinal cord, and medica-tion is injected into the spinal cord. Ideally, one has to be able to talk to the patient during cervical and thoracic epidurals to avoid the potential risk of direct injury to the spinal cord. Similarly, when performing a cervical epidural steroid injection,

deep sedation is risky and has to be avoided. In instances when the patient goes into deep sedation, one has to wait until the patient is more awake until doing procedures, such as cervical and thoracic epidural steroid injections, where valuable feedback from the patient can prevent potential neurologic complications.

The risk of direct cord injury is increased when the injection is performed at the same level as there is severe central stenosis. For instance, if a patient has a severe stenosis at C5-6 level, one should not perform a spinal injection at this level, as the risk of spinal cord injury is high because of narrow epidural space at that level. The injection can be performed at one level below. Baseline neurologic examination is also necessary in case the patient has changes in neurologic status while in the recovery room. A patient can also have a preexisting myelopathy, and physical examination should check for this possibility. The interventional pain management physician should review magnetic resonance imaging films, even though the films may have already been interpreted by a radiologist.

Direct nerve injury

A patient can have a nerve root injury typically after a transforaminal epidural steroid injection and very rarely after an interlaminar injection if the needle strays laterally into the intervertebral foramen. Sedation has to be minimal to get a response from the patient if the nerve root is accidently injured.

Spinal cord infarctions can occur with transforaminal epidural steroid injections.[11] The risk is higher with cervical transforaminal epidural steroid injections, although there is a risk with upper lumbar transforaminal epidural steroid injections as well. These risks can be avoided using a live fluoroscope with digital subtraction techniques to identify vascular uptake. Negative aspiration is not a reliable test to identify if the needle is in a radicular artery.[12] The safe triangle radiologic landmark (the triangle is composed of a roof made up of the pedicle, a tangential base corresponding to the exiting nerve root, and the lateral border of the vertebral body) was used for transforaminal epidural steroid injections for decades. Studies have shown that the "safe triangle"[13] is no longer safe because of potential risks of embolization of the anterior spinal artery; hence, it is safer to inject in the inferior portion of the intervertebral foramen in thoracic and upper lumbar levels.[14–19]

Dural punctures after epidural steroid injections

Patients can have spinal fluid leaks after epidural access for steroid injections[20] or epidural lead placement. This can be a problem with use of large-gauge Touhy needle in epidural lead placement where a 14-gauge needle is used instead of a 20-gauge needle in routine epidural steroid injection use. Post spinal headaches may require fluid hydration, caffeine, nonsteroidal anti-inflammatory drugs, and blood patch if pain is not controlled. Using the Touhy needle with the bevel parallel to the length of the spinal column can split, rather than cut, the dural fibers, potentially reducing the incidence of cerebrospinal fluid leaks.

Epidural hematomas after epidural steroid injections

Epidural hematomas can occur after a translaminar epidural injection for steroid administration or epidural lead placement.[21,22] Anticoagulants need to be stopped before the procedure.[23]

Pneumothorax following trigger point injections

Pneumothorax can occur while performing trigger point injections in the posterior thoracic wall. Use of a fluoroscope can visualize the ribs and the intercostal space to minimize the risk of pneumothorax.[24]

Infections after spinal injections

Epidural abscess, meningitis, discitis, or osteomyelitis is a potential problem with any spinal injection if performed when the sterile barrier is breached.[25] Although most spinal injections do not need antibiotics, they are necessary before advanced procedures, such as discography, intradiscal annuloplasty, nucleoplasty, spinal cord stimulation, and intrathecal opiate trial and pump placement. Although cefazolin is the most common antibiotic used, in patients with an allergy to cefazolin, clindamycin is an alternative. The skin is a potential source for staphylococcal infection and hence it needs to be cleansed with iodine-based dyes. In patients who have allergies to iodine, absolute alcohol can be used instead. Meningitis has been linked to contaminated compounded betamethasone from local pharmacies[26] Sterile drapes are necessary for invasive procedures, such as discography and spinal cord stimulators. Urinary tract infections or respiratory infections are contraindications for spinal injections because of the risk of seeding the bacteria into the site of injection. Skin infections at the site of injections are also a contraindication.

Falls

Patients who are sedated can potentially fall off the narrow table during or after a procedure. Patients who receive sedation need to be positioned on a stretcher or in a recliner and should not be allowed to stand, especially when the spinal injection is done in an office setting. There is also a risk for falls if the fluoroscopy table is not powered on, especially during transfer of a patient from a stretcher to a fluoroscopy table. The ideal table for a spinal procedure is a diving board table with the least amount of hardware possible, especially during a transforaminal approach. Tables that can be placed in a jackknife position are useful when using an interlaminar approach for epidural steroid injections or dorsal column lead placement.

Radiofrequency equipment

The Food and Drug Administration received 628 reports of grounding pad burns between December 1996 and April 1998 from various surgical procedures using grounding pads.[27] In the pain management field, grounding pad injury can potentially occur with improper grounding in several scenarios, such as facet radiofrequency nerve ablation procedures, intradiscal annuloplasty procedures, and use of cautery during a spinal cord stimulator placement.

Radiation safety

In women of childbearing age, urine pregnancy tests are mandatory to avoid fetal radiation exposure. In younger individuals, lead shielding of the table is essential to avoid radiation exposure to the gonads. The shield has to be placed before the patient gets on the table, as the radiation passes from the inferior portion of the table superiorly. One has no control on the lateral-view radiation exposure. Linear collimation and spherical collimation can avoid radiation exposure. Use of pulse mode (8 pps) can drastically reduce fluoroscopic exposure.

Interventional medication toxicity

Steroids Patients receiving steroids as part of the interventional procedure have an increased risk of having elevated blood sugar levels and elevated blood pressure. Steroids have also been linked to vaginal bleeding in women. Appropriate consultation is necessary if the symptoms persist.[28]

Intrathecal morphine trials Patients undergoing an intrathecal morphine trial should have an overnight intensive care unit admission for monitoring of vital signs because of the concern for hypotension. Patients might also require urinary catheterization because of urinary retention.[29]

Local anesthetics Local anesthetics can cause cardiac arrhythmias, especially during a sympathetic block, because of the close proximity to the vascular structures. Cardiac monitoring is necessary before, during, and after the procedure.[30,31]

Allergy

Iodine/iodine contrast/noniodine contrast Patients can have an allergy to contrast. Noniodinated contrast is a useful alternative.[32–34]

Steroid Patients can have allergy to ingredients in the steroid mixture. If the patient has a history of allergies to these ingredients, he or she would need to undergo skin testing to determine the preparation of steroid that is causing allergy.[35]

Latex

Latex allergy is a concern and, if needed, nonlatex gloves should be used. In addition, latex vial tops would also need to be removed so that the needle does not penetrate through the rubber stopper.[36]

Patient identifiers

Wrong patient Wrist bands can be wrongly printed or wrongly attached and one has to verify the name and data on the wrist band before anesthesia.

Wrong side Patients scheduled to receive selective epidurals should have the skin marked on the appropriate side.[37,38]

Wrong procedure Patients often have cervical and lumbar pathologies, and a patient may have a worsening of the cervical pathology on the day a procedure of the lumbar region is scheduled to be performed. It is important to confirm with the patient the type and location of the procedure for the date that it is being performed.

Anesthesia complications

To minimize complications associated with anesthesia, it is recommended that perioperative monitoring occur. The monitoring should include pulse oximetry, blood pressure, temperature, and cardiac telemetry A fully stocked emergency crash cart should be nearby. Peripheral intravenous (IV) access is also recommended. Vasovagal reactions can occur after procedures, and, hence, IV access obtained before the procedure can be used to treat the effects of this type of reaction. Most pain management procedures are performed in prone position, which can increase risk for hypoventilation. Monitoring for this problem is also recommended. Most medications are metabolized via the kidneys and dose adjustment is necessary when using anesthetics.

Aspiration pneumonia

Patients should be advised to fast after midnight before the procedure because of the risk of aspiration pneumonia.

Postprocedure monitoring

Patients need to be monitored before discharge with the length of time depending on the type of anesthesia used (ie, local vs sedation). Patients who received a stellate ganglion block should have their swallowing function monitored. Discharge criteria postprocedure include that the patient should be alert, awake, and able to ambulate as per expectations of the anesthesia. Patients with chronic obstructive pulmonary disease are at risk from an anesthesia standpoint, especially postoperatively, and require close monitoring. Cellulitis can occur at site where peripheral IV access was obtained.

Communication-related issues

Communication among rehabilitation staff, among consultants, and with the family and patient are all critical. Patient expectations of risks, benefits, and alternatives have to be clearly explained to avoid frustration with negative outcomes from pain management procedures.

Organization-related issues: location of the procedure

Hospital-based procedures (versus office and ambulatory procedures) have the added benefit of having medical and surgical specialists and intensive care units available in the event of a postprocedure complication.

Competency of Staff in Providing Care to the Patients

Most hospitals require proof of training in pain management for interventional procedures, either via fellowship training or under mentorship. Most pain management physicians undergo a year of accredited fellowship training, and are certified by the American Board of Medical Specialties. In addition, most hospitals credentialing for pain management require recertification in infection control, radiation safety training, sedation safety training, and basic and advanced life support. Physicians who attend weekend courses for pain management do perform procedures. The American Society of interventional Pain Management is concerned about the risk to patient safety and the real potential for patients experiencing less than optimal clinical outcomes when they are treated by providers who have not successfully completed rigorous specialty medical training.[39] It is important that physicians performing interventional procedures have the proper training and experience to perform them, as well as update their skills and knowledge base on a regular basis. Staff working with the physician should also have the proper training and experience.

PREVENTION STRATEGIES FOR PATIENT SAFETY

Policy and Procedures

It is important to have a clear-cut policy and procedure manual for the pain management department that covers all aspects of pain management. Examples of items that could be included in this manual are (1) clarification on which providers (Anesthesiologists, Pain management specialist, Physiatrist) write orders for pain-controlled analgesia and operate it; and (2) write discharge guidelines following interventional procedures.

Team Rehearsal and Checklists

It is important that team members rehearse the proper procedures to follow in the interventional procedure suite as well as procedures to follow during potential critical events to ensure good communication and coordination of efforts among all team members. Checklists can also be important in avoiding potential problems and have been used by professionals in fields as diverse as engineering, the airline industry, and anesthesiology. Checklists can be used to ensure that (1) patients receive the proper preprocedure and postprocedure instructions, (2) crash carts are kept well stocked, (3) appropriate medications and equipment are available in the interventional procedure suite, and (4) wrong patient/wrong side/wrong procedure mistakes are kept to a minimum.

Quality Assurance and Improvement Process

Errors or "near misses" occur. These are opportunities to learn about what happened and what should have happened, and learn strategies to prevent the event from occurring again. This process should be nonpunitive, include several team members involved the process, and look for systems errors and barriers that prevent successful outcome. Once identified, the team members should identify strategies to implement and then monitor for change in outcomes. The quality improvement process is ongoing.

SUMMARY

Pain management is a field in which patient safety is an important issue. The ramifications of patient error because of medications or injections can be catastrophic. Understanding the areas in which these errors can potentially occur is important. Preventing these errors is the key.

REFERENCES

1. Rasmussen J. Skills, rules, knowledge; signals, signs, and symbols, and other distinctions in human performance models. IEEE Trans Syst Man Cybern 1983; 13:257–66.
2. Fitzgibbon DR, Posner KL, Domino KB, et al. Chronic pain management: American Society of Anesthesiologists Closed Claims Project. Anesthesiology 2004; 100:98–105.
3. Sliwa JA, Makoul G, Betts H. Rehabilitation specific communication skills training: improving physician patient relationship. Am J Phys Med Rehabil 2002;81: 126–32.
4. Abdul-Latif AA. Dropped shoulder syndrome: a cause of lower cervical radiculopathy. J Clin Neurol 2011;7(2):85–9.
5. Cannon DE, Dillingham TR, Miao H, et al. Musculoskeletal disorders in referrals for suspected cervical radiculopathy. Arch Phys Med Rehabil 2007;88(10):1256–9.
6. Carter T, Hall H, McIntosh G, et al. Intertester reliability of a classification system for shoulder pain. Physiotherapy 2012;98(1):40–6.
7. Mizutamari M, Sei A, Tokiyoshi A, et al. Corresponding scapular pain with the nerve root involved in cervical radiculopathy. J Orthop Surg (Hong Kong) 2010; 18(3):356–60.
8. Suri P, Hunter DJ, Katz JN. Bias in the physical examination of patients with lumbar radiculopathy. BMC Musculoskelet Disord 2010;11:275.
9. Papadopoulos EC, Khan SN. Piriformis syndrome and low back pain: a new classification and review of the literature. Orthop Clin North Am 2004;35(1):65–71.
10. You JJ, Gladstone J, Symons S, et al. Patterns of care and outcomes after computed tomography scans for headache. Am J Med 2011;124:58–63.
11. Verrills P, Nowesenitz G, Barnard A. Penetration of a cervical radicular artery during a transforaminal epidural injection. Pain Med 2010;11(2):229–31.
12. Furman MB, Giovanniello MT, O'Brien EM. Incidence of intravascular penetration in transforaminal cervical epidural steroid injections. Spine 2003;28(1):21–5.
13. Lee IS, Kim SH, Lee JW, et al. Comparison of the temporary diagnostic relief of transforaminal epidural steroid injection approaches: conventional versus posterolateral technique. AJNR Am J Neuroradiol 2007;28(2):204–8.
14. Neal JM. Anatomy and pathophysiology of spinal cord injuries associated with regional anesthesia and pain medicine. Reg Anesth Pain Med 2008;33:423–34.
15. Benny B, Azari P, Briones D. Complications of cervical transforaminal epidural steroid injections. Am J Phys Med Rehabil 2010;89(7):601–7.
16. Weinstein SM, Herring SA, NASS. Lumbar epidural steroid injections. Spine J 2003;3(Suppl 3):37S–44S.
17. Abram SE, O'Connor TC. Complications associated with epidural steroid injections. Reg Anesth 1996;21(2):149–62.

18. Atluri S, Sudarshan G, Yerramsetty P. Time to understand "safe triangle technique" for transforaminal epidural steroid injections. Pain Physician 2011;14(5):E459–60.
19. Glaser SE, Shah RV. Root cause analysis of paraplegia following transforaminal epidural steroid injections: the 'unsafe' triangle. Pain Physician 2010;13(3):237–44.
20. Ortiz de la Tabla González R, Martínez Navas A, Echevarría Moreno M. [Neurologic complications of central neuraxial blocks]. Rev Esp Anestesiol Reanim 2011;58(7):434–43 [in Spanish].
21. Friedrich JM, Harrast MA. Lumbar epidural steroid injections: indications, contraindications, risks, and benefits. Curr Sports Med Rep 2010;9(1):43–9.
22. Snarr J. Risk, benefits and complications of epidural steroid injections: a case report. AANA J 2007;75(3):183–8.
23. Horlocker T, Wedel D, Rowlingson J, et al. Regional anesthesia in the patient receiving antithrombotic or thrombolytic therapy: American Society of Regional Anesthesia and Pain Medicine Evidence-Based Guidelines. Reg Anesth Pain Med 2010;35(1):64–101.
24. Criscuolo CM. Interventional approaches to the management of myofascial pain syndrome. Curr Pain Headache Rep 2001;5(5):407–11.
25. Kerwat K, Wulf H, Morin A. [Hygiene standards for spinal anaesthesia]. Anasthesiol Intensivmed Notfallmed Schmerzther 2010;45(3):196–8 [in German].
26. Civen R, Vugia DJ, Alexander R, et al. Outbreak of Serratia marcescens infections following injection of betamethasone compounded at a community pharmacy. Clin Infect Dis 2006;43(7):831–7.
27. Mann D. Reducing the hazard of burns and bovie pads. Plast Reconstr Surg 2000;106(4):947.
28. Marinangeli F, Ciccozzi A, Donatelli F, et al. Clinical use of spinal or epidural steroids. Minerva Anestesiol 2002;68(7-8):613–20.
29. Gerber HR. Intrathecal morphine for chronic benign pain. Best Pract Res Clin Anaesthesiol 2003;17(3):429–42.
30. Wolfe JW, Butterworth JF. Local anesthetic systemic toxicity: update on mechanisms and treatment. Curr Opin Anaesthesiol 2011;24(5):561–6.
31. Jeng CL, Torrillo TM, Rosenblatt MA. Complications of peripheral nerve blocks. Br J Anaesth 2010;105(Suppl 1):i97–107.
32. Boyden TF, Gurm HS. Does gadolinium-based angiography protect against contrast-induced nephropathy? A systematic review of the literature. Catheter Cardiovasc Interv 2008;71(5):687–93.
33. Maliborski A, Zukowski P, Nowicki G, et al. Contrast-induced nephropathy— a review of current literature and guidelines. Med Sci Monit 2011;17(9): RA199–204.
34. Pan JJ, Draganov PV. Adverse reactions to iodinated contrast media administered at the time of endoscopic retrograde cholangiopancreatography (ERCP). Inflamm Allergy Drug Targets 2009;8(1):17–20.
35. Eisenach JC, Curry R, Hood DD, et al. Phase I safety assessment of intrathecal ketorolac. Pain 2002;99(3):599–604.
36. Harding LJ, Vaughan RS. Latex allergy—potentially a painful postoperative problem. Anaesthesia 2000;55(7):723–4.
37. Devine J, Chutkan N, Norvell DC, et al. Avoiding wrong site surgery: a systematic review. Spine (Phila Pa 1976) 2010;35(Suppl 9):S28–36.
38. Wong DA, Watters WC 3rd. To err is human: quality and safety issues in spine care. Spine (Phila Pa 1976) 2007;32(Suppl 11):S2–8.
39. Available at: http://www.asipp.org/documents/physician-statement-062507a.pdf. Accessed March 27, 2012.

APPENDIX A: INTERVENTIONAL PAIN MANAGEMENT PROCEDURE INSTRUCTIONS/ CHECKLIST FOR PATIENTS

Before Procedure
- Understand all the risks/benefits/alternatives explained.
- Do not take ANY blood-thinning medications before the procedure.
  - Aspirin-7 days
  - Coumadin-3 days
  - Plavix-7 days
  - Motrin/Relafen- 3days.

Day of Procedure
- Do not eat or drink after 12 midnight.
- Done at ———— Surgical Center. Address ————————————
- If you require heart or blood pressure medications, you may take these with sips of water at least 3 hours before the scheduled time of the procedure.
- Need an escort to take you home after the procedure.
- Sometimes there can be a delay in the start time.
- If you need to cancel the procedure, please call ———— and speak to the operator.

After Procedure Instructions
- Resume all medications after the procedure.
- Do not drive or work for that day.
- Resume work next day.
- Relief takes at least 24 hours after the procedure.
- You may need more than one injection.

APPENDIX B: PAIN MANAGEMENT CART SUPPLIES

Epidural Kit			Date	Date	Date	Date	Date	Date
Kenalog	40 mg/mL	1 mL						
Marcaine Vial	0.50%	10 mL						
Marcaine Vial	0.25%	10 mL						
Lidocaine Vial	1%	10 mL						
Omnipaque		10 mL						
Spinal Needle	22G	3.5						
Spinal Needle	22G	5						
Spinal Needle	25G	3.5						
Touhy Needle	20G	3.5						
Touhy Needle	20G	6"						
Needle	18G	1.5						
Needle	25G	1.5						
Alcohol wipes								
Betadine								
4 × 4 Dressings								
LOR Syringe	Glass	5 mL						

Safety Considerations During Cardiac and Pulmonary Rehabilitation Program

Yelena Suler, MD[a],*, Laurentiu Iulius Dinescu, MD[b]

KEYWORDS

- Complications during cardiac rehabilitation
- Precautions during cardiac rehabilitation
- Karvonen method • SBAR technique
- Sexual counseling during cardiac rehabilitation
- Patient education during cardiac rehabilitation
- Secretion mobilization • Airway clearance
- Glossopharyngeal breathing

As more and more patients with cardiac and pulmonary diseases are living longer lives, the need for cardio-pulmonary rehabilitation continues to grow. The goal of this article is to provide clinicians of rehabilitation medicine with an overview of the safety concerns and strategies to implement in the rehabilitation of patients with cardiac and/or pulmonary disorder.

CARDIAC REHABILITATION

Cardiovascular disease is a leading cause of morbidity and mortality in the United States, but advances over the last several decades in diagnosis and treatment have resulted in a definite trend of decreasing the mortality rates associated with it.

Improvement in the technology used in interventional cardiology and cardiac surgery has increased the survival rates of patients who suffered from acute myocardial infarction or underwent, cardiac surgeries, and cardiac interventional procedures. Current pharmacologic, surgical, dietary, and educational methods allow early recognition and treatment of cardiovascular disease. These advances have resulted in an

[a] Department of Physical Medicine and Rehabilitation, Coler Goldwater Specialty Hospital and Nursing Facility, 1 Main Street, Roosevelt Island, New York, NY 10044, USA
[b] Department of Physical Medicine and Rehabilitation, Kingsbrook Jewish Medical Center, 585 Schenectady Avenue, Brooklyn, NY 11203, USA
* Corresponding author.
E-mail address: yelena.suler@nychhc.org

Phys Med Rehabil Clin N Am 23 (2012) 433–440
doi:10.1016/j.pmr.2012.02.013
1047-9651/12/$ – see front matter © 2012 Elsevier Inc. All rights reserved.

pmr.theclinics.com

increase in the number of potential candidates referred to cardiac rehabilitation (CR) programs.

Participation in a CR program has shown a decrease in the rates of morbidity and mortality for patients with cardiovascular disease. Patients who has the following cardiovascular conditions can benefit from CR programs: (1) myocardial infarction; (2) cardiovascular surgeries, such as coronary artery bypass graft, cardiac transplant, cardiac valve replacement or repair, major vessel repair (ie, aortic aneurysm repair); (3) congestive heart failure (CHF) exacerbation due to ischemic or nonischemic cardiomyopathy.

Most patients can begin a CR program soon after the completion of a procedure or as soon as they are medically stable after an acute cardiac event with no symptoms of CHF, cardiac ischemia, or arrhythmia.[1–5]

CR is divided into 4 phases, and each phase has specific goals and safety considerations for patients[6–8]:

Phase I (Inpatient CR or Acute Phase of CR)

In this phase of CR, patients are trained to safely perform self-care activities and household ambulation . The patient's functional activity gradually increases from bedside activities to ambulation on flat surfaces and stairs. The CR program begins while the patient is still in the cardiac care unit and then continues in the acute rehabilitation unit, till the patient reaches a level of independence (or modified independence) with self-care activities and household ambulation and can be safely discharged home. These activities require less than 4.0 metabolic equivalents (METs) and should not increase the patient's heart rate to more than 20 beats per minute (BPM) from resting heart rate.

Monitoring for complications

Phase I of the CR program is conducted when the patient is susceptible to major complications, such as bleeding, myocardial infarction, pulmonary embolism, deep vein thrombosis (DVT), cardiac arrhythmias, stroke, wound dehiscence, wound infection, CHF, hypotension/hypertension, electrolyte disturbance, and cardiac tamponade. The physiatrist involved in CR must be familiar with the procedure performed and its complications to adequately monitor the symptoms and understand the meaning of the clinical presentation. Careful monitoring of blood pressure, heart rate, oxygen (O_2) saturation, and respiratory rate at rest and during physical activities helps with early diagnosis of these complications. Some of the complications include

1. Dyspnea, tachycardia, and a sudden decrease in a previously normal O_2 saturation to less than 90%, can be caused by a variety of conditions, such as pulmonary embolism, exacerbation of CHF, pneumonia, increasing pleural effusion, and atelectasis. The workup commonly includes chest radiograph, arterial blood gas analysis, venous Doppler scan (to rule out DVT), and spiral computed tomography (to rule out pulmonary embolism).
2. Fever might be due to urinary tract infection (UTI), pneumonia, surgical wound infection, endocarditis, sepsis caused by intravenous catheters, DVT, or pulmonary embolism.
3. Hypotension, which is a frequent clinical finding during CR, is commonly medication induced. Combination of high doses of diuretics, β-blockers, and ACE inhibitors is recommended for the treatment of acute cardiac events, which often induces hypotension during rehabilitation. Observation of orthostatic hypotension during exercises can be a sign of hypovolemia (due to diuretics). The usage of

high doses of β-blockers can cause hypotension along with bradycardia. Dose adjustments of these medications can often be accomplished in a rehabilitation setting. If medication-induced hypotension is ruled out as a cause of hypotension, the loss of postural reflexes due to prolonged bed rest or autonomic dysfunction is considered as the potential cause (especially for patients with diabetes mellitus).

4. Hypertension increases the workload of the heart and must be treated promptly to decrease the chance of cardiac injury.

Exercise program

Absolute contraindications for inpatient or outpatient exercise program as per American College of Sport Medicine include[6–8] (1) unstable angina, (2) exacerbation of CHF, (3) uncontrolled tachycardia (more than 100 BPM), (4) uncontrolled arrhythmia, (5) second- or third-degree atrioventricular (AV) block without pacemaker, (6) ST segment displacement for more than 3 mm at rest, (7) resting blood pressure more than 200/110 mm Hg, (8) moderate-to-severe aortic stenosis, (9) active myocarditis or pericarditis, (10) fever with temperature above 100°F or acute systemic illness, (11) dissecting aneurysm, (12) idiopathic hypertrophic subaortic stenosis, (13) recent embolism or thrombophlebitis, and (14) significant drop in resting systolic blood pressure (more than 20 mm Hg).

Precautions

1. Sternal precautions must be specified in the rehabilitation prescription for therapy if the patient had a sternotomy.[6–8] Patients should avoid pushing, pulling, or lifting weight more than 4.5 kg for approximately 6 weeks after surgery. After the patient is discharged home, the patient is restricted from driving a car for approximately 6 weeks after the sternotomy. Patient must be instructed not to twist his/her body, and take small steps while turning.
2. Restriction of isometric exercises must be specified because of the increase in heart rate.
3. Raising legs above the heart level should be avoided to prevent a potential increase of preload.
4. Performing Valsalva maneuver should be avoided due to the potential of induction of an arrhythmia.
5. Heart rate should be maintained less than 100 BPM or is not allowed to increase more than 20 BPM above the resting level during exercise for patients on β-blockers.
6. Systolic blood pressure is maintained less than 200 mm Hg and diastolic blood pressure less than 110 mm Hg during exercise. Exercise must be stopped if systolic blood pressure drops more than 20 mm Hg below the resting level during activities.
7. O_2 saturation must be maintained above 92% at rest and with physical exertion.
8. Activity-induced changes in electrocardiogram (ECG) have to be monitored. Activities have to be stopped if patient has ST segment displacement greater than 2 to 3 mm, ventricular tachycardia, new onset of left bundle branch block, second- or third-degree AV block, frequent multifocal premature ventricular contractions (PVCs).
9. Exercise sessions have to start with warm-up activities and end with a cooldown period to prevent exercise-induced hypotension.

Medications

Accurate and timely information about the patient's medications is very important in the management of the patient undergoing CR. A complete list of medications has to be available at the time of the patient's admission to the CR unit. Attention must be paid to medications with potentially serious side effects. Such medications include

1. Warfarin for patients with mechanical or mitral valve replacement or repair
2. Clopidogrel for patients who underwent cardiac stent placement
3. Diuretics for the treatment and prevention of CHF
4. Digoxin for the management of atrial fibrillation.

Information about the most recent dose and recommendations for the future use of these medications have to be stated in the discharge summary. In addition, information regarding discontinued medications and the reasons for their discontinuation (eg, side effects, such as gastrointestinal hemorrhage, hemorrhagic stroke while on anticoagulants, severe bradycardia or hypotension in response to β-blockers or deterioration of kidney function while on diuretics) must be provided at the time of transfer of patient to the rehabilitation unit.

Communication between medical providers

The care for the cardiac patient is carried out by a chain of medical providers: primary care physician, medical and surgical consultants, nursing staff, dieticians, laboratory services, physical and occupational therapists, and other allied health professionals. Without reliable communication between all members of the team, it is very difficult to provide safe care to the cardiac patient.

The SBAR (situation, background, assessment, and recommendation) technique for the exchange of information among clinicians was introduced recently.[9] This communication technique can be very helpful in ensuring that complete information is shared between clinical staff. In SBAR, situation refers to the problem that needs to be addressed; background provides key information and a context for the problem; assessment refers to the clinician's understanding of the problem in the context of the patient's condition; recommendation is the clinician's recommended course of action.

Example: Information about nontherapeutic international normalized ratio (INR) may be endorsed from one clinician to another as: "INR is not therapeutic today, follow INR tomorrow." Using the SBAR method, the message can be delivered in the following manner:

S (Situation): INR is 1.5 and not in therapeutic range today.

B (Background): Patient underwent aortic valve replacement with mechanical valve 2 weeks ago. Patient is on warfarin with a target INR between 2.5 and 3.5;

A (Assessment): Patient underwent aortic valve replacement and requires warfarin to maintain INR between within 2.5 and 3.5; however, the current INR indicates that it is not in the therapeutic range. He is currently receiving warfarin, 4 mg, which was started 2 days ago. Heparin was started today;

R (Recommendation): Follow-up INR level tomorrow. If INR is within therapeutic range, discontinue Heparin. If INR is not therapeutic, increase Coumadin dose to 5 mg and repeat INR in 1 day.

The SBAR method creates a more complete message about the patient's situation and helps the next provider to avoid serious mistakes in further management.

Phase II of CR (Outpatient Supervised Program)

The goal of phase II is to gradually improve the patient's endurance, establish healthy lifestyle, control modifiable risk factors for cardiovascular disease, monitor and improve psychological adjustment of the patient to his/her illness, and resume social roles and activities in his family, work, and community.[5]

Exercise program

Exercise activities in phase II are higher in metabolic demand compared with phase I, and require even more supervision in the cardiac gym. At the beginning of phase II, a submaximal stress test is usually done. Depending on the results of the test and patient's risk, the physiatrist generates an individualized prescription for the intensity, duration, and frequency of exercise within safe parameters. The Karvonen method may be used in this situation together with the *Guidelines for Risk Stratification of Cardiac Patients* created by American Association of Cardiovascular and Pulmonary Rehabilitation.[8] The age-adjusted method to calculate the target exercise heart rate can also be used; however, it is less specific and accurate for the patient with multiple comorbidities. The cardiac risk stratification guidelines must be applied to determine the program's intensity that the patient can safely tolerate (low, low-to-moderate, or moderate intensity).[4,8] Contraindications for the exercise program in phase II are the same as those in phase I of CR.

Sexual counseling

The safety of sexual activities after cardiac events or surgery must be discussed with the patient while he/she is still in the hospital. From the authors' observation, the medical provider is often the initiator of this conversation. In general, it is recommended to avoid sexual activities for approximately 4 to 6 weeks after cardiac surgery. The patient must be taught simple self-testing techniques to assess his/her readiness to resume sexual activities safely. The ability to walk for 10 minutes at a speed of 3 miles per hour, followed by climbing 2 flights of stairs (approximately 22 steps) with each stair 17 cm in height within 10 seconds (or 2 steps/s), provides evidence that the patient may safely tolerate sexual activity.[10,11]

Return to work considerations

Returning to work is an important goal of CR if the patient was working before the cardiac event, and plans to return back to work. The ability to safely return back to work should be evaluated by the end of phase II of the CR program.

Patients often return to their previous work, with the exception of heavy manual labor. In these cases, modification of duty or altering the nature of the job needs to be considered.

Phase III and Phase IV of CR (Training and Maintenance)

In these phases, the goal is to improve the general fitness level of the cardiac patient, which is usually accomplished in a setting that requires less supervision. During these phases, the cardiac patient continues his/her exercise program, adheres to healthy lifestyle, and works on minimizing cardiac risk factors. The safety considerations regarding exercise program and control of risk factors are the same as for phase II.

Patient education

Education of the cardiac patient is imperative for the rehabilitation team. The educated patient becomes a conscious member of the team and an active participant. Education improves the patients' understanding of his/her cardiac disease, and improves compliance with their medications, diet, and exercise. The topics for education are

1. Cardiac risk modification program, which includes hyperlipidemia control, hypertension control, diet modification, smoking cessation, diabetes mellitus control, stress management, adherence to exercise program.
2. Each patient must have a working knowledge of his/her medications, their indications, dosing schedule, and side-effects.
3. Education about the symptoms of CHF, such as shortness of breath, weight gain, lower extremity edema, and cardiac pain, helps to alert the patient and prevent major deterioration of his/her medical condition.
4. Sternal precautions.
5. Education of safe sexual practice after cardiac event.

From the authors' experience, teaching conducted in small groups of participants with similar diagnoses and experiences improves the learning ability of patients and promotes open discussions of common problems encountered by cardiac patients and exchange of ideas about "healthy lifestyle."

PULMONARY REHABILITATION

Patients with pulmonary problems can be divided into 2 major groups[12–15]:

1. Patients with impaired oxygenation (chronic obstructive pulmonary disease [COPD]).
2. Patients with impaired ventilation (chronic restrictive disease).

The documented benefits of pulmonary rehabilitation are (1) improvement in the quality of life, (2) reduction in number of hospitalizations, (3) improvement in symptoms, and (4) improvement in exercise tolerance.

Safety During Exercise Program

Improvement in endurance and ability to complete simple activities of daily living safely (without dropping O_2 saturation below 90% or increasing heart rate more than 120 BPM) is one of the goals of pulmonary rehabilitation program.

The monitoring of heart rate and O_2 saturation is mandatory during the pulmonary rehabilitation program, especially for patients with coexistent cardiac disease. Heart rate during exercise may increase by 20% to 30% of resting rate. Exercises must be stopped if the patient develops chest pain, severe dyspnea, heart rate of more than 120 BPM, or frequent PVCs (more than 6 per minute) in the ECG. For patients with neuromuscular diseases (multiple sclerosis, post-polio syndrome), exercises should not be continued to the point of fatigue. The heart rate must return to the level that was before activity within 5 to 10 minutes.

Oxygen Supplementation

Oxygen requirements have to be assessed at rest, during activities, and during sleep. Patients with Pao_2 less than 55 to 60 mm Hg benefit from oxygen supplementation. Multiple studies showed that oxygen therapy results in decreased dyspnea, enhanced performance and prolonged survival, as well as improved pulmonary hypertension and reduced polycythemia. Oxygen must be provided with caution to patients with hypercapnia. Oxygen supplementation has to be carefully titrated to avoid increasing the Pco_2 level.

Nocturnal hypoxemia must be considered if the patient has persistent erythrocytosis, cor pulmonale or mental impairment. Assessment with nocturnal oximetry and/or capnography is easy to perform and helps to make an adjustment in oxygen supplementation.

Nutritional Therapy

Nutritional status assessment and adjustment of diet is essential for patients with chronic pulmonary disease (especially with COPD and ventilator-dependent patients). Prevention of weight loss results in decreased morbidity and mortality in patients with COPD. It also improves patient's endurance and subjective well being. Teaching patients feeding strategies to avoid early satiety, bloating, dyspnea after meal, and constipation, is one of the most important elements in pulmonary rehabilitation.

Common recommendations are: (1) eat small, but frequent meals, (2) eat high-calorie food first, (3) eat cold food first, (4) avoid gas-forming food, (5) rest before meal, (6) increase dietary fat level in daily consumption for patients with hypercapnia, (7) limit liquid consumption during meal time (sip liquid 1 hour after meals), (8) control constipation.

Special Safety Considerations for Patients with COPD During Rehabilitation Program

Secretion management is one of the major modalities used during rehabilitation, which helps by preventing the development of new atelectasis and pneumonia.

1. Secretion mobilization by postural drainage, percussion, and vibration, and then
2. Airway clearance with controlled cough technique, assisted cough, or huffing, are usually used to maintain an airway adequately open.

Special Safety Considerations During Rehabilitation of Patients with Restrictive Pulmonary Disease Due to Weakness of Respiratory Muscles

Patients with very weak diaphragm, who require mechanical ventilation, but have preserved oral musculature, would benefit from learning glossopharyngeal breathing. This technique of propelling boluses of air by rhythmic movements of the tongue, lips, and soft palate allows maintaining ventilation up to several hours. In case of ventilator failure, this technique may help the patient to survive until mechanical ventilation is restored. Patients with tetraplegia are good candidates to learn this breathing technique.

REFERENCES

1. Kodama S, Saito K, Tanaka S, et al. Cardiorespiratory fitness as a quantitative predictor of all-cause mortality and cardiovascular events in healthy men and women: a meta-analysis. JAMA 2009;301:2024.
2. Fletcher BJ, Lloyd A, Fletcher GF. Outpatient rehabilitative training in patients with cardiovascular disease: emphasis on training method. Heart Lung 1988;17:199.
3. Douglas P. Exercise and fitness in prevention of cardiovascular disease. UpToDate; 2012.
4. Gupta S, Rohatgi A, Ayers CR, et al. Cardiorespiratory fitness and classification of risk of cardiovascular disease mortality. Circulation 2011;123:1377.
5. Fletcher BJ, Thiel J, Fletcher GF. Phase II intensive monitored cardiac rehabilitation for coronary artery disease and coronary risk factors—a six-session protocol. Am J Cardiol 1986;57:751.
6. Wenger NK, Hellerstein HK, editors. Rehabilitation of the coronary patient. 3rd edition. New York: Churchill Livingstone; 1992.
7. Mahler DA, American College of Sports Medicine Staff, ACSM. ACSM Guidelines for exercise testing and prescription. 5th edition. Philadelphia: Lea & Febiger; 1995. p. 78.

8. American Association of Cardiovascular and Pulmonary Rehabilitation (AACVPR). Guidelines for cardiac rehabilitation programs. Champaign (IL): Human Kinetics Publishers; 1995. p. 34.

9. Velji K, Baker GR, Fancott C, et al. Effectiveness of an adapted SBAR communication tool for a rehabilitation setting. Healthc Q 2008;(Spec):72–9.

10. Hellerstein HK, Friedman EH. Sexual activity and the postcoronary patient. Arch Intern Med 1970;125:987–99.

11. Larson JL, McNaughton MW, Kennedy JW, et al. Heart rate and blood pressure reponse to sexual activity and a stair-climbing test. Heart Lung 1980;9:1025–30.

12. Alba AS. Concepts in pulmonary rehabilitation. In: Braddom RL, editor. Physical medicine and rehabilitation. Philadelphia: W.B. Saunders; 1996. p. 671–86.

13. Bach JR. Rehabilitation of the patient with respiratory dysfunction. In: DeLisa JA, editor. Rehabilitation: principles and practice. 2nd edition. Philadelphia: Lippincot Williams & Wilkins; 1993. p. 952–72.

14. Bach JR. Pulmonary rehabilitation: the obstructive and paralytic conditions. Philadelphia: Hanley & Belfus; 1996.

15. Rogers RM, Donahoe M. Nutrition in pulmonary rehabilitation. In: Fishman AP, editor. Pulmonary rehabilitation. New York: Marcel Dekker; 1996. p. 543–64.

Patient Safety in Cancer Rehabilitation

Adrian Cristian, MD, MHCM[a],*, Andy Tran, MD[b],
Karishma Patel, MD[c]

KEYWORDS

• Patient safety • Cancer rehabilitation

It has been estimated that there are 1.5 million people diagnosed with cancer each year and that there are 13 million cancer survivors in the United States as of 2010.[1] More than 60% of those diagnosed are surviving 5 years or more.[1] This is due to a combination of factors, such as earlier diagnosis and advances in the treatment of various types of cancer. Cancer survivors, however, often have to live with the long-term effects of their underlying disease as well as effects of treatments, such as surgery, chemotherapy, and radiation therapy (RT), on their bodies. Rehabilitation professionals have a great deal to offer these survivors and provide rehabilitative services for them throughout their life span, including periods of acute hospitalizations for surgical and medical treatments, acute and subacute inpatient rehabilitation admissions, outpatient rehabilitation programs, and rehabilitation in the home setting as well as the end-stages of their disease. Given the complexity of the medical care rendered to these patients, it is important for rehabilitation professionals to provide these services in a safe manner. The goal of this article is to describe the basic principles of patient safety in the delivery of cancer rehabilitation services. An excellent resource on the topic of cancer rehabilitation in general as well as patient safety in the care of cancer patients is available for interested readers.[2]

WHY IS THE CANCER PATIENT AT RISK DURING REHABILITATION?
Cancer-Related Complications

Depending on the type of cancer, its location, and extent of metastasis, there are many specific cancer-related complications of which rehabilitation professionals should be aware. They range from general in nature to organ or organ system specific.

Disclosure: The authors have no financial disclosures.
[a] Department of Rehabilitation Medicine, Kingsbrook Rehabilitation Institute, Kingsbrook Jewish Medical Center, 585 Schenectady Avenue, Brooklyn, NY, USA
[b] Department of Medical Education, Kingsbrook Jewish Medical Center, 585 Schenectady Avenue, Brooklyn, NY, USA
[c] 3420 Avenue North, Brooklyn, NY 11234, USA
* Corresponding author.
E-mail address: acristian@kingsbrook.org

Phys Med Rehabil Clin N Am 23 (2012) 441–456
doi:10.1016/j.pmr.2012.02.015
1047-9651/12/$ – see front matter © 2012 Elsevier Inc. All rights reserved.

Pulmonary complications

The lung is a common site of both primary cancer and metastatic disease for cancers of the breast, colon, kidney, and gastrointestinal tract. The location of the cancer can be a cause of bronchial obstruction, pleural effusion, pneumothorax, and phrenic nerve paralysis. Metastatic disease to the ribs also is a source of pain with inspiration. Other complications include pulmonary embolisms (PEs) and pneumonia. Patients with a history of exposure of lungs to RT for the treatment of cancer can have radiation pneumonitis or pulmonary fibrosis. These complications are compounded in patients with history of chronic obstructive pulmonary disease. The significance of these complications in the rehabilitation setting is decreased exercise capacity, shortness of breath, and pain.[3]

Cardiac complications

Pericardial effusions and involvement of the pleura secondary to cancer can be a cause of constrictive pericarditis. Patients with a history of RT or chemotherapy may also have sustained injury to the heart muscle and the coronary arteries. Patients may present in the rehabilitation setting with symptoms of angina on exertion.[4]

Gastrointestinal complications

Depending on the type of cancer, complications include dysphagia, nausea, vomiting, poor nutritional intake and appetite, bowel obstruction, and diarrhea. The diarrhea may also be related to infections of the gastrointestinal tract.[5]

Renal complications

Fluid and electrolyte disorders are a significant source of morbidity in cancer patients. These disorders may be due to an underlying cancer (eg, multiple myeloma, lymphoma, or leukemia) or its treatments (eg, bone marrow transplant). Hypercalcemia and changes in potassium and sodium levels can present with altered mental status and weakness. Hypovolemia has several sources and may present with orthostatic hypotension, which contributes to falls.[6]

Endocrine complications

The syndrome of inappropriate secretion of antidiuretic hormone (SIADH) is the second most common paraneoplastic endocrine disorder.[7] It is seen in patients with small cell lung cancer and is a complication of chemotherapeutic medications (vincristine, vinblastine, cisplatin, and cyclophosphamide). Rehabilitation professionals should be aware of its presentation—changes in mental status, nausea, vomiting, weakness, muscle cramps, and seizures. Thyroid dysfunction, such as hypothyroidism, is seen in patients with a history of thyroid cancer or RT to the neck region for cancer. The clinical presentation includes cognitive slowing, fatigue, cold intolerance, and pleural/pericardial effusions. Cancer patients with diabetes deserve special mention because the combination of tight glycemic control and inadequate nutritional intake can lead to symptomatic hypoglycemia while patients undergo rehabilitation. Rehabilitation professionals should be aware of the clinical presentation of hypoglycemia, which includes sweating, anxiety, tremor, nausea, and fatigue and can progress to altered mental status, syncope, and seizures.[7]

Hematological complications

Bone marrow infiltration from cancer can have a profound effect on cancer patients, which in turn affects their rehabilitation program. Anemia manifests through decreased exercise tolerance, angina symptoms, dizziness, and tachycardia. Neutropenia predisposes to infections and thrombocytopenia increases the risk of hemorrhages. Hyperviscosity syndrome characterized by erythrocytosis, leukocytosis, and thrombocytosis can lead to intracranial hemorrhaging and respiratory failures.[8]

Infectious disease complications

Cancer patients are at increased risk of infections secondary to their underlying cancer diagnosis as well as its treatment (eg, bone marrow transplant). Common examples are pneumonia, urinary tract infection, gastrointestinal infections, and cellulitis. These infections have implications for their rehabilitation, including reduced ability to tolerate a rehabilitation program. For example, pneumonia is associated with shortness of breath and decreased oxygen saturation during therapy sessions.

Venous thromboembolic events

Between 3% and 18% of cancer patients have venous thrombosis.[9,10] There is a significant increase in mortality among cancer patients with a venous thromboembolic event.[11] The increased risk is often associated with a hypercoagulable state, decreased mobility, presence of varicose veins, fractures, use of oral corticosteroids, oral contraceptives, central venous catheters, and certain chemotherapy medications (cyclophosphamide, methotrexate, tamoxifen, and thalidomide).[12,13]

Orthopedic complications

There are several types of cancer that metastasize to bone with breast, lung, prostate, renal, and thyroid being the most common sites of origin.[14] Metastasis is the most common malignant process affecting the bones. Of all the new cases of invasive carcinoma diagnosed annually in the United States, approximately 50% eventually metastasize to bones.[14] These metastatic lesions and other destructive processes affecting bones, such as myeloma and lymphoma, predispose the bone to an impending fracture. A pathologic fracture in these settings exposes patients to extreme pain, urgent hospitalization, and the risk of surgery in less than ideal circumstances. Mirels proposed a scoring system to classify pathologic fracture risk based on 4 characteristics[1]: site of lesion (upper limb, lower limb, or peritrochanter)[3]; type of lesion (blastic, mixed, or lytic)[4]; size of lesion relative to the diameter of the bone (<1/3; 1/3–2/3; >2/3); and[5] pain (mild, moderate, or functional). Each of these characteristics was assigned progressive scores ranging from 1 to 3. The highest scores were for lytic lesions in the peritrochanter region, greater than two-thirds in size relative to the diameter of the bone and pain with function.[15,16] Functional pain is caused by muscles contracting around a lesion. A patient's inability to perform a straight leg raise may indicate an impending pathologic fracture of the hip.[17] The rate of pathologic fracture was 0% for lesions less than one-third the size of the cortex, 5% for lesions between one-third and two-thirds the size of the cortex, and 81% for lesions occupying more than two-thirds of the cortex.[16] Harrington[18] suggests that both lytic and blastic long bone metastases are at risk for developing pathologic fractures in instances where greater than 50% of the circumferential cortical bone has been destroyed or where the pain with weight-bearing stresses persists, increases, or recurs despite adequate local irradiation. Moreover, lesions of the proximal femur are at a high risk for fracture if they are in excess of 2.5 cm in any dimension or if they are associated with avulsion of the lesser trochanter. In a study done by Fidler,[19] fractures were highly unlikely to occur (2.3%) when less than 50% of the cortex was destroyed and most likely to occur (80%) when greater than 75% of the cortex was destroyed. Pain was the only subjective variable in this classification system. Mild, moderate, or functional pain was assigned a score from 1 to 3, respectively. Rate of fracture was only 10% among patients with mild to moderate pain. All the patients with functional pain, however, progressed to a fracture.[16]

Nervous system complications

Cancer patients with metastatic disease to the brain or those with primary brain tumors can have seizures, communication disorders secondary to aphasia, swallowing dysfunction, hemiparesis, and impaired balance. Cognitive deficits in sustained attention, short-term and delayed recall, processing speed, executive function, organizational skills, self-awareness, and mental fatigue can have a significant impact on the rehabilitation program. Fluctuating cognition and arousal due to underlying disease and treatments also affect rehabilitation.[20,21]

Communication and swallowing complications

Head and neck cancer patients can have significant impairments in communication and swallowing function, including increased risk of aspiration secondary to the underlying cancer or its treatments. RT can lead to fibrosis of key muscles and structures used in the swallowing mechanism, such as base of the tongue, epiglottis, hypopharynx, and larynx,[22] increasing the risk of aspiration as well as having an adverse effect on overall oral nutritional intake and hydration.

Impact on the Cancer Patient

Medical debility

Cancer patients can be significantly debilitated due to location, type, and extent of involvement of the cancer as well as treatments rendered, such as surgery, chemotherapy, and RT. Because cancer occurs in 76% of adults over age 55,[1] cancer patients often have additional comorbidities from other medical diagnoses, such as coronary artery disease and diabetes, as well as the impact from earlier treatments for a recurrence of the cancer or other cancers. Many patients also receive steroids as part of their treatment protocols, which can cause a myopathy, furthering their already debilitated state as well as increasing the risk of fractures due to the demineralizing effect on bone.

Metastatic disease

There is a significant number of cancers that often metastasize to different parts of the body, such as bone, brain, lungs, and spinal cord. The presence of metastatic disease can pose safety risks to patients undergoing rehabilitation depending on its location. Examples are (1) metastasis to bone that increases the risk of pathologic fractures in vertebral bodies and long bones and (2) metastasis to the brain, which can lead to cognitive and physical impairments, such as memory loss, impaired judgment, hemiparesis, aphasia, and impaired balance, leading to increased risk of falling and difficulty understanding and following medical instructions as well as patients' ability to advocate for their needs. Metastatic disease can also compress peripheral and central nervous system tissues, such as the brachial and lumbosacral plexus, peripheral nerves, and spinal cord, all of which have a profound effect on patients undergoing rehabilitation.[23,24] It has been estimated that 25% to 30% of all cancer patients have metastatic disease to the lung[25] and metastasis to the pleura occurs in 12% of breast cancer patients and 7% to 15% of lung cancers patients. Metastasis to the heart occurs in 8.4% of cancer patients.[1] All of these pose an increased safety risk to patients undergoing rehabilitation programs.

Chemotherapy

There are myriad chemotherapeutic agents used in the treatment of cancer, often combined for maximal antineoplastic effects. These treatments, however, are often associated with significant toxicities in both the short term and long term of a patient's life. Short-term generalized toxicities are varied; examples are nausea, vomiting, alopecia, mouth sores, and fatigue. Some toxicities have direct effects on organs: (1) doxorubicin and daunorubicin have direct effect on the heart, causing cardiomyopathy; (2) platins (cisplatin, carboplatin, and oxaliplatin), vinca alkaloids (vincristine and vinblastine), and taxanes (paclitaxel and docetaxel) cause damage to peripheral nerves; and (3) bleomycin, busulfan, methotrexate, and carmustine are linked with pulmonary fibrosis.[1] Other toxicities have more generalized effects that are important in the rehabilitation setting. Examples are (1) infections, such as pneumonias secondary to a compromised immune system; (2) decreased hemoglobin, affecting the ability to tolerate an aerobic exercise program; and (3) decreased platelet counts, increasing the risk of bleeding.[8]

Radiation therapy

RT has both short-term and long-term effects seen in the rehabilitation setting. Short-term effects include nausea, vomiting, alopecia, fatigue, localized skin irritation and blisters, loss of appetite, and mouth sores, all of which can affect a patient's ability to tolerate a rehabilitation program. Long-term effects include myelopathy, plexopathy, encephalopathy, lymphedema, pulmonary fibrosis, accelerated atherosclerosis, osteoporosis, delayed healing, and osteonecrosis. Radiation fibrosis can cause injuries to peripheral nerve as well as injuries to muscles, bones, and connective tissues, in turn leading to contractures in limbs with an increased risk of falling if RT effects are in the lower extremities.[26] Cognitive impairments also are seen in patients undergoing RT to the brain, in turn leading to impaired judgment or memory loss, which also increases safety risks, such as falls and difficulty understanding medical instructions.[27]

Surgical treatments

Surgical treatments for cancer can alter a patient's anatomy by removal of both diseased and healthy tissue, including bone, muscles, peripheral nerves, and connective tissues, in turn leading to significant impairments and disabilities. Lack of knowledge about the type of surgery performed as well as specific precautions after it places patients at risk.

Pain management

Pain is common in cancer patients. It has been estimated that 28% of newly diagnosed patients, 50% to 70% of patients receiving antineoplastic therapy, and 64% to 80% patients with advanced disease experience pain.[1] Opioid medications are commonly used to treat pain in the cancer patient population; however, side effects from opioids can lead to drowsiness, impaired cognition, and falls. Invasive procedures, such as injections and nerve blocks used to treat cancer pain, pose their own safety risks.

Access to rehabilitative services

Access to rehabilitative services also is limited by lack of cancer-specific rehabilitative expertise, depleted financial reserves, limited medical insurance, and fragmented social support systems.

PATIENT ASSESSMENT WITH AN EMPHASIS ON PATIENT SAFETY
Medical History

The medical history is an important communication tool between rehabilitation clinicians caring for cancer patients as patients move along the continuum of care. The key elements of this document are (1) cancer diagnosis—type of cancer and stage and extent of metastatic disease (based on radiology and pathology reports); (2) complications related to the cancer infections, deep vein thrombosis (DVT), and anemia as well as treatments for the complications; and (3) treatments: chronology of all the treatments rendered, including surgeries, chemotherapy, and RT. Description of surgeries should include (1) type of surgery; (2) diseased and nondiseased structures removed, including bone, muscles, and peripheral nerves[21]; (3) postoperative precautions and instructions; (4) contact information for the surgeon who performed the surgery; and (5) future planned surgeries. Description of chemotherapy protocols should include (1) chemotherapeutic agents used in the past and present; (2) number of cycles and dates of chemotherapy cycles; (3) complications associated with the chemotherapy; and (4) diagnostic reports for key organs that may have been affected by the chemotherapy (eg, echocardiogram for patients with cardiomyopathy, pulmonary function tests for patients with pulmonary disease, and nerve conduction studies for patients with peripheral neuropathy). Description of RT treatments should include (1) structures that were irradiated, (2) total amount of radiation delivered to the structures in the past (remote and distant), (3) dates of the radiation treatments in the past and number of treatments planned for the future, and (4) side effects or long-term effects of the RT. Pain assessment includes (1) location, duration, quality, intensity, radiation, aggravating factors, and alleviating factors and (2) treatments rendered—medications, procedures, and their side effects. Other important information includes (1) past medical and surgical history (eg, diabetes, heart disease, and pulmonary disease); (2) allergies; (3) medications; (4) review of systems; (5) social and functional status; (6) pertinent laboratory values—hemoglobin, white blood cell, and platelet count; (7) pertinent radiology reports; (8) contact information for all key clinicians in a patient's care—hematologist/oncologist, radiation oncologist, surgeon, primary care and physical therapists, occupational therapists, and speech pathologists who worked with the patient in the past as well as hospitals where the patient received treatments.

Physical Examination

The physical examination should focus on specific organ systems affected by the cancer. Key components are (1) vital signs, such as, temperature, respiratory rate, and oxygen saturation; it is useful to obtain heart rate and blood pressure readings in the supine, sitting, or standing position; (2) cardiopulmonary assessment; (3) neurological assessment: (a) cranial nerves, speech, and swallow; (b) brief cognitive evaluation that includes, at minimum, orientation to person, place, and time; immediate and delayed recall; and ability to follow instructions; (c) motor strength testing of key muscle groups; (d) sensory testing—light touch, pinprick, temperature, position sense, and vibration; (e) muscle stretch reflexes; (f) trunk control; and (g) gait; (4) musculoskeletal system: range of motion for all the key joints and spine and presence of contractures; and (5) skin: evidence of pressure ulcers and myofascial restrictions to movement.

TYPES OF PATIENT SAFETY RISKS IN REHABILITATION MEDICINE AS THEY APPLY TO THE CANCER PATIENT

Patient safety risks in cancer patients are grouped into 4 broad categories: (1) communication and coordination of care, (2) diagnosis, (3) treatment, and (4) monitoring.

Communication and Coordination of Care

The rehabilitation of cancer patients and survivors does not occur in a vacuum. Patients are often cared for by several medical, surgical, nursing, and allied health personnel. This care is provided along a continuum of care that often includes acute hospitalizations, care in both acute and subacute rehabilitation facilities, outpatient treatment centers, and home setting. Fragmented care at transition points in which key elements of a patient's medical and surgical history are not communicated in a timely fashion can have a significant adverse effect on the patient's rehabilitation and well-being. Limited information between care providers regarding changes in medical status, disease progression, and infectious disease precautions poses safety risks to cancer patients.

Diagnosis

Type and stage of cancer, extent of metastasis, and prognosis are key factors in determining the rehabilitation program of cancer patients. Additionally, accurately diagnosing conditions commonly seen in this population by rehabilitation clinicians ensures timely initiation of treatment. Examples are (1) DVT in the upper and lower extremities; (2) PE; (3) spinal cord compression; (4) plexus involvement secondary to metastatic disease or RT; (5) pathologic fractures of the spine and long bones; (6) cognitive impairments and neurologic compromise secondary to primary brain tumors or metastatic disease; (7) misdiagnosing cancer recurrence and bone metastasis in patients with musculoskeletal complaints, such as lower back, shoulder, or hip pain; and (8) radiation fibrosis.

Treatment

Once a diagnosis of one or more of the above-mentioned conditions has been made, timely initiation of appropriate treatments by medical, surgical, nursing, and rehabilitation personnel is essential. The treatments can pose their own safety risks to patients, however. Examples are (1) injections into musculoskeletal structures that have been altered as a result of treatments, such as surgery and radiation, (2) adverse effects of exercises, soft tissue mobilization techniques, and modalities. (3) application of modalities over insensate areas and areas with poor vascular supply or known history of underlying malignancy; (4) inaccurate weight-bearing precautions in patients with metastatic disease to bones and risk of pathologic fractures; (5) exercise parameters that do not take into account the impairments associated with chemotherapy, RT, or surgical treatments rendered (eg, pulmonary fibrosis, cardiomyopathy, and limited cardiopulmonary reserve); and (6) chest physical therapy over ribs that have been affected by metastatic disease. The competency of rehabilitation clinicians in the care of cancer patients is also important because not all rehabilitation clinicians have the same level of expertise in the treatment of this complex and fragile population. Lack of adequate staffing levels of rehabilitation professionals in the continuum of rehabilitative care also poses a safety risk to patients.

Monitoring

Limited monitoring of cancer patients and survivors undergoing rehabilitation also poses safety risks. Examples are (1) cancer patients with new complaints of musculoskeletal pain, (2) cancer patients with new-onset cognitive impairments, and (3) reactions to chemotherapeutic and RT.

STRATEGIES TO MAXIMIZE PATIENT SAFETY IN THE REHABILITATION OF THE CANCER PATIENT

To maximize patient safety in the rehabilitation of cancer patients, the most competent and experienced providers should provide the care under optimal circumstances based on a detailed knowledge of a patient's medical condition and using the most appropriate equipment and knowledge available.

COMMUNICATION AND COORDINATION OF CARE
Handoffs and Transition Points

Cancer patients pose a specific safety risk due to the multiple caregivers involved in their care and the numerous points of care in the health care continuum. This continuum often involves (1) inpatient hospitalizations in various units of a medical center—intensive care units and surgical, medical, and rehabilitative wards; (2) outpatient clinics; (3) nursing homes; and (4) patient home via visiting nursing and therapy services. Communication and coordination of care are especially important patient safety considerations for rehabilitation professionals. Some key strategies are as follows:

1. Exchange of information between physicians, therapists, and nurses should occur in quiet areas where there are minimal distractions and interruptions.
2. The information should be collected following a structured checklist to ensure that all key information is made available from the sender to the receiver. A sample checklist is enclosed in **Box 1**.
3. Use verbal repeat back communication in which the sender states the information concisely and the receiver repeats it back. This gives the sender the opportunity to check for understanding and clarify content if necessary.[28] This technique can also be used after an educational session with a patient.
4. Use critical language that everyone agrees on when there is confusion about the information communicated. Some possible phrases are (1) "I need a little clarity regarding/I am concerned about whether or not this patient should undergo ambulation training given the low platelet count." Alternative phrasing is, "I am concerned about the safety of ambulation in this patient given the low platelet count."[29]
5. Ensure adequate flow of rehabilitation information along the continuum of rehabilitative care. For example, weight-bearing and range-of-motion precautions in limbs at risk for pathologic fractures should be reported between (1) nursing shifts; (2) physiatrists, therapists, surgeons, and oncologists; and (3) therapists and

---

Box 1
Cancer specific structured communication tool for transition points in care

a. Type, location, stage, and location of metastasis

b. Treatments rendered and dates of treatments

    i. Chemotherapy

    ii. RT

    iii. Surgeries

c. Medical and surgical complications

d. Medications

e. Allergies

f. Contact information of key physicians, nurses, and therapists involved in care

g. Imaging and pathology reports

h. Laboratory results (hemoglobin, white blood cell and platelet counts, calcium, international normalized ratio, potassium and sodium levels)

i. Precautions (eg, weight bearing)

physiatrists working with patients on different days and in different settings (eg, acute, subacute, outpatient, and home settings) using a standardized checklist instrument.

6. Use a double-check system for key information that affects a patient's care (eg, clarification regarding exercise protocols and use of modalities in patients with low hemoglobin and low platelet counts). In this system, two individuals confirm the accuracy of the information.

7. Use structured communication techniques, such as the SBAR technique developed by Michael and colleagues.[30] In this technique, the sender of information presents the information in a structured format that includes the following: (1) situation (brief description of the situation), (2) background (key information about the background of the patient to provide context), (3) assessment, and (4) recommendations for action. For example, in a patient with a risk of a pathologic fracture, the SBAR communication includes

   a. Situation: large metastatic lesion in shoulder identified on imaging study
   b. Background: patient with history of metastatic breast cancer; patient was evaluated by oncological orthopedist and range-of-motion precautions clarified
   c. Assessment: active and passive range of motion of the limb poses increased risk of pathologic fracture
   d. Recommendation: avoid active and passive range of motion to the limb.

This information can then be distributed to all clinicians involved in a patient's care as well as passed on to other points in the rehabilitation continuum of care.

Delivery of Rehabilitation Services

Some key points in the safe delivery of rehabilitative services to cancer patients are as follows:

1. Standardize rehabilitation protocols and minimize variability in care. Simplify protocols, remove unnecessary steps, and use technology to reduce reliance on human memory (eg, electronic medical records).

2. Evaluate the delivery of rehabilitation services for potential breakdown. Some areas of potential breakdown are staff related:
   a. Increased workload for rehabilitation providers leading to workarounds with less emphasis on safety.
   b. Loss of providers with specific expertise in the rehabilitation of cancer patients (eg, physical therapist with significant expertise in lymphedema therapy).
   c. Use of new technology without appropriate and sustained training of all staff (eg, electronic medical record system).
   d. Provider burnout. Caring for cancer patients can be challenging for staff members, which in turn results in increased staff turnover. Having systems in place to provide support and counseling to staff members helps rehabilitation providers in caring for this population.
   e. Minimize fatigue in rehabilitation providers, such as physicians, therapists, and nursing staff. When fatigued, clinicians experience reduced decision-making ability, prolonged response time, impaired memory, and difficulty concentrating and communicating.[31]
   f. Emergency equipment should be up to date and emergency care protocols should be in place and rehearsed on a regular basis by rehabilitation professionals (eg, protocols for the management of the unresponsive patient or the patient who sustained a fall).

g. Orientation and mentoring of less-experienced clinical staff by more experienced clinical staff. Rehabilitation of cancer patients is a subspecialty of rehabilitation medicine that requires physicians, therapists, and rehabilitation nursing staff to develop and practice a unique set of clinical skills in assessment and treatment.

h. Treating clinicians should take the time to discuss and rehearse the treatment plan before applying it to the patient.

i. Implement a formal process, such as a root cause analysis (RCA), to evaluate near misses, close calls, and adverse events with an emphasis on system errors. RCAs are used to answer 4 basic questions: (1) What happened? (2) How did it happen? (3) What should have happened? and (4) What can be done to prevent this from happening again. The Institute for Healthcare Improvement provides on-line instruction on how to perform an RCA.[32]

j. Identify and minimize barriers that limit access to rehabilitative care. Some of these barriers are architectural, attitudinal, physical, knowledge based, transportation related, and financial.

k. The physical environment in which patients receive rehabilitative care should minimize the risk of injury to the patient. The space should be well lit and free of clutter, provide an ambient temperature, and take into account the infection control requirements of cancer patients. This is especially important in the treatments of certain subsets of cancer patients (eg, bone marrow transplant patients).

DIAGNOSIS AND TREATMENT-RELATED CONSIDERATIONS

Rehabilitation providers often spend a considerable amount of time with their cancer patients and thus are in a position of making diagnoses or alerting appropriate clinicians to key signs and symptoms that can then be used to make a diagnosis. It is important not to delay in making an accurate diagnosis because this may either cause a delay in treatment or provide inappropriate treatment. Rehabilitation clinicians should be vigilant for changes in a patient's condition because these may represent a progression of the underlying disease or an adverse reaction to a treatment. Rehabilitation professionals should be aware of the signs and symptoms of disorders commonly seen in cancer patients undergoing rehabilitation. Some of these are provided in **Box 2**.

Physiatrists commonly use a variety of treatments to treat cancer-related impairments. Many of these are grouped into 3 main categories: (1) medications, (2) interventional procedures, and (3) rehabilitation therapies. Physiatrists should be knowledgeable

---

Box 2
Common diagnoses and conditions seen in the rehabilitation setting by clinicians

DVT of the lower and upper extremities

PE

Seizure disorder

Pathologic fractures

Infections—cellulitis, urinary tract infection, pneumonia, gastrointestinal infections

Electrolyte imbalances—potassium, calcium, sodium

Orthostatic hypotension

about the benefits and risks of these interventions, have the competencies to perform them, and adequately educate their patients about them. Although a detailed description of each of these interventions is beyond the scope of this article, some general concepts as they apply to patient safety are addressed.

Medications

When prescribing medications, the physiatrist should have a working knowledge of the medication's mechanism of action, pharmacokinetics, significant drug-drug interactions, and side effects. The medication prescription should ideally be written in a quiet area that is free of interruptions and distractions. The correct medication, the correct dose, and the correct unit of measurement should be written. The physiatrist should obtain information about patient allergies as well as kidney and liver function. Attention should also be given to using the appropriate abbreviation for the medication.

Procedures

There are a variety of procedures used by physiatrists in the care of cancer patients. Examples are (1) botulinum toxin injections (for the treatment of radiation fibrosis), (2) trigger point injections, and (3) peripheral joint injections. Interventional physiatrists often use spinal injections in the management of pain syndromes. From a patient safety perspective, clinicians with the appropriate competency and the most experience available should perform the procedure. A thorough understanding of the anatomy subjected to the procedure is essential. The anatomy in cancer patients may be altered from the underlying cancer as well as by treatments, such as surgery, chemotherapy, and RT. Common safety procedures are (1) double-checking patient identification, (2) identification of the body part that will undergo the procedure, including right versus left considerations, and (3) use of time-out before the procedure. Rehearsals of the injection protocol by the physiatrist and team also are helpful. The physician should discuss with the patient the various aspects of the procedure, including what will actually be done; who will be performing the procedure; the risks, benefits, and alternatives; and postinjection instructions of care.

Rehabilitation Prescription

The rehabilitation prescription is a key communication tool in ensuring the safety of cancer patients undergoing a rehabilitation program. Key precautions considerations include the following.

Infectious Disease Precautions

(1) Wash hands between patient treatments. (2) Clarify infection control precautions for patients with treating physicians and follow infection control protocols for medical center or clinic. (Note: some patients may require mask, gown, and gloves and reverse isolation rooms.) (3) Avoid compressive therapy in patients with evidence of cellulitis in an extremity that is treated for lymphedema. (4) Follow medical center or clinic infection control protocols.

Modalities

Avoid application of superficial and deep heat modalities over insensate body parts, body parts with poor circulation, sites at risk for bleeding, and sites where tumors are located. Avoid application of traction in areas of malignancy or at risk of pathologic fractures.[33]

Exercise Precautions

(1) During periods of acute illness, exercise program should be limited or held until the acute illness is resolved. (2) Vital signs: blood pressure, pulse, respiratory rate, and pulse oximetry should be obtained before and during exercise session. It is also a good idea to obtain blood pressure and heart rate readings in the supine, sitting, and standing positions before inception of exercise to check for orthostatic changes. (3) Range-of-motion and resistive exercise precautions in patients with risk of pathologic fractures—check with oncological orthopedist on specific precautions or limitations on use of passive or active assisted range-of-motion or resistive exercises in the affected limbs. (4) Weight-bearing status should be clarified with an oncological orthopedist before inception of exercises that involve a limb at risk for pathologic fractures; this should be reassessed if a patient complains of pain in the affected limb at rest or with activity. (5) Fall risk: there is an increased risk of falling in cancer patients due to a cancer-related impairment (eg, hemiplegia secondary to a brain tumor) or cancer treatment (eg, chemotherapy-related neuropathy or steroid-induced myopathy).

Cardiac Precautions

(1) Monitor for symptoms of chest pain, rate of perceived exertion, and dizziness before, during, and after exercise program.[4] (2) In high-risk patients, cardiology work-up and clearance before inception of exercise program are advised, including obtaining the results of an echocardiogram and/or stress test and modifying the exercise program based on the results.

Pulmonary Precautions

(1) Monitor for symptoms, such as dizziness and shortness of breath; (2) monitor oxygen saturation before, during, and after exercise sessions and maintain oxygen saturation greater than 90%; (3) clarify with patient's oncologist if patient can receive supplemental oxygen during rehabilitation sessions given chemotherapy medications (eg, contraindicated in patients treated with bleomycin); and (4) avoid chest physical therapy over ribs that have metastatic disease involvement.[34]

Hematological Precautions

It is important to review hemoglobin, white blood cell count, and platelet count before initiation and during the rehabilitation program. Values relevant to the practice of rehabilitation medicine are described in the literature.[8]

Venous Thromboembolic Events

A significant concern in the rehabilitation of cancer patients with DVT is the possibility of a potential fatal complication, such as a PE associated with early ambulation after the diagnosis of the DVT. The literature on the appropriate timing to begin ambulation is thus far inconclusive. There are no clear protocols to show that early ambulation of a patient once diagnosed with DVT either improves or worsens the risk for PE.[35] Investigators have suggested that early ambulation is safe for the majority of patients with DVT, once adequate treatment, such as unfractionated heparin or low molecular weight heparin and compression stockings, has been implemented.[35] Clinicians should consider the following questions before deciding to start ambulation in a patient with DVT: (1) Is the patient receiving adequate medical treatment for DVT? (2) Will ambulation place the patient at increased risk of acute PE? (3) Should a PE occur during the patient's rehabilitation, would he/she be able to survive the event? (4) Will continued bed rest place the patient at increased risk of propagation of the DVT and at increased risk for other complications of bed rest? and (5) Does the patient have evidence of PE before beginning ambulation?[34] to date there is limited information concerning range-of-motion or exercise restrictions in patients with upper-extremity DVT.

Wound and Surgery-Related Precautions

Check with treating physician or surgeon before initiating rehabilitation program over areas that have wound related or recent surgeries because certain rehabilitation techniques may affect the healing of the wounds or be contraindicated after certain types of surgeries (eg, lifting precautions after certain type of breast reconstruction surgeries).

Seizures Risk

Some cancer patients have an increased risk of seizures and the antiseizure medication regimen should be optimized before inception of an exercise program. Rehabilitation team members should be aware of a patient's seizure risk and have emergency care protocols that are activated if a seizure occurs.

Cognitive and Communication Impairments

It is important for rehabilitation clinicians to know if their cancer patients have an underlying cognitive and/or communication impairment secondary to their cancer or its treatment. These impairments can have a negative impact on the ability of patients to safely participate in a rehabilitation program and follow through on recommended treatments.

Preventive measures to maximize patient safety	
Condition	**Preventive Measure**
DVT and PE	Prevention with antiembolic stockings, low molecular weight heparin, and sequential compression devices
Impending pathologic fractures	Do not perform manual muscle testing, passive range of motion, or active range of motion in limb with a potential for impending pathologic fracture or chest physical therapy; percussion over ribs with metastatic involvement.[21] Range-of-motion restrictions in joints near grafts and/or incisions (avoid wound dehiscence). Avoid progressive resistive exercises in a limb with a risk for pathologic fracture—use assistive devices to unload that limb. Rule out rib fractures before performing chest physical therapy, vibration, massage, or percussion. Spinal precautions in patients with bone metastasis—avoid excessive flexion, extension rotation. Speak to spine surgeon on specific precautions. Monitor patient for pain. Pain in limb or spine of patient with a history of cancer may be an indicator of cancer recurrence or metastatic disease.
Infections	Wash hands in-between patient treatments using technique recommended by local medical center protocols. Use infection control recommendations that are specific to the patient. Disinfect equipment used by cancer patients per local medical center policy.
Orthostatic hypotension Head and neck cancer patients	Antiembolism stockings, replenish fluids if volume depleted, abdominal binders, tilt table Evaluation of swallowing function for possibility of aspiration

Education of Patients and Their Caregivers

Well-educated patients and their caregivers are important components of rehabilitation programs that emphasize patient safety. Patients and their caregivers should be educated (1) in their native language, (2) at an appropriate reading level, (3) taking into account any cognitive impairments, and (4) in a manner they can easily understand. Educational strategies should include (1) clear instructions on risks, benefits, expected outcomes, and alternatives of rehabilitation treatments that are recommended and (2) the functional impact of the recommended plans. Clinicians providing the education should check for understanding. When providing education on medications, the following information should be included: (1) name and dose of medication and (2) risks, benefits, side effects, significant adverse effects, and drug-drug interactions.

SUMMARY

Given the complexity of medical issues facing cancer survivors, patient safety is a cornerstone in their rehabilitative care. Rehabilitation clinicians should have a thorough understanding of the impact of the cancer and its treatments on cancer survivors in their diagnosis and treatment plans.

REFERENCES

1. Cheville A. Cancer rehabilitation. In: Braddom RL, editor. Physical medicine and rehabilitation. 4th edition. Philadelphia: Elsevier-Saunders; 2011.
2. Stubblefield MD, Odell MW, editors. Cancer rehabilitation, principles and practice. New York: Demos Medical; 2009.
3. Bartels MN, Freeland ML. Pulmonary complications of cancer. In: Stubblefield MD, Odell MW, editors. Cancer rehabilitation, principles and practice. New York: Demos Medical; 2009. p. 331–47.
4. Bartels MN, Leight M. Cardiac complications of cancer. In: Stubblefield MD, Odell MW, editors. Cancer rehabilitation, principles and practice. New York: Demos Medical; 2009. p. 349–58.
5. Han J, Smith RG, Fox K, et al. Gastrointestinal complications of cancer. In: Stubblefield MD, Odell MW, editors. Cancer rehabilitation, principles and practice. New York: Demos Medical; 2009. p. 358–76.
6. Stern M, Sun P. Renal complications of cancer. In: Stubblefield MD, Odell MW, editors. Cancer rehabilitation, principles and practice. New York: Demos Medical; 2009. p. 377–81.
7. Khowong J. Endocrine complications of cancer. In: Stubblefield MD, Odell MW, editors. Cancer rehabilitation, principles and practice. New York: Demos Medical; 2009. p. 383–91.
8. Stampas A, Smith RG, Savodnik A, et al. Hematologic complications of cancer. In: Stubblefield MD, Odell MW, editors. Cancer rehabilitation, principles and practice. New York: Demos Medical; 2009. p. 393–403.
9. Grudeva-Popova J. Cancer and venous thromboembolism. J BUON 2005;10(4): 483–9.
10. Prandoni P, Piccioli A. Thrombosis as a harbinger of cancer. Curr Opin Hematol 2006;13(5):362–5.
11. Semrad TJ, O'Donnell R, Wun T, et al. Epidemiology of venous thromboembolism in 9489 patients with malignant glioma. J Neurosurg 2007;106(4):601–8.

12. Durica SS. Venous thromboembolism in the cancer patient. Curr Opin Hematol 1997;4(5):306–11.
13. Lin J, Molnar A. Thromboembolic complications of cancer. In: Stubblefield MD, Odell MW, editors. Cancer rehabilitation, principles and practice. New York: Demos Medical; 2009.
14. Buckwalter JA, Brandser EA. Metastatic disease of the skeleton. Am Fam Physician 1997;55(5):1761–8.
15. Mirels H. Metastatic disease in long bones: a proposed scoring system for diagnosing impending pathological fractures. Clin Orthop Relat Res 2003;(Suppl 415): S4–13.
16. Jawad MU, Scully SP. In brief: classifications in brief: Mirels' classification: metastatic disease in long bones and impending pathologic fracture. Clin Orthop Relat Res 2010;468(10):2825–7.
17. O'Toole GC, Boland P, Herklotz M. Bone metastasis. In: Stubblefield MD, Odell MW, editors. Cancer rehabilitation, principles and practice. New York: Demos Medical; 2009. p. 773–82.
18. Harrington KD. Impending pathologic fractures from metastatic malignancy: evaluation and management. Instr Course Lect 1986;35:357–81.
19. Fidler M. Incidence of fracture through metastases in long bones. Acta Orthop Scand 1981;52(6):623–7.
20. Veramonti T, Meyers CA. Cognitive dysfunction in the cancer patient. In: Stubblefield MD, Odell MW, editors. Cancer rehabilitation, principles and practice. New York: Demos Medical; 2009. p. 989–1000.
21. Fitzpatrick TW. Principles of physical and occupational therapy in cancer. In: Stubblefield MD, Odell MW, editors. Cancer rehabilitation, principles and practice. New York: Demos Medical; 2009. p. 785–96.
22. Ho ML. Communication and swallowing dysfunction in the cancer patient. In: Stubblefield MD, Odell MW, editors. Cancer rehabilitation, principles and practice. New York: Demos Medical; 2009. p. 941–58.
23. Ferrante MA. Plexopathy in cancer. In: Stubblefield MD, Odell MW, editors. Cancer rehabilitation, principles and practice. New York: Demos Medical; 2009. p. 567–89.
24. Mckinley W. Rehabilitation of patients with spinal cord dysfunction in the cancer setting. In: Stubblefield MD, Odell MW, editors. Cancer rehabilitation, principles and practice. New York: Demos Medical; 2009. p. 533–50.
25. Dahele M, Skipworth RJ, Wall L, et al. Objective physical activity and self-reported quality of life in patients receiving palliative chemotherapy. J Pain Symptom Manage 2007;33:676–85.
26. Stubblefield MD. Radiation fibrosis. In: Stubblefield MD, Odell MW, editors. Cancer rehabilitation, principles and practice. New York: Demos Medical; 2009. p. 723–45.
27. Yamada Y. Principles of radiotherapy. In: Stubblefield MD, Odell MW, editors. Cancer rehabilitation, principles and practice. New York: Demos Medical; 2009. p. 73–9.
28. Michael L. Communication during time of transition. Available at: http://www.ihi.org. Accessed February 15, 2012.
29. Michael L. Patient safety-teamwork and communication: basic tools and techniques. Available at: http://www.ihi.org. Accessed February 15, 2012.
30. Michael L, Bonacum D, Graham S. SBAR technique for communication: a situational briefing model. Available at: http://www.ihi.org. Accessed February 15, 2012.

31. Federico F. Human factors and safety. Available at: http://www.ihi.org. Accessed February 15, 2012.
32. Huber S, Ogrinc G. RCA helps us learn from errors. Available at: http://www.ihi.org. Accessed February 15, 2012.
33. Wing J. Therapeutic modalities in cancer. In: Stubblefield MD, Odell MW, editors. Cancer rehabilitation, principles and practice. New York: Demos Medical; 2009. p. 797–801.
34. Bunting RW, Shea B. Bone metastasis and rehabilitation. Cancer 2001;92(4): 1029–38.
35. Partsch H, Blatter W. Compression and walking versus bed rest in the treatment of proximal deep venous thrombosis with low molecular weight heparin. J Vasc Surg 2000;32:861–9.

Index

Note: Page numbers of article titles are in **boldface** type.

Phys Med Rehabil Clin N Am 23 (2012) 457–474
doi:10.1016/S1047-9651(12)00034-4
1047-9651/12/$ – see front matter © 2012 Elsevier Inc. All rights reserved.

pmr.theclinics.com

Moving?

Make sure your subscription moves with you!

To notify us of your new address, find your **Clinics Account Number** (located on your mailing label above your name), and contact customer service at:

Email: journalscustomerservice-usa@elsevier.com

800-654-2452 (subscribers in the U.S. & Canada)
314-447-8871 (subscribers outside of the U.S. & Canada)

Fax number: 314-447-8029

Elsevier Health Sciences Division
Subscription Customer Service
3251 Riverport Lane
Maryland Heights, MO 63043

*To ensure uninterrupted delivery of your subscription, please notify us at least 4 weeks in advance of move.

Printed and bound by CPI Group (UK) Ltd, Croydon, CR0 4YY

03/10/2024

01040456-0007